GYNECOLOGIC CANCERS - BASIC SCIENCES, CLINICAL AND THERAPEUTIC PERSPECTIVES

Edited by **Samir A. Farghaly**

Gynecologic Cancers - Basic Sciences, Clinical and Therapeutic Perspectives
http://dx.doi.org/10.5772/59526
Edited by Samir A. Farghaly

Contributors

Atara I Ntekim, Janica C. Wong, Priyatham Gorjala, Benjamin Costantino, Ronald Fiscus, Ana Fernández Montes, Coralia Bleotu, Angelo Di Giorgio, Bernice Robinson-Bennett, Mark Williams, John Villeneuve, Carlos Telleria, Fernando Anschau, Manoel Afonso Guimarães Gonçalves, Rapoport, Melissa Teo, Jens Hahne, Arnd Honig, Jörg Engel, Nicola Valeri, Andrea Lampis, Srinivas, Ignacio Zapardiel, Carmen G. Ponce

Published by InTech

Janeza Trdine 9, 51000 Rijeka, Croatia

Notice

Publishing Process Manager Sandra Bakic

Technical Editor InTech DTP team

Cover InTech Design team

First published March, 2016

Printed in Croatia

Additional hard copies can be obtained from orders@intechopen.com

Gynecologic Cancers - Basic Sciences, Clinical and Therapeutic Perspectives , Edited by Samir A. Farghaly

p. cm.

ISBN 978-953-51-2254-8

For EU product safety concerns:
IN TECH d.o.o., Prolaz Marije Krucifikse Kozulić 3, 51000 Rijeka, Croatia,
info@intechopen.com or visit our website at intechopen.com.

Meet the editor

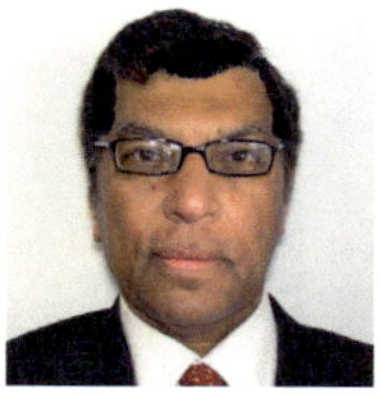

Samir A. Farghaly is a Physician / Scientist and expert in Obstetrics and Gynecology at Joan and Sanford I. Weill College of Medicine, and the New York Presbyterian Hospital / Weill Cornell Medical Center, Cornell University, New York, USA. He received his M.D. and his PhD degree in molecular biology from London University. Dr. Farghaly received several national and international clinical and research awards. He has been an invited speaker at several national and international conferences on Women's health, Molecular genetic of female cancers, and Gynecological cancer and oncologic radical surgical techniques. Dr. Farghaly is a member of several national and international societies, organizations, and foundations of Women health and cancer. He is the founder and Editor-in Chief of Enliven: Challenges in Cancer Detection and Therapy Journal, Current Trends in Gynecologic Oncology, and The International Journal of Gynecological, Obstetrical and Reproductive Medicine Research. He acts as Senior Editor / Editor and member of editorial boards, editorial advisory boards of 18 international medical journals on Gynecological Cancers, Gene Expression and Therapy, Women's Health and Gynecology. Dr. Farghaly has published 99 articles in reputed peer review journals, written several book chapters, and is an author and editor of 4 books.

Contents

Preface

Worldwide, the number of new gynecological cancer cases in 2012, was 1,085,900 and 417,600 deaths from all cancers of the female genital tract. In the USA in 2015, there were 98,280 women diagnosed with gynecologic cancers and 30,440 died from it. In the United States, ovarian cancer is the leading cause of gynecologic cancer–related morbidity and mortality due to the difficulty in detecting early-stage disease. Early recognition of symptoms and regular gynecologic screening are the best tools for women to maintain gynecologic health. Over the last 10 years or so, the treatment of gynecologic cancers has evolved. New scientific and clinical advances have modified the standard of care and led to improved patient oncologic outcomes. The treatment of gynecologic cancers requires comprehensive review and assessment of multiple issues including genetics, radiology, surgery, molecular diagnostics, and chemotherapy. A multidisciplinary team approach is crucial in providing the best care to patients and ensuring successful treatment, and optimal quality of life.

The purpose of this book is to provide a broad background of several aspects of basic sciences, clinical, and therapeutic aspects of gynecological cancers. It provides state-of-the-art information on the molecular genetics and biology of cancers of the female genital tract and new approaches to its diagnosis and management. Better understandings of the molecular events that underlie gynecologic cancers development are very much needed.

The contributors of this book come from several renowned academic medical institutions in the USA, Germany, Italy, Spain, Romania, South Africa, Brazil, Singapore, India and Nigeria.

The role of BRCA1 gene mutation and EMR protein in the development of metastatic breast cancer is discussed in Chapter 1. The interaction between genetic and epigenetic alterations leading to the malignant phenotype presentation in gynecological cancers is presented in Chapter 2. The anti-angogenic therapy as a targeted molecular therapy for epithelial ovarian cancer is covered in Chapter 3. The comprehensive review and in depth analysis of peritonectomy and hyperthermic intraperitoneal chemotherapy (HIPEC), in patients with locally advanced epithelial ovarian cancer is discussed in Chapter 4. The molecular aspects, and the targeted molecular therapy of patients with BRCA1 and BRCA2 genes hereditary ovarian cancer is reviewed in Chapter 5. The outcome of the cancer Genome Atlas (TCGA) related to high grade serous ovarian cancer (HGSOG) in reference to redefinition of ovarian cancer pathology, its propagation pattern, and the characteristics of histological subtypes of epithelial ovarian cancer is reviewed In Chapter 6. Overview of the PI3K/AKT/ mTOR signaling network in ovarian and endometrial cancer, in addition to the rationale for targeting this pathway is discussed in Chapter 7. Clinical, current management, and future directions in research related to recurrent ovarian cancer is covered in Chapter 8. The role of cytoreductive surgery and hyperthermic intraperitoneal chemotherapy in patients with recurrent ovarian cancer, who have peritoneal metastasis is presented in Chapter 9. The anti-angiogenic effects by targeting the protein kinase G type- I- alpha signaling pathway and its downstream effects on expression of inhibition of apoptosis proteins in epithelial ovarian cancer is reviewed in Chapter 10. Analysis of risk factors, diagnostic methods, and characteristics of women with endometrial cancer, and recommended current innovative therapy is presented in Chapter 11. The conventional surgical management of endometrial cancer, advantages of robotic surgery in those patients, comparison of outcome between open surgery, laparoscopic, and assisted robotic surgery for this disease is reviewed in Chapter 12. The pathophysiogy of Human Immunodeficiency Virus infection, clinical aspects, and management of uterine cervical cancer in HIV positive patients is reviewed in Chapter 13. The feasibility of sentinel lymph node detection in uterine cervical cancer, its techniques and clinical advantages are discussed in Chapter 14. Clinical presentation, histopathological classification, prognosis, recurrence factors and treatment of cancer of the vulva is reviewed in Chapter 15.

This book volume is intended for all clinicians and basic medical scientists caring for women with gynecologic cancers, including attending surgeons and physicians, clinical fellows, and residents in the disciplines of gynecologic oncology, radiotherapy, surgical oncology, medical oncology, and primary care. Also, PhD students and post-doctoral fellows in basic medical sciences.

I would like to acknowledge the assistance of Janell Mensinger, PhD of the University of Drexel, Philadelphia, USA for her valuable contribution to the book, in reviewing the biostatistical data of some of the book chapters.

I hope that you find this book very useful, and benefit from the extensive experience of the knowledgeable team of contributors who have authored its contents.

This book is dedicated to my beloved children Raied and Tamer, and the memory of my mother Amina, and father Aly, who had a great influence on me, and my academic and professional medical career. Also, to my sisters Sorya, Nadia, and brother Rafat and their families, my late siblings Nabil, and Magdy and their families. In addition to my late nephew, Islam.

Samir A. Farghaly, M.D., PhD
Joan and Sanford I. Weill Medical College / The Graduate School of Medical Sciences
The New York Presbyterian Hospital / Weill Cornell Medical Center,
Cornell University,
New York, NY, USA

Chapter 1

Role of BRCA1 in Breast Cancer Metastasis

S. Satheesh Kumar, K.H. Sreelatha,
Revathy Nadhan and Priya Srinivas

Additional information is available at the end of the chapter

http://dx.doi.org/10.5772/60787

Abstract

The role of BRCA1 in breast cancer metastasis is a less explored area that might have importance in increased aggressiveness of BRCA1 defective triple negative cancers. The possible influence of BRCA1 on apico basal polarity and ezrin, radixin and meosin (ERM) proteins are discussed in this review as a reason for cell metastasis. This might help in developing antimetastatic drugs that could help for better prognosis in BRCA1 defective breast cancers.

Keywords: BRCA1, ezrin, radixin, moesin, apicobasal polarity

1. Introduction

Breast cancer is the second largest cancer and the fifth major cause of death. There are many factors involved in breast cancer development and metastasis. Among the tumor suppressors that play a critical role in hereditary breast cancers, BRCA1 mutations are highly frequent, whereas loss of BRCA1 expression by promoter hyper methylation or allelic loss has frequently been noted in sporadic breast cancer [1, 2]. Mutation or loss of the functional BRCA1 expression in breast cancer is usually accompanied with TP53 mutations, ER/PR/HER2 negativity, and loss of ATM/CHK2, which, in turn, leads to a highly aggressive basal phenotype, which clearly possesses a therapeutic challenge [2, 3]. Specific malignant changes caused by BRCA1 mutations in the breast and the ovary remain a mystery till date.

2. BRCA1

BRCA1 is a multifunctional protein that is well known to be involved in multiple cellular processes by shuttling between nucleus and cytoplasm. Structurally, BRCA1 has three domains: (a) the RING domain; (b) the serine cluster domain (SCD); and (c) the BRCT domain. Potentially, four mutations are considered to be deleterious (5382insC, 5396 + 1G>A, 185delAG, and 2288delT) in the BRCA1 gene among the many mutations reported [4, 5]. The tumor suppressor function of BRCA1 is mainly attributed to the RING and BRCT domains of BRCA1, as women with hereditary breast cancer mainly possess mutations in one of the two domains.

Functionally, the RING domain of BRCA1 along with BARD1 possesses E3-ligase-mediated tumor suppressor activity, and any mutation in this domain would severely affect the heterodimerization and the stability of BRCA1 and BARD1, which, in turn, affects the tumor suppressor activity of BRCA1 [5]. The C-terminal BRCT domain is a phospho-protein binding domain known to interact with several partners and is reported to be critical for the localization of BRCA1 at the DNA damage site [6]. Furthermore, the tumor suppressor activity of the BRCT domain of BRCA1 has been reported using mouse models, although the exact mechanism is still debatable [7]. In short, functionally, BRCA1 is known to regulate multiple cellular processes such as DNA double strand repair, check point regulation, ubiquitination, and transcriptional regulation.

The RING domain, discovered as Really Interesting New Gene, spans from exon 2–7 of 24 exons of the BRCA1 gene. The RING domain of BRCA1 with a ring finger consists of seven cysteine and one histidine residues critically coordinate with Zn atoms, which actually stabilizes the RING structure [8, 9]. BARD1, a protein that is structurally homologous to the BRCA1 RING domain, interacts with the RING domain of BRCA1 and is critically important for the ubiquitin ligase activity, and it is reported to ubiquitinate several target proteins for degradation such as ER alpha, progesterone receptor, histone H2A, and CtIP [10-12]. It also modulates the nuclear import and export of BRCA1 [13, 14].

The core domain, which spans exons 11–13, is the largest domain of BRCA1 and is often called the serine cluster domain (SCD). It has two nuclear localization signals (NLSs), which control the nuclear import of BRCA1. Numerous proteins are reported to interact with this domain, and some of the notable binding partners are the retinoblastoma protein (RB), cMyc, PALB2, Rad50, and Rad51. The interaction between BRCA1 and RB is critically important for the BRCA1-mediated cell cycle regulation, as mutation in the binding region of BRCA1 failed to arrest the cell cycle progression [15]. PALB2, RAD50, and RAD51 interactions with BRCA1 are crucial for the BRCA1-mediated DNA repair. RAD50 and RAD51 mainly play a role in both homologous recombination (HR) and nonhomologous end joining (NHEJ) mediated by BRCA1, whereas PALB2 plays a role mainly in HR [16-18]. Mutations in any of the binding portions of this molecule severely affect the DNA repair capacity of BRCA1. Furthermore, BRCA1 is known to regulate the transcriptional activity of few oncogenic proteins reported till date. The well-studied example is that BRCA1 is known to downregulate the oncogenic transcriptional factor cMyc [19]. In addition, the serine clusters in this domain are reported to be phosphorylated by several kinases, including ATM/ATR during DNA damage, and this phosphorylation is mandatory for the assembly of BRCA1 to the DNA damage site, and again, any mutation affecting the phosphorylation of BRCA1 could severely affect the DNA repair ability [20].

Finally, the BRCA1 C terminal domain (BRCT) is reported to modulate its interactions with phosphoproteins that are critically important for the tumor suppressor activity of BRCA1 in particular nuclear localization and assembly at the DNA damage sites [21]. Several mutations have been reported in the BRCA1 gene portion that interfere with several cellular processes, and sometimes, they can be highly lethal [22]. Interestingly some of the mutations in the BRCA1 gene portion (for example, C61G RING mutation) are hypomorphic, i.e., it does not lose its complete DNA repair ability but still maintains the residual unknown DNA repair mechanism [5, 23]. From the therapeutic point of view, BRCA1 mutations with residual tumor suppressor activity clearly pose a complexity in the treatment compared with BRCA1-proficient or BRCA1-deficient breast/ovarian tumors.

3. BRCA1 defect and pathological condition

Clinically, BRCA1 is reported to be functional in different organs of the body apart from its cardinal role in the breast and the ovary. Recently, BRCA1 has been reported to play an immense role in brain development [24]. In addition, its role as a regulator of metabolic function in skeletal muscles has been reported [25]. It also plays a huge role in Alzheimer disease, although the exact role is still unclear [26]. Recently, BRCA1 has been reported to act as a transcriptional cofactor during HIV infection [27]; again, the evidence is still preliminary. The function of BRCA1 as a tumor suppressor is crucial in the breast and ovarian tissue, and mutations in BRCA1 usually predispose to breast or ovarian cancer as discussed earlier. Apart from that, BRCA1 mutations are also reported to develop cancers in the prostate, fallopian tube, peritoneal, and pancreas, the specificity being unclear [28, 29]. Acute myeloid leukemia and the Fanconi anemia subtype has been reported if BRCA1 mutations are inherited from both parents [30-32]. Although BRCA1 has been studied for 20 years, its multiple facets are still undiscovered to a larger extent, which makes BRCA1 the molecule of attraction in current research. The role of BRCA1 in metastasis is one of the novel functions evidenced very recently.

4. BRCA1 in migration/invasion

Although there are no evidencing reports regarding the role of BRCA1 in ovarian cancer metastasis, its role in breast cancer metastasis is clearly an emerging subject with a few reports. The RING and BRCT domain of BRCA1 has been reported to be critically important for controlling the cancer cell migration and motility in the breast or the ovary [7, 33], although the complete mechanism is ill understood. In addition, restoration of full-length BRCA1 in 3450delCAAG mutated breast cancer cells is reported to block the cell invasion and motility induced by that particular mutation [34]. Furthermore, BRCA1 has been implicated to play a key role in epithelial to mesenchymal transition, again the exact mechanism being unclear [35]. In this review, we discuss the possible mechanistic role of BRCA1 in the migration and invasion of BRCA1-defective breast tumors, which is less explored till date. Currently, there are two evident mechanisms through which BRCA1 could control the migration and invasion of breast cancers that will have immense potential in the futuristic breast cancer treatments. First, the mechanism deals with the role of BRCA1 in maintaining the apicobasal polarity. The second mechanism deals with the role of BRCA1 in regulating the ERM complex that maintain the cytoskeleton.

4.1. BRCA1 and apicobasal polarity

Apicobasal polarity is a unique polarity feature of the epithelial cells that refers to the apical membrane on one side and the basolateral membrane on other side, separated by tight junctions. It is a critical feature of cytoskeletal reorganization in the epithelium of the breast and plays a key role in maintaining the integrity of cell-cell connections by maintaining the adherent junctions through microtubule organization [36]. In addition, it is known to be regulated by several signaling pathways such as WNT signaling, TGFβ, and integrin-mediated signaling. Furthermore, it is critically important for the differentiation of the breast epithelium, whereas the loss of epithelial polarity is often considered a hallmark of EMT and cancer [37-39]. Frequently, the loss of expression or mislocalization of the molecules of polarity complex such as SCRIB, Crumbs, and PAR has been implicated in the carcinogenesis of the breast [40-42]. Recently, BRCA1 has been reported to play a key role in the cytoskeletal organization and polarity of the breast tissue [43]. Probably, the loss of polarity in BRCA1-mutated breast tumors results in the loss of cell–cell adhesion and, hence, the movement of cancer cells from the primary to the distant site.

Mechanistically, BRCA1 regulates the polarity and, hence, the differentiation of breast cancer cells by regulating the expression of Hyaluronan-Mediated Motility Receptor (HMMR), a low-penetrance breast cancer susceptibility gene product that is usually over expressed in BRCA1-related tumors and results in poor prognosis [43-45]. The early report comes from a linkage association study where the genetic variation at chromosome 5q33–34, which is actually the gene location of HMMR, is clearly associated with the risk of breast cancer among BRCA1 mutation carriers [46]. Furthermore, it was confirmed by a pilot study conducted in Spain and Italy, where HMMR rs299290 variation among BRCA1 mutation carriers clearly posed a risk of breast cancer [47]. In addition, BRCA1-related breast cancers, which are generally ER negative but not ER positive, are associated with the HMMR genetic variation. Further knockdown of BRCA1 has clearly impaired the polarization by modulating the cytoskeletal components and its organization. For instance, the cytoskeletal molecule vimentin is increased, and CCD49f is decreased upon BRCA1 knockdown. Maxwell et al. (2011) have shown that BRCA1, through the non-centrosome-dependent assembly of microtubules, maintains the polarity of the breast epithelium and the loss of BRCA1 clearly impair the cytoskeletal reorganization, as observed by increased levels of intermediate filament proteins such as vimentin. Furthermore, BRCA1 is reported to maintain the polarization of breast epithelium by directing the proteosome-mediated degradation of the BRCA1 target, HMMR [47]. Supporting evidence shows that proteosome inhibition and BRCA1 depletion clearly induced the expression of HMMR, which might be the probable reason why an overexpression of HMMR and polarity loss is frequently observed in BRCA1-related breast cancer than BRCA1-unrelated breast cancer [47]. Further accumulation of microtubule-associated factors TUBG1 by HMMR at the centromere in BRCA1-mutated breast tumors was reported to have impaired the polarity and hence induced the basal phenotype [43, 48]. Overexpression of TUBG1 and HMMR has clearly impaired the polarization, even in the presence of BRCA1, suggesting that the upregulation of microtubule-associated factors together with the depletion or mutation of BRCA1 and proteosome inhibition is the prime event in the loss of polarity in BRCA1-related breast tumors. Further overexpression of Aurora kinase A (AURKA) is reported to regulate the HMMR-mediated polarity loss, and HMMR is shown to negatively regulate AURKA. The depletion of AURKA is also known to reduce the abundance of HMMR, and the abundance is restored to the normal level in AURKA- and BRCA1-depleted conditions [43]. Clearly, a strict balance exists between BRCA1, HMMR, and AURKA, and probably, the polarity is completely dependent on the interactions between these molecules.

PAR is a polarity complex of par3, par6, and aPKC known to regulate cell plasticity by localizing at the tight junction [14]. Par6 is critically regulated by TGFβ signaling, and its misregulation leads to the highly aggressive breast tumorigenesis. Further correlation of the par6 expression and BRCA1 mutation has recently been reported. Although no direct regulation has been established between par6 and BRCA1, par6 has been shown to be over expressed in BRCA1-mutated breast tumors, which, in turn, have been linked with the high expression of basal markers such as cytokeratin 5/14 and vimentin. Alternatively, a positive association was reported between the activation of PAR6 pathway and the expression of basal cytokeratins in BRCA1-mutated breast tumors [40, 49, 50].

Starita et al. (2004) have shown that BRCA1 inhibits the expression of gamma tubulin by direct ubiquitination and is reported to maintain the centrosome number, and probably, the mutation in BRCA1 has readily increased the tubulin expression and polymerization and, hence, might induce the metastasis of breast cancer cells.

It clearly shows that BRCA1 sustains the polarity of breast cancer cells by maintaining a tight regulation with centrosome pathway components and the loss of BRCA1 in BRCA1-mutated breast tumors, leading to impaired polarization, which, in turn, results in the basal-like phenotype of breast cancer cells. Furthermore, the loss of polarity induces the EMT process [51-53], which might promote the migration and invasion of BRCA1-related breast cancer cells. Here comes the question of how the cancer cell migrates in a condition where BRCA1 is a wild type. Probably, the epigenetic silencing of BRCA1 as reported in many sporadic breast tumors might prevail in such situations, which needs future experimentations.

4.2. BRCA1 and ERM complex

Ezrin, radixin, and moesin, together known as ERM, are three functionally homologous adapter proteins consisting of an N-terminal FERM domain and a C-terminal ERM associated the F-actin-binding domain (C-ERMAD) that is linked to the N-terminal FERM domain through the intermediate alpha helical region. Activation of ERM has been reported as an important process in the functioning of ERM. ERM remains in the closed conformation until it is activated by the phosphorylation of threonine residues in ezrin, moesin, and radixin [54]. Activated ERM helps in linking the actin cytoskeleton to the plasma membrane through the FERM and F-actin-binding domain [55]. Further activated ERM is reported to interact with transmembrane proteins such as receptor kinases, CD43, and CD44 [56]. Functionally, ERM has been critically implicated in the normal physiological as well as in the cancer conditions. In particular, ERM is known to be involved in three key events: (a) epithelial morphogenesis; (b) migration; and (c) adhesion. Changes in the above-mentioned events are observed during cancer, and it is a clear indication of cancer. Basically, polarity is maintained by ERM in normal physiological conditions and the overexpression of ERM during cancerous conditions leads to a more mesenchymal nature of the cells, and hence, it promotes the event of metastasis by probably interacting with EGFR, CD44, and HGFR [57, 58].

Abnormal expression and localization of ERM has been reported in different types of cancer, and it is clearly known to regulate the cellular signaling and the cytoskeleton during cancer progression, which, in turn, affects the migration and motility behavior of cancer cells. The ERM complex is known to be directly or indirectly phosphorylated by many kinases, which, in turn, activate many signaling pathways involved in cell adhesion, migration, morphology, and proliferation during tumorigenesis [58, 59]. Further overexpression of ERM molecules together or individually was reported to be a clear indication of the EMT process [60, 61]. All the above-mentioned activities of ERM were also highly pronounced in breast cancer [62-64]. In addition, moesin was associated with poor relapse-free survival in breast cancer patients. Although the role of ERM in breast cancer progression was well studied over the years, its relation with BRCA1 during metastasis was ill understood, with only a few recent reports [33]. ERM has been reported to be associated with the ER-negative basal phenotype, and the expression of ERM was also reported to be high in BRCA1-related basal breast tumors compared with BRCA1-unrelated or sporadic breast tumors [65], which, in turn, could contribute to the migration and invasion of cancer cells. Recently, its relation with BRCA1 during migration has been revealed in breast cancer cell lines. Although ERM acts through multiple pathways to promote cancer cell migration and invasion, the presence or absence of BRCA1 was found to be highly significant in ERM-mediated cell motility and migration of breast cancer cells [33]. As previously discussed, the tumor suppressor activity of BRCA1 mainly lies in the BRCT domain, as the mutation of BRCA1 leading to the expression of truncated protein is frequently associated with breast and ovarian cancers [7]. Interestingly, BRCA1 was found to localize at the leading edges and focal adhesion sites of the plasma membrane and reported to control the breast cancer cell spreading and cell motility [33]. Furthermore, the BRCT domain of wild-type BRCA1 was found to co-localize with F-actin, ezrin, moesin, and radixin in the plasma membrane of breast cancer cells and hence controls the breast cancer cell motility in an unknown manner. In addition, a detailed study on this will give an idea on the exact localization of BRCA1 in the plasma membrane and its contributions to inhibit metastasis. Further stable expression of the BRCT coding domain of BRCA1 in breast cancer cells was found to co-localize with ERM and F-actin along with wild-type BRCA1. The BRCT coding domain acts as a dominant negative factor by gradually displacing the endogenous wild-type BRCA1 at leading edges and focal adhesion sites, thus promoting the motility and migratory capacity of breast cancer cells. Probably, BRCA1, by interacting through its BRCT domain, might reduce the ERM protein levels by ubiquitinating it through the E3 ubiquitin ligase activity and hence reduce the motility of breast cancer cells. Alternatively, mutation in the BRCA1 gene at the BRCT domain fails to reduce the levels of ERM at the leading edges, and hence, the motility behavior of breast cancer cells was increased. In addition, this might be one of the reasons why ERM is highly overexpressed in BRCA1-related basal breast tumors than BRCA1-unrelated tumors [65]. It was also reported that not only the BRCT domain but also the E3 ubiquitin ligase activity of BRCA1 are required for complete tumor suppressor function [33], further supporting the above-mentioned speculation, although it was contradictory to previous reports. This will have immense potential in tumor metastasis in BRCA1-defective cancers which the researchers have overlooked. Further studies are warranted to elucidate the exact signaling pathways and the biological consequences associated with ERM in BRCA1-related and BRCA1-unrelated breast tumors.

5. Screening and diagnosis of BRCA1 mutated breast and ovarian cancers

The major annoying fact about BRCA1/2 mutation is that the inheritance of BRCA1/2 mutation increases the risk for breast cancer by about 20–25% [66, 67]. Women who inherit BRCA1 mutation have 55–65% risk of getting breast cancer [68, 69]. In addition, BRCA1 mutations are quite frequent among a particular ethnic population; e.g. Ashkenazi Jews have a high prevalence of BRCA1 mutation than any other population. Particularly, 2288delT and 5382insC mutation in the gene portion of BRCA1 is highly prevalent in Ashkenazi Jews, with a frequency of 1.1% and 0.1–0.15%, respectively [22, 70]. High prevalence has also been reported among the Dutch and Norwegian populations. In addition, the prevalence highly varies within the population, e.g., the US population based on their different ethnic origin [22, 71, 72]. Early clinical breast examination is the best possible method of diagnosing and treating breast tumors [73]. There are many screening tools in the current scenario that particularly assess the family history and its probable association with BRCA1 mutation [74]. However, the screening is mainly recommended for those who have a family history of breast/ovarian cancers [74]. The other specific tissue where inherited BRCA1 mutations usually predispose cancer is the ovary. Estimated data show that women who inherit BRCA1 mutations have 39% of developing ovarian cancer [68, 69]. Women with Ashkenazi Jewish heritage or familial history of breast cancer have increased risk of three to six times than the general public, and women with BRCA1 mutations have more than six times greater risk than the general population to develop ovarian cancer. Screening is usually done by analyzing serum markers such as CA-125 and/or transvaginal ultrasound, and in the case of BRCA1-related ovarian cancer, the screening starts early at the age of 30.

6. Management and therapy of BRCA1 mutated cancers

Surprisingly, a survival advantage for BRCA1 mutation carriers is growing now, although it is still under controversy. An improvement in the survival rate was observed in BRCA1 mutation carriers of the Ashkenazi ethnicity upon platinum-based chemotherapy compared with BRCA1 non-mutated patients [75]. In addition, many studies from different parts of the world have substantiated the survival advantage among BRCA1 mutation carriers of ovarian origin, although the exact reason is not yet clear [76-78]. However, there are reports which indicates in the case of breast cancer, BRCA1 mutation does not pose any survival advantage; instead, it poses a clear challenge to chemotherapy. In the treatment point of view, the hormone therapy usually fails as BRCA1-mutated breast and ovarian cancer tends to be triple negative in general. The commonly used drugs are either insensitive or have developed resistance in BRCA1-mutated conditions. The only promising drug that is effective in treating BRCA1-mutated breast and ovarian cancer is the PARP inhibitor. The well-studied PARP inhibitor, Olaparib, has been found to be effective in treating BRCA1-mutated breast, ovarian, pancreatic, and prostate cancer. The loss of DNA repair by homologous recombination in BRCA1-mutated conditions activates the alternate method of single-strand DNA repair by poly(ADP-ribose)polymerase [79-81]. The rescue of DNA repair by PARP clearly imposes a chemotherapeutic challenge, and the inhibition of PARP during this condition has improved the benefit rate by 63% [82, 83]. Although it is not completely evaluated as a drug for treating BRCA-related cancers, significant clinical activity has been demonstrated in BRCA1-mutated breast and ovarian cancer during phase trials. There was suspicion that the PARP inhibitor alone or in combination could be an effective drug alternative in treating BRCA1-mutated breast and ovarian cancer. However, recent information has shown that the PARP inhibitor may not be clinically successful as drug resistance against the PARP inhibitor is also observed. As of now, we do not have an effective treatment for BRCA1-related cancers. Designing drugs considering BRCA1 interaction with metastasis-related proteins would be an effective strategy to treat BRCA1-related cancers.

7. Conclusions

It is very clear that BRCAl is a multifunctional protein that exerts its function from the nucleus to the cytoplasm to the plasma membrane. BRCA1, by controlling apicobasal polarity and by interacting with ERM proteins, is supposed to be involved in cancer cell metastasis. If the link between BRCA1 and migration/invasion is completely unraveled, then we could revolutionize the treatment modalities for controlling metastasis in BRCA1-defective breast tumors.

Acknowledgements

This work was supported by an intramural grant from the Rajiv Gandhi Centre for Biotechnology, Kerala State Council for Science Technology and Environment (No. 016/SRSHS/2011/CSTE), a grant-in-aid from the Board of Research in Nuclear Sciences *(No. 2009/37/5/BRNS/1620 and No.37(1)/14/16/2014)* and Indian Council of Medical Research (*No.3/2/2/215/2013/NCD-III*) to P. S. The authors also acknowledge the University Grants Commission (UGC), Government of India, for the Senior Research Fellowship to Satheesh Kumar S., the Indian Council for Medical Research (ICMR), Government of India, for the Senior Research Fellowship to Sreelatha K H; and the Council for Scientific and Industrial Research (CSIR), Government of India, for the Senior Research Fellowship to Revathy Nadhan.

Author details

S. Satheesh Kumar, K.H. Sreelatha, Revathy Nadhan and Priya Srinivas*

*Address all correspondence to: priyasrinivas@rgcb.res.in

Cancer Research Program , Rajiv Gandhi Centre for Biotechnology3, Thycaud PO, Thiruvananthapuram, Kerala, India

References

[1] Bal, A., et al., BRCA1-methylated sporadic breast cancers are BRCA-like in showing a basal phenotype and absence of ER expression. Virchows Arch, 2012. 461(3): p. 305-12.

[2] Tung, N., et al., Prevalence and predictors of loss of wild type BRCA1 in estrogen receptor positive and negative BRCA1-associated breast cancers. Breast Cancer Res, 2010. 12(6): p. R95.

[3] McAlpine, J.N., et al., BRCA1 and BRCA2 mutations correlate with TP53 abnormalities and presence of immune cell infiltrates in ovarian high-grade serous carcinoma. Mod Pathol, 2012. 25(5): p. 740-50.

[4] Elstrodt, F., et al., BRCA1 mutation analysis of 41 human breast cancer cell lines reveals three new deleterious mutants. Cancer Res, 2006. 66(1): p. 41-5.

[5] Drost, R., et al., BRCA1 RING function is essential for tumor suppression but dispensable for therapy resistance. Cancer Cell, 2011. 20(6): p. 797-809.

[6] Sobhian, B., et al., RAP80 targets BRCA1 to specific ubiquitin structures at DNA damage sites. Science, 2007. 316(5828): p. 1198-202.

[7] Shakya, R., et al., BRCA1 tumor suppression depends on BRCT phosphoprotein binding, but not its E3 ligase activity. Science, 2011. 334(6055): p. 525-8.

[8] Lipkowitz, S. and A.M. Weissman, RINGs of good and evil: RING finger ubiquitin ligases at the crossroads of tumour suppression and oncogenesis. Nat Rev Cancer, 2011. 11(9): p. 629-43.

[9] Bienstock, R.J., et al., Molecular modeling of the amino-terminal zinc ring domain of BRCA1. Cancer Res, 1996. 56(11): p. 2539-45.

[10] Heine, G.F. and J.D. Parvin, BRCA1 control of steroid receptor ubiquitination. Sci STKE, 2007. 2007(391): p. pe34.

[11] Calvo, V. and M. Beato, BRCA1 counteracts progesterone action by ubiquitination leading to progesterone receptor degradation and epigenetic silencing of target promoters. Cancer Res, 2011. 71(9): p. 3422-31.

[12] Ma, Y., et al., BRCA1 regulates acetylation and ubiquitination of estrogen receptor-alpha. Mol Endocrinol, 2010. 24(1): p. 76-90.

[13] Brzovic, P.S., et al., Structure of a BRCA1-BARD1 heterodimeric RING-RING complex. Nat Struct Biol, 2001. 8(10): p. 833-7.

[14] Rodriguez, J.A. and B.R. Henderson, Identification of a functional nuclear export sequence in BRCA1. J Biol Chem, 2000. 275(49): p. 38589-96.

[15] Aprelikova, O.N., et al., BRCA1-associated growth arrest is RB-dependent. Proc Natl Acad Sci U S A, 1999. 96(21): p. 11866-71.

[16] Ballal, R.D., et al., BRCA1 localization to the telomere and its loss from the telomere in response to DNA damage. J Biol Chem, 2009. 284(52): p. 36083-98.

[17] Zhong, Q., et al., Association of BRCA1 with the hRad50-hMre11-p95 complex and the DNA damage response. Science, 1999. 285(5428): p. 747-50.

[18] Sy, S.M., M.S. Huen, and J. Chen, PALB2 is an integral component of the BRCA complex required for homologous recombination repair. Proc Natl Acad Sci U S A, 2009. 106(17): p. 7155-60.

[19] Wang, Q., et al., BRCA1 binds c-Myc and inhibits its transcriptional and transforming activity in cells. Oncogene, 1998. 17(15): p. 1939-48.

[20] Cortez, D., et al., Requirement of ATM-dependent phosphorylation of brca1 in the DNA damage response to double-strand breaks. Science, 1999. 286(5442): p. 1162-6.

[21] Nelson, A.C. and J.T. Holt, Impact of RING and BRCT domain mutations on BRCA1 protein stability, localization and recruitment to DNA damage. Radiat Res, 2010. 174(1): p. 1-13.

[22] Petrucelli, N., M.B. Daly, and G.L. Feldman, Hereditary breast and ovarian cancer due to mutations in BRCA1 and BRCA2. Genet Med, 2010. 12(5): p. 245-59.

[23] Tassone, P., et al., BRCA1 expression modulates chemosensitivity of BRCA1-defective HCC1937 human breast cancer cells. Br J Cancer, 2003. 88(8): p. 1285-91.

[24] Pao, G.M., et al., Role of BRCA1 in brain development. Proc Natl Acad Sci U S A, 2014. 111(13): p. E1240-8.

[25] Jackson, K.C., et al., BRCA1 is a novel regulator of metabolic function in skeletal muscle. J Lipid Res, 2014. 55(4): p. 668-80.

[26] Evans, T.A., et al., BRCA1 may modulate neuronal cell cycle re-entry in Alzheimer disease. Int J Med Sci, 2007. 4(3): p. 140-5.

[27] Irene Guendel1, B.W.M., Alan Baer1, Seth M Dever23, Kristoffer Valerie2, Jia Guo1, Yuntao Wu1 and Kylene Kehn-Hall1*, BRCA1 functions as a novel transcriptional co-factor in HIV-1 infection. Virology Journal 2015. 12:40.

[28] Brose, M.S., et al., Cancer risk estimates for BRCA1 mutation carriers identified in a risk evaluation program. J Natl Cancer Inst, 2002. 94(18): p. 1365-72.

[29] Finch, A., et al., Salpingo-oophorectomy and the risk of ovarian, fallopian tube, and peritoneal cancers in women with a BRCA1 or BRCA2 Mutation. JAMA, 2006. 296(2): p. 185-92.

[30] Howlett, N.G., et al., Biallelic inactivation of BRCA2 in Fanconi anemia. Science, 2002. 297(5581): p. 606-9.

[31] Alter, B.P., Fanconi anemia and the development of leukemia. Best Pract Res Clin Haematol, 2014. 27(3-4): p. 214-21.

[32] Sawyer, S.L., et al., Biallelic mutations in BRCA1 cause a new Fanconi anemia subtype. Cancer Discov, 2015. 5(2): p. 135-42.

[33] Coene, E.D., et al., A novel role for BRCA1 in regulating breast cancer cell spreading and motility. J Cell Biol, 2011. 192(3): p. 497-512.

[34] Yasmeen, A., et al., BRCA1 mutations contribute to cell motility and invasion by affecting its main regulators. Cell Cycle, 2008. 7(23): p. 3781-3.

[35] Bai, F., et al., BRCA1 suppresses epithelial-to-mesenchymal transition and stem cell dedifferentiation during mammary and tumor development. Cancer Res, 2014. 74(21): p. 6161-72.

[36] Meng, W., et al., Anchorage of microtubule minus ends to adherens junctions regulates epithelial cell-cell contacts. Cell, 2008. 135(5): p. 948-59.

[37] Royer, C. and X. Lu, Epithelial cell polarity: a major gatekeeper against cancer? Cell Death Differ, 2011. 18(9): p. 1470-7.

[38] Khursheed, M. and M.D. Bashyam, Apico-basal polarity complex and cancer. J Biosci, 2014. 39(1): p. 145-55.

[39] Furuta, S., et al., Depletion of BRCA1 impairs differentiation but enhances proliferation of mammary epithelial cells. Proc Natl Acad Sci U S A, 2005. 102(26): p. 9176-81.

[40] Zhan, L., et al., Deregulation of scribble promotes mammary tumorigenesis and reveals a role for cell polarity in carcinoma. Cell, 2008. 135(5): p. 865-78.

[41] Roh, M.H., et al., The Crumbs3-Pals1 complex participates in the establishment of polarity in mammalian epithelial cells. J Cell Sci, 2003. 116(Pt 14): p. 2895-906.

[42] Cunliffe, H.E., et al., PAR6B is required for tight junction formation and activated PKCzeta localization in breast cancer. Am J Cancer Res, 2012. 2(5): p. 478-91.

[43] Maxwell, C.A., et al., Interplay between BRCA1 and RHAMM regulates epithelial apicobasal polarization and may influence risk of breast cancer. PLoS Biol, 2011. 9(11): p. e1001199.

[44] Assmann, V., et al., The pattern of expression of the microtubule-binding protein RHAMM/IHABP in mammary carcinoma suggests a role in the invasive behaviour of tumour cells. J Pathol, 2001. 195(2): p. 191-6.

[45] Bieche, I., et al., Identification of a three-gene expression signature of poor-prognosis breast carcinoma. Mol Cancer, 2004. 3(1): p. 37.

[46] Nathanson, K.L., et al., CGH-targeted linkage analysis reveals a possible BRCA1 modifier locus on chromosome 5q. Hum Mol Genet, 2002. 11(11): p. 1327-32.

[47] Pujana, M.A., et al., Network modeling links breast cancer susceptibility and centrosome dysfunction. Nat Genet, 2007. 39(11): p. 1338-49.

[48] Tolg, C., et al., RHAMM promotes interphase microtubule instability and mitotic spindle integrity through MEK1/ERK1/2 activity. J Biol Chem, 2010. 285(34): p. 26461-74.

[49] Nolan, M.E., et al., The polarity protein Par6 induces cell proliferation and is overexpressed in breast cancer. Cancer Res, 2008. 68(20): p. 8201-9.

[50] Viloria-Petit, A.M., et al., A role for the TGFbeta-Par6 polarity pathway in breast cancer progression. Proc Natl Acad Sci U S A, 2009. 106(33): p. 14028-33.

[51] Moreno-Bueno, G., F. Portillo, and A. Cano, Transcriptional regulation of cell polarity in EMT and cancer. Oncogene, 2008. 27(55): p. 6958-69.

[52] Coradini, D., et al., Cell polarity, epithelial-mesenchymal transition, and cell-fate decision gene expression in ductal carcinoma in situ. Int J Surg Oncol, 2012. 2012: p. 984346.

[53] Huang, R.Y., P. Guilford, and J.P. Thiery, Early events in cell adhesion and polarity during epithelial-mesenchymal transition. J Cell Sci, 2012. 125(Pt 19): p. 4417-22.

[54] Niggli, V. and J. Rossy, Ezrin/radixin/moesin: versatile controllers of signaling molecules and of the cortical cytoskeleton. Int J Biochem Cell Biol, 2008. 40(3): p. 344-9.

[55] Pearson, M.A., et al., Structure of the ERM protein moesin reveals the FERM domain fold masked by an extended actin binding tail domain. Cell, 2000. 101(3): p. 259-70.

[56] Orian-Rousseau, V., et al., Hepatocyte growth factor-induced Ras activation requires ERM proteins linked to both CD44v6 and F-actin. Mol Biol Cell, 2007. 18(1): p. 76-83.

[57] Fehon, R.G., A.I. McClatchey, and A. Bretscher, Organizing the cell cortex: the role of ERM proteins. Nat Rev Mol Cell Biol, 2010. 11(4): p. 276-87.

[58] Clucas, J. and F. Valderrama, ERM proteins in cancer progression. J Cell Sci, 2014. 127(Pt 2): p. 267-75.

[59] Arpin, M., et al., Emerging role for ERM proteins in cell adhesion and migration. Cell Adh Migr, 2011. 5(2): p. 199-206.

[60] Haynes, J., et al., Dynamic actin remodeling during epithelial-mesenchymal transition depends on increased moesin expression. Mol Biol Cell, 2011. 22(24): p. 4750-64.

[61] Wang, C.C., et al., Differential expression of moesin in breast cancers and its implication in epithelial-mesenchymal transition. Histopathology, 2012. 61(1): p. 78-87.

[62] Mak, H., et al., Ezrin phosphorylation on tyrosine 477 regulates invasion and metastasis of breast cancer cells. BMC Cancer, 2012. 12: p. 82.

[63] Ma, L. and T. Jiang, Clinical implications of Ezrin and CD44 coexpression in breast cancer. Oncol Rep, 2013. 30(4): p. 1899-905.

[64] Li, J., et al., Role for ezrin in breast cancer cell chemotaxis to CCL5. Oncol Rep, 2010. 24(4): p. 965-71.

[65] Charafe-Jauffret, E., et al., Gene expression profiling of breast cell lines identifies potential new basal markers. Oncogene, 2006. 25(15): p. 2273-84.

[66] Easton, D.F., How many more breast cancer predisposition genes are there? Breast Cancer Res, 1999. 1(1): p. 14-7.

[67] Campeau, P.M., W.D. Foulkes, and M.D. Tischkowitz, Hereditary breast cancer: new genetic developments, new therapeutic avenues. Hum Genet, 2008. 124(1): p. 31-42.

[68] Antoniou, A., et al., Average risks of breast and ovarian cancer associated with BRCA1 or BRCA2 mutations detected in case Series unselected for family history: a combined analysis of 22 studies. Am J Hum Genet, 2003. 72(5): p. 1117-30.

[69] Chen, S. and G. Parmigiani, Meta-analysis of BRCA1 and BRCA2 penetrance. J Clin Oncol, 2007. 25(11): p. 1329-33.

[70] Petrucelli, N., M.B. Daly, and G.L. Feldman, BRCA1 and BRCA2 Hereditary Breast and Ovarian Cancer, in GeneReviews(R), R.A. Pagon, et al., Editors. 1993: Seattle (WA).

[71] Malone, K.E., et al., Prevalence and predictors of BRCA1 and BRCA2 mutations in a population-based study of breast cancer in white and black American women ages 35 to 64 years. Cancer Res, 2006. 66(16): p. 8297-308.

[72] John, E.M., et al., Prevalence of pathogenic BRCA1 mutation carriers in 5 US racial/ethnic groups. JAMA, 2007. 298(24): p. 2869-76.

[73] Burke, W., et al., Recommendations for follow-up care of individuals with an inherited predisposition to cancer. II. BRCA1 and BRCA2. Cancer Genetics Studies Consortium. JAMA, 1997. 277(12): p. 997-1003.

[74] Moyer, V.A. and U.S.P.S.T. Force, Risk assessment, genetic counseling, and genetic testing for BRCA-related cancer in women: U.S. Preventive Services Task Force recommendation statement. Ann Intern Med, 2014. 160(4): p. 271-81.

[75] Cass, I., et al., Improved survival in women with BRCA-associated ovarian carcinoma. Cancer, 2003. 97(9): p. 2187-95.

[76] Aida, H., et al., Clinical features of ovarian cancer in Japanese women with germ-line mutations of BRCA1. Clin Cancer Res, 1998. 4(1): p. 235-40.

[77] Tan, D.S., et al., "BRCAness" syndrome in ovarian cancer: a case-control study describing the clinical features and outcome of patients with epithelial ovarian cancer associated with BRCA1 and BRCA2 mutations. J Clin Oncol, 2008. 26(34): p. 5530-6.

[78] Chetrit, A., et al., Effect of BRCA1/2 mutations on long-term survival of patients with invasive ovarian cancer: the national Israeli study of ovarian cancer. J Clin Oncol, 2008. 26(1): p. 20-5.

[79] Farmer, H., et al., Targeting the DNA repair defect in BRCA mutant cells as a therapeutic strategy. Nature, 2005. 434(7035): p. 917-21.

[80] Patel, A.G., J.N. Sarkaria, and S.H. Kaufmann, Nonhomologous end joining drives poly(ADP-ribose) polymerase (PARP) inhibitor lethality in homologous recombination-deficient cells. Proc Natl Acad Sci U S A, 2011. 108(8): p. 3406-11.

[81] Tong, W.M., U. Cortes, and Z.Q. Wang, Poly(ADP-ribose) polymerase: a guardian angel protecting the genome and suppressing tumorigenesis. Biochim Biophys Acta, 2001. 1552(1): p. 27-37.

[82] Fong, P.C., et al., Inhibition of poly(ADP-ribose) polymerase in tumors from BRCA mutation carriers. N Engl J Med, 2009. 361(2): p. 123-34.

[83] Turner, N., A. Tutt, and A. Ashworth, Hallmarks of 'BRCAness' in sporadic cancers. Nat Rev Cancer, 2004. 4(10): p. 814-9.

Chapter 2

Interplay of Epigenetics with Gynecological Cancer

Coralia Bleotu, Demetra Socolov, Mariana Anton, Anca Botezatu, Adriana Plesa, Iulia Virginia Iancu, Lorelei Irina Brasoveanu, Gabriela Anton and Carmen Cristina Diaconu

Additional information is available at the end of the chapter

http://dx.doi.org/10.5772/61032

Abstract

Recent data on the cell deregulation that occurs during the progression to cancer underlines the cooperation between genetic and epigenetic alterations leading to a malignant phenotype. Unlike genetic alterations, the epigenetic changes do not affect the DNA sequence of the genes, but determine the regulation of gene expression acting upon the genome. Moreover, unlike genetic changes, epigenetic ones are reversible, making them therapeutic targets in various conditions in general and in cancer disease in particular. The term *epigenetics* includes a series of covalent modifications that regulate the methylation pattern of DNA and posttranslational modifications of histones. Gene expression can also be regulated at the posttranscriptional level by microRNAs (miRNAs), a family of small noncoding RNAs that inhibit the translation of mRNA to protein. miRNAs can act as 'oncomiRs', as tumor suppressors, or both. In this chapter, we will (1) summarize the current literature on the key processes responsible for epigenetic regulation: DNA methylation, histone modifications and posttranscriptional gene regulation by miRNAs; (2) evaluate aberrant epigenetic modifications as essential players in cancer progression; (3) establish the roles of microenvironment-mediated epigenetic perturbations in the development of gynecological neoplasia; (4) evaluate epigenetic factors involved in drug resistance.

Keywords: Epigenetic, biomarker, gynecological cancer

1. Introduction

1.1. Key processes responsible for epigenetic regulation

Epigenetics could be broadly defined as the sum of cellular and physiological trait variations that are not caused by changes in the DNA sequence. Epigenetic mechanisms are essential for the normal development and maintenance of tissue-specific gene expression patterns in mammals. Disruption of epigenetic processes can lead to altered gene function resulting in imprinting disorders, developmental abnormalities and cancer. The epigenetic mechanisms that will be presented in this chapter are (1) DNA methylation, (2) chromatin and histone modifications, and (3) regulatory noncoding RNAs.

1.1.1. DNA methylation

DNA methylation is a biochemical process characterized by the addition of a methyl group especially at the C5 position of cytosine from CpG dinucleotides and is accomplished by two classes of DNA methyltransferases involved in maintenance and *de novo* methylation [1]. CpG dinucleotides are not randomly distributed across the human genome but are found in short CpG-rich DNA sequences called 'CpG islands.' CpG islands are found in regions of large repetitive sequences (e.g. centromeric repeats, retrotransposon elements, rDNA) [2, 3] and in 60% of human gene promoters [4]. Some CpG islands are methylated, whereas the majority of them usually remain unmethylated during development and in differentiated tissues [5]. CpG islands' promoters become methylated during development (imprinted genes, chromosome X inactivation) [2]. Another role of CpG island methylation is to silence noncoding DNA and transposable DNA elements to prevent chromosomal instability by heavy methylation of repetitive sequences [5]. DNA methylation leads to gene silencing by either preventing or promoting the recruitment of regulatory proteins to DNA. Methylation of CpG islands can block the access of transcription factors to the transcription sites [6, 7], or by recruiting methyl-binding domain proteins (MBDs), which can mediate gene repression through interactions with histone deacetylases (HDACs) [8, 9]. This epigenetic modification does not change the DNA sequence, but enhances the stability and chromosome integrity and promotes genome organization into transcriptionally active or silenced regions. DNA methylation at the whole genome level provides a specific global methylation pattern [2, 10] that plays an important role in regulating gene expression (e.g. development and cell-specific gene expression) in association with chromatin-associated proteins. The maintenance of a cell-specific methylation pattern after every cellular DNA replication cycle provides a stable gene-silencing mechanism that plays an important role in regulating gene expression. The maintenance methyltransferase DNMT1 is responsible for copying DNA methylation patterns to the daughter strands during DNA replication, whereas DNMT3a and DNMT3b are *de novo* methyltransferases that establish the methylation patterns early in development [11]. DNMT3L, a homologous protein to other DNMT3s, increases the ability of DNM3a and 3b to bind to DNA, stimulating their activity. Some problems in the establishment of methylation biomarkers in gynecologic cancers, especially in cervical cancer [12], come from the fact that: (1) the extent of methylation across the various CpG sites in a promoter can be rather heterogeneous and consequently, the assay outcome is likely to be influenced by the region of CpGs that is targeted; (2) the distinct levels of background methylation due to differences in cell type composition between cervical tissue samples that can contain substantial amounts of nonepithelial (stromal) cells and cervical scrapings that are enriched in superficial epithelial cells. For this reason, the methylation results obtained from tissue samples may not be directly extrapolated to cervical scrapings [13]. In addition, while the methylation of tumor suppressor' promoters is an early and frequent alteration in carcinogenesis [14] and, on the other hand, is widespread in the human genome, only a subset of affected loci play critical roles in tumorigenesis [15]. CpG hypermethylation is gene- and cancer type–specific [16, 17, 18, 19], providing a useful signature for tumor diagnosis and prognosis [18] that must be established accurately.

1.1.2. *Covalent histone modifications*

Mammalian genome represents a highly structured complex comprised of compacted DNA and proteins that can adopt different three-dimensional conformations dependent of nuclear context and biochemical changes present in the genome and at the histone level [20]. At first glance, the chromatin is present in two forms: transcriptionally active euchromatin and more condensed and transcriptionally inactive heterochromatin. In the genome, there are some structural regions (such as centromeres) containing constitutive heterochromatin; others may go through an open conformation to a compact one—optional heterochromatin. These transitions, vital to the establishment of necessary transcriptional various models of embryonic development, growth, and adult life, are under epigenetic control. Nucleosomes form the repetitive fundamental units of the chromatin and are designed to pack the huge eukaryotic genome in the nucleus (mammalian cells contain approximately 2 m of linear DNA wrapped in a core size of 10 μm in diameter) [20]. The nucleosomes in turn are compacted and form the chromosomes. The nucleosomal core consists of approximately 147 base pairs wrapped around a histone octamer made up of two copies of the histones H2A, H2B, H3, and H4. Histone H1 (linker histone) and its isoforms are involved in chromatin compaction underlying nucleosome condensation. Decondensed nucleosomes look like a bead wrapping a DNA molecule [21]. Histone covalent modifications (epigenetic changes) represent important regulatory elements that influence chromatin interactions by structural changes either by electrostatic interactions and recruitment of nonhistone proteins [22].

Histones can undergo a variety of posttranslational modifications at the N-terminus (like acetylation, methylation, phosphorylation, sumoylation, ubiquitination, and ADP-ribosylation) that can alter the DNA–histone interaction, with a major impact on chromatin structure and key cellular processes such as transcription, replication, and repair [20]. The histone code may be transient or stable. The mechanism of inheritance of this histone code is not fully understood. The patterns of histone modifications are specific to each cell type and play a key role in determining cellular identity [23, 24]. In contrast with stem cells, differentiated cells acquire a more rigid chromatin structure, which is important for maintaining cell specialization [23]. Epigenetic regulation mediated by histone modification is a dynamic process. Lysine residue methylation using histone methyltransferase (HMT) is correlated either with transcriptional activation or repression, whereas lysine acetylation correlates with transcriptional activation [25]. Histone methyltransferases (HMTs) and demethylases (HDMs) work in tandem to determine the degree of methylation of the lysine residue [26]. Histone H3 lysine 4 trimethylation (H3K4me3) correlates with euchromatin and gene transcription activation. Histone H3 lysine 27 trimethylation and/or lysine 9 (H3K27me3/H3K9me3) is correlated with the transcriptional repression of heterochromatin and H3K27me3 modification is critical for stem cells; demethylation at this level is correlated with differentiation [27, 28, 29, 30, 31]. These two modifications represent the main silencing mechanisms in mammalian cells, H3K9me3 working in concert with DNA methylation and H3K27me3 largely working exclusive of DNA methylation [32]. Histone acetylation is one of the histone modifications that have been studied extensively. The two homonymous enzymes that are involved in maintaining a specific profile are histone acetyltransferases (HATs) and histone deacetylases (HDACs) [26]. Generally, the level of histone acetylation correlated with transcriptional activation and deacetylation correlates with transcriptional repression. H3 histone acetylations at lysine 9 (H3K9ac) and lysine 4 to 16 are characteristic euchromatin changes located in regions where genes are actively transcribed. Although histone modifications act mainly by altering the architecture of some modifications (H3K4me3 and H3K9ac) mediates gene regulation by recruiting other proteins involved in chromatin remodeling [33, 34]. Histone modifications and DNA methylation interact with each other at multiple levels to determine gene expression status, chromatin organization, and cellular identity [35]. Several HMTs, including G9a, SUV39H1, and PRMT5, methylate DNA to specific genomic targets recruiting DNA methyltransferases (DNMTs) [36, 37, 38]. In addition, DNMTs may recruit HDACs and methyl-binding proteins to achieve gene silencing and chromatin condensation [8, 9]. DNA methylation can also be established via H3K9 methylation, such as MeCP2, thereby establishing a repressive chromatin state [39]. Recent studies showed that the main chromatin changes that occurs during tumorigenesis are characterized by a global loss of acetylated H4 lysine 16 (H4K16ac) and H4 lysine 20 trimethylation (H4K20me3) [40]. HDACs were found overexpressed in various types of cancer [41, 42] (becoming a major target for epigenetic therapy), along with HATs, whose expression can also be altered in cancer. MOZ, MORF, CBP, and p300 (HATs) may be targets for chromosomal translocations, especially in leukemia [43]. Changes in histone methylation patterns (deregulation of HMTs) are associated with aberrant gene silencing in cancer, and an effective cancer treatment strategy targeting HDMs represents a promising treatment option.

1.2. Posttranscriptional gene regulation by noncoding RNAs

Noncoding RNAs are involved in fundamental processes, such as chromatin dynamics and gene silencing, and their transcripts outnumber the group of protein transcripts. It is well known that the initiation of X-chromosome inactivation is regulated by noncoding RNAs (Xist function) and the noncoding RNAs molecules are also involved in imprinting, suggesting that antisense RNA can induce transcriptional silencing [44, 45, 46]. The characterized noncoding RNA family consists of a large group of small regulatory microRNAs (about 1400 microRNAs in humans) [47].MicroRNAs (miRNAs) are short noncoding RNAs of 20–24 nucleotides that play important roles in virtually all biological pathways in mammals like differentiation and growth control. Based on computer predictions, it was proposed that miRNAs may regulate many cell cycle control genes [48]. miRNAs influence numerous cancer-relevant processes such as proliferation, cell cycle control, apoptosis, differentiation, migration, and metabolism. The key processes of miRNA biogenesis pathways have been characterized. Primary miRNA transcripts are transcribed from separate transcriptional units or embedded within the introns of protein coding genes by RNA polymerase II. Primary miRNA transcripts are processed by a complex formed by RNase III enzyme and Drosha, resulting in a pre-miRNA hairpin that is subsequently exported from the nucleus to the cytoplasm by exportin 5 (XPO5). Further pre-miRNA molecules are processed by another protein complex, including DICER and TRBP, to produce the single-stranded mature miRNA (ssmiRNA). ssmiRNA is subsequently incorporated in RNA induced silencing complex (RISC), along with key proteins such as AGO2 and GW182. The role of mature miRNA (as part of the RISC) is to induce posttranscriptional gene silencing by complementary sequence motifs to the target mRNAs predominantly found within the 3′ untranslated regions (UTRs) [47, 49, 50]. One specific miRNA may target up to several hundred mRNAs; therefore, a miRNA may silence various genes while a specific mRNA may be targeted by several miRNAs. Aberrant miRNA expression may interfere with gene transcription and influence cancer-related signaling pathways [51, 52, 53].New data are added to decipher the role of miRNAs in normal physiology and pathology. Several microarray expression studies performed on a wide spectrum of cancer types have proved that deregulated miRNAs expression is the rule rather than the exception in cancer [54, 55, 56, 57]. Animal models featuring miRNA overexpression or knock-down have demonstrated the relation between miRNAs and cancer development, thus proposing miRNAs as potential biomarkers and putative therapeutic targets [58]. In addition, since miRNAs were discovered, many researchers focused their interest on identifying miRNAs generated by viruses. Several data support this hypothesis mainly based on miRNA size, which allows them to avoid the immune system but also to be supported by the small size of viral genome. It is not unexpected that many miRNAs encoded by viruses have been discovered, most of them transcribed from double-stranded DNA viruses [59]. miRNAs can regulate the expression of viral genes that are involved in controlling viral replication. It is supposed that these miRNAs might influence viral gene expression in a differentiation-dependent manner by targeting viral transcripts. On the other hand, different hrHPV types have different oncogenic potentials, viral miRNA being considered one of the factors involved in oncogenic regulation; some conserved miRNAs are involved in the switch from HPV productive to transforming infections.

2. Evaluation of aberrant epigenetic modifications as essential players in cancer progression

Normally, evolution and morphological state of genital organs are in close interdependence with hormonal status that is different in different periods: childhood, sexual maturity, climacterium, and menopause. On the other hand, there is an increasing interest in the identification of diagnostic biomarkers and biomarkers able to predict both response to treatment and survival. For an optimal planning of therapeutic strategy in high-risk patients, a close association between biological variables and (epi)genetic profiles associated with aggressive clinical behavior could be useful. Therefore, many cellular changes should be analysed in this context.

Benign tumors of the vulva can be developed from epithelial components (papillomas and warts) mezenchimatos tissue (fibroma, leiomyoma, lipoma, hemangioma, and lymphangioma), and local glands (Bartholin gland cysts or cysts of sweat glands). *Vulvar cancer* is a rare malignant disease accounting for less than 5% of gynecological malignancies [60, 61, 62]. The most common vulvar cancers are epidermoid carcinoma and rarely adenocarcinomas that are developed in the Bartholin glands or sweat glands. Approximately 20%–40% of vulvar squamous carcinomas are often associated with papilloma virus infection [60 - 66] and are more frequent in young people. Non-HPV vulvar cancers occur in the elderly and are associated with somatic mutations, especially in TP53 [60 - 63, 65, 66]. Tumors harbouring a mutation have a worse prognosis than vulvar squamous cancers without (epi)genetic changes [67 - 70]. However, allelic imbalances seem to occur in both groups and the cumulative number of epigenetic changes increases from dysplasia to cancer [71]. The data with respect to epigenetic changes in vulvar cancer progression is limited to a few articles on DNA hypermethylation but not to chromatin remodeling or histone modifications. This data is presented in Table 1. Hypermethylation seems to be more frequent in vulvar squamous cancers than in vulvar intraepithelial neoplasia, but more studies are needed. Taking into account the existence of two etiological categories of vulvar carcinomas (related or not to HPV), the miRNA signature in these two types of vulvar carcinomas were evaluated [72]. Some miRNAs had lower expression in HPV-positive tumors (miR-1291, miR-342-3p, miR-193a-5p, miR-29c#-, miR-106b#, miR-22#, miR-365, miR-151-5P, miR-144#, miR-125b-1#, miR-519b-3p, miR-26b, miR-19b-1, and miR-1254) and other microRNAs had higher expression in HPV-positive tumors (miR-1274B, miR-142-3p, miR-21, miR-708, miR-16, miR-660, miR-29c, miR-1267, miR-454, and miR-186) [72]. In HPV-negative samples, we observed an association between lymph node metastases with decreased expression of miR-223-5p and miR-19b-1-5p, vascular invasion with decreased expression of miR-100-3p and miR-19b-5p-1, and advanced tumor staging (FIGO IIIA, IIIB, and IIIC) with expression of microRNAs miR-519b-1-5p and miR-133a. In addition, de Melo Maia and collaborators (2013) built a network between miRNA expression profiles and putative target mRNAs (TP53, RB, PTEN, and EGFR) based on prediction algorithms, demonstrating that the evaluated miRNAs can be involved in vulvar cancer progression, thereby providing biomarkers for the establishment of prognostic and predictive values of response to novel targeting therapies in vulvar cancer [72].

The vagina is a fibromuscular tubular organ, which histologically consists of three layers of tissue: (1) an outer layer consisting of fibro-elastic connective tissue; (2) vaginal muscles with a longitudinal outer layer and an inner layer of fibers circularly arranged in a spiral; and (3) Malpighian mucosa, covered by squamous epithelium. The vaginal epithelium undergoes changes in relation to the period of the woman's life and depending on hormonal stimulus. Histological changes are reflected in vaginal cytology. Vaginal epithelium responds to ovarian stimuli through proliferation, differentiation and desquamation. Thus, in adult women, under the action of estrogen during the proliferative phase, vaginal mucosa proliferates and differentiates morphologically and functionally, and later, during the luteal phase, under the action of progesterone, superficial cell layer desquamation occurs. The action of estrogen on the vaginal mucosa is exercised on the epithelium as well as on the subjacent stroma.

Vaginal cancer is also a rare malignancy, accounting for about 2%–3% of all gynecologic cancers [73, 74]. The squamous cell carcinomas (SCC) are more frequent (80%–90%) than adenocarcinomas. If the risk factors linked to vaginal squamous cell carcinoma are smoking, immunosuppression, high number of sexual partners, papillomavirus and history of cervical precancerous and cancerous lesions [75, 76, 77], in the case of the vaginal adenocarcinomas, particularly clear cell adenocarcinomas, exposure to an antiabortive drug diethylstilbestrol (DES) was incriminated [78, 79, 80]. On the other hand, if squamous vaginal cancer tends to occur more commonly in the proximal third of the vagina, especially the posterior vaginal wall, the adenocarcinomas are mostly seen in the anterior upper vaginal wall [74]. Human papillomaviruses have been also linked to vaginal cancers, HPV prevalence in 2/3 lesions of vaginal intraepithelial neoplasia and invasive vaginal cancer being over 90% and 70%, respectively [81, 82]. The HPV oncogenic transformation has been associated with high levels of E6 and E7 viral oncoproteins in the epithelia that can be achieved by two mechanisms: (1) increased production of E6 and E7 after the loss of E2 (the normal regulator of E6 and E7 expression) during viral integration [83]; (2) methylation of the E2-binding sites (E2BS) in the viral LCR in the region close to the early promoter that could inhibit E6 and E7 transcription [84]. Therefore, HPV16-related integration, methylation in E2BS3 and 4, and viral load may represent different viral characteristics driving vaginal and vulvar carcinogenesis [85].The adverse health outcomes induced by DES exposure during fetal development include infertility, early menopause, and breast cancer, along with a rare form of vaginal adenocarcinoma in adolescent girls [86, 87]. While animal models show an association of early exposure to estrogens with the expression levels of several genes [88, 89, 90] and epigenetic changes, including DNA methylation and histone modifications [91, 92, 93], the first study that evaluates the possible effects of *in utero* DES exposure on genome wide DNA methylation in humans cannot find evidence of large persistent effects of *in utero* DES exposure on blood DNA methylation [94].

The uterus is a hollow organ, in which the product of conception is developed. It consists of three parts: body, isthmus, and cervix. The corpus presents a mucosa (endometrium), muscular wall (myometrium), and serous peritoneal surface. The endometrium is a specialized tissue, particularly receptive to the influence of sex hormones that differs from a histological point of view at prepubertal periods, sexual maturity, and menopause. Also, the uterine mucosa is in constant transformation during menstrual cycles, sexual maturity, growth processes, functional maturation, and regression. Similar risk factors for endometrial cancers were incriminated: adult obesity [95], first-degree family history of endometrial cancer, or colorectal cancer [96]. Nulliparity and infertility appeared to independently contribute to endometrial cancer risk [97]. The endometrium is extremely sensitive to hormones, the estrogen and progesterone being two key regulators of proliferation and differentiation in reproductive tissues [98]. The two isoforms of the progesterone receptor, PRA and PRB, required for endometrial differentiation [99], are generated by alternative transcription and translation from the same gene with the addition of 164 amino acids in the N-terminus sequences of PRB [98] that makes them functionally different [99]. A shift in the estrogen–progesterone balance is the major cause for the development of endometrial cancer [100]. Progesterone is an important inducer of endometrial differentiation and an inhibitor of tumorigenesis because the addition of progestin (synthetic progesterone) can prevent endometrial cancer induced by an excess of estrogens from endogenous sources (e.g., adipose tissue storage of estrogen and with polycystic ovarian syndrome) or from exogenous sources in therapeutic administration [100]. While progestin therapy achieves promising outcomes with early stage endometrial cancer, advanced and recurrent disease has only minor effects. This is due to the fact that in advanced endometrial cancer, the progesterone receptor is lost but it has been demonstrated that reestablishing progesterone signaling in these cells can inhibit endometrial cancer cell proliferation and invasion and increase sensitivity to apoptotic stimuli [100]. The epigenetic restoration of progesterone receptor expression could result in resensitization of endometrial tumors to progestin therapy. The functional role of epigenetic factors in endometrial cancer development began to be evaluated. A study by Jones and collaborators (2013) emphasizes the role of HAND2 hypermethylation, which is a key step in endometrial carcinogenesis [101]. HAND2 is a basic helix-loop-helix transcription factor and developmental regulator [102], expressed in the normal endometrial stroma. The physiological function of HAND2 is to suppress the production of fibroblast growth factors that mediate the paracrine mitogenic effects of estrogen on the endometrial epithelium [103]. HAND2 is under progesterone regulation [104, 105], entering in the progesterone-mediated suppression of estrogen-induced pathways. Consequently, the methylation of HAND2 is able to predict the response to progesterone [101]. HAND2 methylation is the most common molecular alteration in endometrial cancer and, on the other hand, is an early event in endometrial carcinogenesis that makes it a sensitive test to correctly identify endometrial cancer patients amongst those women who present with postmenopausal bleeding [101].

Histologically, *the cervix* shows mucosa, muscle wall, and the peritoneal serosa. The mucosa of the cervix has an exocervical portion (covered by squamous epithelium, nonkeratinized) and one endocervical (covered by a single-layered cylindrical epithelium, mucus secreting, which contains a small number of ciliated cells, basal stem cells and racemic, tubular, or branched type glands). Cancer of the uterine cervix is the major cause of death from gynecological cancers and in over 90% of cases is associated with high-risk human papilloma virus (hrHPV). Etiological factors include cigarette smoking, impairment of cell-mediated immunity, and long-term estrogen–progestin use [106, 107, 108]. But the main etiological factor of squamous cell carcinoma (that accounts for about 80% of the cases) as well as adenocarcinoma are human papilloma virus infections [109]. The role of other sexually transmitted infections (*Chlamydia trachomatis* and herpes simplex virus) is still unclear [108, 110].In cervical cancer, tumorigenesis of both squamous cell carcinoma and adenocarcinoma is HPV-related [109]. The transforming potential of E6 and E7 viral oncoproteins is based on their numerous actions on cellular proteins, mainly on p53 and pRB tumor suppressors, which are degraded and inactivated, respectively. In addition to the already reported genomic alterations in cervical cancer development by hrHPV, many studies underline the involvement of epigenetic alteration in host cell genes or at the levels of RNA. In order to find some diagnostic and prognostic biomarkers, the methylation of host cell genes and methylation of viral genes were evaluated [12]. The CpG hypermethylation of promoters of tumor suppressor genes, an early and frequent alteration in carcinogenesis, affects all important pathways: cell adhesion (cell adhesion molecule 1 (CADM1)) [13], E-cadherin [111, 112], apoptosis (DAPK, a proapoptotic serine/threonine kinase [113, 114]), cell cycle (cyclin A1 methylation [114, 115]), fragile histidine triad (FHIT) [116], cell signaling pathways (retinoic acid receptor [117], Ras association domain family 1 isoform A (RASSF1) [118]), Wnt/β catenin pathway (adenomatous polyposis coli (APC) [119] and PTEN [120]), p53 signaling pathway (p73 [121]), and DNA repair (O6 methylguanine DNA methyltransferase (MGMT) [113, 122]).For cervical scrapings, some methylation marker panels of host genes, with sensitivities of over 80% for CIN3+ were evaluated: SOX1/PAX1, SOX1/LMX1A, SOX1/NKX6-1, PAX1/LMX1A; PAX1/NKX6-1, LMX1A/NKX6-1 [123], JAM3/EPB41L3/TERT/C13ORF18 [124], and CADM1/MAL [13, 125], etc. Host gene methylation analysis might be an alternative for hrHPV DNA detection because aberrant methylation can be detected in cervical smears up to 7 years prior to the diagnosis of cervical cancer [126]. On the other hand, for methylation analysis, cervical scrape samples as well as self-collected cervico-vaginal lavage samples can be used [127].As accurate predictor tests, the measurement of DNA methylation in HPV genomes, in certain early (E) and late (L) open reading frames (ORF) as well as in parts of the upstream regulatory region (URR), may have diagnostic value. The hypermethylation in the L1 region was a common feature of cervical cancer but not of CIN induced by HPV16 [128], or HPV18 [129]. But the DNA methylation on multiple CG sites in the L1, L2, E2, and E4 ORFs were significantly associated with CIN2+ after accounting for multiple testing [130]. Some studies have contradictory results because most were quite small and heterogeneous and did not always include (1) comparable sets of specimens (cancer, high-grade CIN, cell lines), (2) exactly the same CG sites, or (3) the same methodology [12]. Overall, as cervical cancer prevention moves to DNA testing methods, DNA-based biomarkers, such as HPV methylation could serve as a reflex strategy to identify women at high risk for cervical cancer [131], but the region with the best predictive value must be established.In addition to the already reported genomic alterations in cervical cancer development by hrHPV, many studies underline the involvement of viral or cellular miRNAs, mainly based on the fact that some RNA micromolecules target transcriptional factors that modulate both cellular and viral gene expression [132, 133].In HPV infection, E6 decreases miR-34a [132, 134], which is a target of p53, thus the effect of E6 on miRNA-34a is mediated by decreased p53 [132,134]. On the other hand, one of the targets of miR-34a is p18Ink4c [135], an inhibitor of CDK4/6 that promotes the cell cycle. E7 decreases miR-203 during keratinocyte differentiation, which is a tumor suppressor and thus increases carcinogenesis [136] through an increase of cell survival targeting antiapoptotic protein bcl-w [137], induction of G1 cell cycle arrest targeting survivin [138], inhibition of migration and invasion targeting LIM and SH3 protein [139]. E7 upregulates miR-15a, miR-15b, and miR-15b through E2F1 and E2F3 [140, 141] and in turn, these miR decrease cyclin E1, leading to cell cycle arrest [142]. A lot of other miRs are upregulated or decreased by virus oncogenes inducing changes in cellular signaling pathways, some of these have not yet been elucidated [143].

Ovaries, paired organs, constitute the female sexual gland with endocrine lunette and also produce ova. The ovary is covered by germinal epithelium (formed from cuboid or cylindrical cells) and subjacent is a thin layer of dense connective tissue. The ovary presents a cortical area (comprised of follicles, corpus luteum, and stroma) and a medulla. Starting from puberty till menopause, there is a growth and maturation of one ovarian follicle during each menstrual cycle and the formation of one corpus luteum after rupture of the follicle and oocyte removal. If the egg is not fertilized, the corpus luteum regresses, undergoes progressive sclerosis forming a hyaline. If the egg is fertilized, the corpus luteum becomes more voluminous and luteal cells increase, constituting the corpus luteum of pregnancy. Ovarian stroma is formed from fibroblastic and mesenchymal cells. Stromal cells present both characters of connective cells and steroid activity (secreting androgens and estrogens). Ovarian medulla consists of lax connective tissue containing blood and lymph vessels, nerves, and embryonic elements. The growth and development of the follicle during the ovarian cycle are driven by two gonadotrophic hormones, secreted by the anterior pituitary: follicle-stimulating hormone (FSH) and luteinising hormone (LH). Both FSH and LH are under the control of gonadotrophin-releasing hormone (GnRH) secreted by the hypothalamus through negative feedback carried out by estrogens that are secreted by thecal cells of the follicle.

Ovarian cancer ranks second after cervical cancer worldwide. On the other hand, ovarian cancer is in seventh place in terms of incidence among malignant tumors in women and eighth with respect to death due to malignant tumors in women worldwide [144]. If approximately 90% of ovarian cancers arise from epithelial cells, 3% are from germ cells and 7% from granulosa-theca cells. Ovarian cancer comprises different types of tumors with widely differing clinicopathologic features and behaviors. Based on clinicopathologic and molecular genetic studies, two histologic types of epithelial ovarian serous carcinomas were established: low-grade serous carcinomas (LGSCs) and high-grade serous carcinomas (HGSCs) [145]. Although they are developed independently along different molecular pathways, both types develop from fallopian tube epithelium and involve the ovary secondarily. Type I tumors (LGSCs) are comprised of low-grade serous, low-grade endometrioid, mucinous, and clear cell carcinomas; typically present as large cystic masses confined to one ovary; have a relatively indolent course; and are relatively genetically stable being associated with mutations in KRAS, BRAF, PTEN, PIK3CA, CTNNB1, ARID1A, and PPP2R1A [146, 147] that perturb signaling pathways. Type II tumors (HGSCs) are composed of high-grade serous, high-grade endometrioid, undifferentiated carcinomas and malignant-mixed mesodermal tumors; clinically aggressive and typically present at an advanced stage, which contributes to their high fatality [148]; at the time of diagnosis, they demonstrate marked chromosomal aberrations but over the course of the disease these changes remain relatively stable [149]; approximately 60% of HGSC have the fallopian tube as the origin of serous tumors [150], because the expression profiles of ovarian HGSCs more closely resemble fallopian tube epithelium than the ovarian surface epithelium [151]; they harbor TP53 mutations in over 95% of cases [152, 153], but rarely harbor the mutations detected in the low-grade serous tumors; another possible origin of HGSC is from inclusion cysts through a process of implantation of tubal (müllerian-type) tissue rather than by a process of metaplasia from ovarian surface epithelium (mesothelial). Hypermethylation has been found to be associated with the inactivation of almost every pathway involved in ovarian cancer development, including DNA repair, cell cycle regulation, apoptosis, cell adherence, and detoxification pathways [154]. Complete or partial inactivation of the BRCA1 gene through hypermethylation of its promoter has been reported in 15% of sporadic ovarian tumors [155, 156], 31% of carcinomas but not in the benign or borderline tumors [157], or in the hereditary type of the disease, nor in samples from women with a germ line BRCA1 mutation [158, 159]. On the other hand, hypermethylation of BRCA1 was detected at a significantly higher frequency in serous carcinomas than in tumors of the other histological types [160]. The homeobox genes (HOX), a family of transcription factors that function during embryonic development and control pattern formation, differentiation, and proliferation [161] was associated with ovarian cancers [162]. In addition, based on the high percentage of methylation of the HOXA9 gene observed in 95% of patients with high-grade serous ovarian carcinoma [163, 164], it has been suggested that the methylation status of HOXA9 and HOXAD11 genes may serve as potential diagnostic and prognostic biomarkers [163,164]. Some other genes found hypomethylated were associated with progression towards cancer: LINE-1 elements [165], SNGG (synucelin-γ), encoding an activator of the MAPK and Elk-1 signaling cascades [166, 167], etc. Overall, DNA hypomethylation may promote tumorigenesis by transcriptional activation of proto-oncogenes and on the other hand loss of imprinting or genomic instability. DNA hypermethylation predisposes to gene mutation because the methylated cytosines are often deaminated and converted to thymine leading to inactivation of tumor suppressor genes. However, these phenomena deregulate the main functions of gynecological cancer cells (Figure 1 and Table 1).

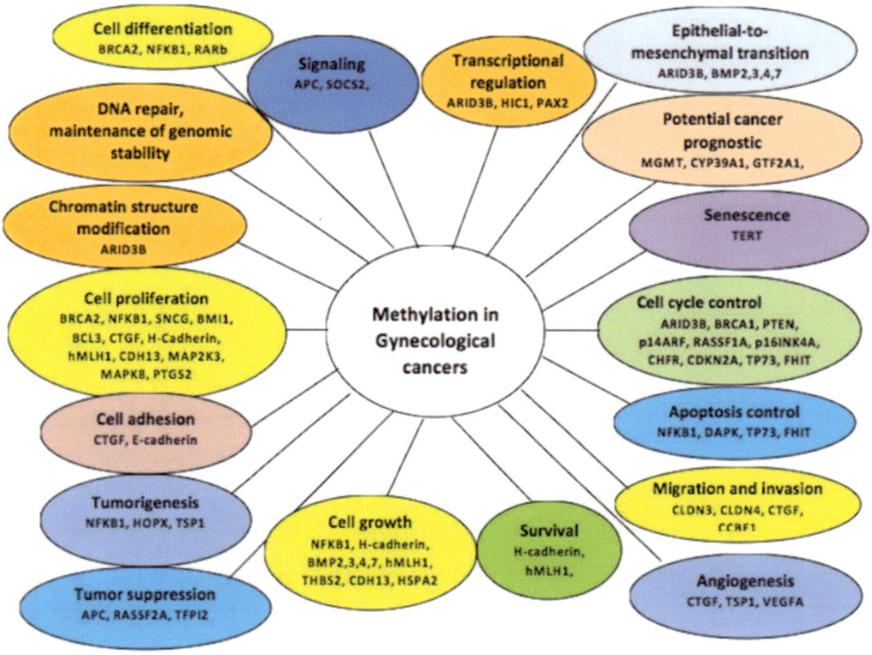

Figure 1. Biological functions influenced by alterations of DNA methylation in gynecological cancers.

	Genes	Functions	Expression change	Epigenetic regulation	References
Ovarian cancer	*BRCA2*	Cell proliferation and differentiation	Overexpression	Hypomethylation	168, 169
	CLDN3;CLDN4	Migration and invasion	Overexpression	DNA hypomethylation, H3 acetylation; Loss of repressive histone modifications	170, 171, 172

Genes	Functions	Expression change	Epigenetic regulation	References
HOXA10 *HOXA11*	Fertility, embryo viability, regulation of hematopoietic lineage commitment; regulation of uterine development and is required for female fertility	Overexpression	DNA hypomethylation/ hypermethylation	164, 173, 174, 175
MAL	Formation, stabilization and maintenance of glycosphingolipid-enriched membrane microdomains	Overexpression	Hypomethylation	176
NFKB1	Cell proliferation; Inflammation, immunity, differentiation, cell growth, tumorigenesis, and apoptosis	Overexpression	miR-9 downregulation	177
SNCG	Cell proliferation	Overexpression	DNA hypomethylation	167
BMI1	Cell proliferation	Overexpression	miR-15a and miR-16 down regulation	178
TUBB3	Taxane drug resistance	Overexpression	DNA hypomethylation, chromatin acetylation	179
ARID3B	Epithelial-to-mesenchymal transition; Embryonic patterning, cell lineage gene regulation, cell cycle control, transcriptional regulation and possibly in chromatin structure modification	Overexpression	miR-125a downregulation via EGFR signaling	180
BCL3	Cell proliferation, tumorigenesis	Overexpression	miR-125b downregulation	181
BRCA1	DNA repair, cell cycle checkpoint control, and maintenance of genomic stability	Overexpression	Hypermethylation	182
PTEN, *p14ARF*	Cell cycle regulation	Overexpression	Hypermethylation	182
DAPK	Regulator of programmed cell death	Overexpression	Hypermethylation	182
RASSF1A	Negative regulator of cell proliferation through inhibition of G1/S-phase progression	Overexpression	Hypermethylation	159,182, 183
p16INK4A	Cell cycle regulation	Overexpression	Hypermethylation	183
APC	Tumor suppression by antagonizing the WNT.	Overexpression	Hypermethylation	159, 183

	Genes	Functions	Expression change	Epigenetic regulation	References
	CTGF	Cell adhesion, migration, proliferation, angiogenesis	Overexpression	Hypermethylation	184
	CCBE1	Extracellular matrix remodeling and migration	Overexpression	Hypermethylation	185
	HIC1	Transcription factor	Overexpression	Hypermethylation	159
	RARb	Cell differentiation	Overexpression	Hypermethylation	183
	E-cadherin	Cell adhesion		Hypermethylation	183
	H-cadherin	Regulation of cell growth, survival and proliferation	Overexpression	Hypermethylation	183
	hMLH1	Regulation of cell growth, survival and proliferation DNA mismatch repair	Overexpression	Hypermethylation	186, 187, 188
	GSTP1	Detoxification	Overexpression	Hypermethylation	189
	MGMT	Potential prognostic cancer	Overexpression	Hypermethylation	187,188
	CYP39A1	Potential prognostic cancer	Overexpression	Hypermethylation	190
	GTF2A1, FOXD4L4, EBP	Potential prognostic cancer	Overexpression	Hypermethylation	190
	HAAO	Potential prognostic cancer	Overexpression	Hypermethylation	190
Endometrial cancer	*BMP2,3,4,7*	Cell growth and EMT	Overexpression	Hypomethylation	191
	SOX4	Prognosis	Overexpression	miR-129-2 downregulation by DNA hypermethylation	192
	hMLH1	Regulation of cell growth, survival and proliferation; DNA mismatch repair		Hypermethylation	193, 194
	RASSF1A	Negative regulator of cell proliferation through inhibition of G1/S-phase progression		Hypermethylation	195, 196, 197
	CHFR	Regulates progression of the cell cycle		Hypermethylation	198, 199
	APC	Signaling and intracellular adhesion		Hypermethylation	200
	THBS2	Inhibitor of tumor growth and angiogenesis		Hypermethylation	201
	p16INK4A	Cell cycle regulation		Hypermethylation	202
	PTEN	Cell cycle regulation		Hypermethylation	203

	Genes	Functions	Expression change	Epigenetic regulation	References
	PER1	Cells circadian rhythms maintenance; cancer development		Hypermethylation	204
	HOPX	Tumorigenesis		Hypermethylation	205
	CDH13	Regulation of cell growth, survival and proliferation		Hypermethylation	206
	HSPA2, MLH1	Regulation of cell growth		Hypermethylation	206
	SOCS2	Cytokine-inducible negative regulators of cytokine signaling		Hypermethylation	206
	PAX2	Transcriptional factor		Hypomethylation	207
Vulvar cancer	*CDKN2A*	Cell cycle regulation		Hypermethylation	208, 209
	MGMT	Potential prognostic cancer		Hypermethylation	210
	RASSF2A	Tumor suppressor gene		Hypermethylation	210
	RASSF1A	Negative regulator of cell proliferation through inhibition of G1/S-phase progression		Hypermethylation	210
	TERT	Cellular senescence		Hypermethylation	209
	TSP1	Platelet aggregation, angiogenesis, and tumorigenesis		Hypermethylation	210
	TFPI2	Tumor suppressor gene		Hypermethylation	209
	TP73, FHIT	Cell cycle regulation; apoptosis		Hypermethylation	211
	TSLC-1			Hypermethylation	212
Cervical cancer	*CAGE*	RNA processing	Overexpression	Hypomethylation	213
	MAP2K3	Cell proliferation	Overexpression	miR-214 downregulation	177
	MAPK8	Cell proliferation	Overexpression	miR-214 downregulation	177
	PTGS2	Cell proliferation, migration, invasion	Overexpression	miR-101 downregulation	214
	SERPINH1	Metastasis	Overexpression	miR-29a downregulation	215
	VEGFA	Tumor growth, angiogenesis	Overexpression	miR-203 downregulation by DNA hypermethylation	216

Table 1. Altered DNA methylation in gynecological cancer

miRNA as key players in cell fate decisions are strongly linked to gynecological cancer. But, although the methods to discover miRNA were improved, research is still in progress. Some of these miRNA that have been associated with gynecologic cancers are shown in Figure 2 and Table 2.

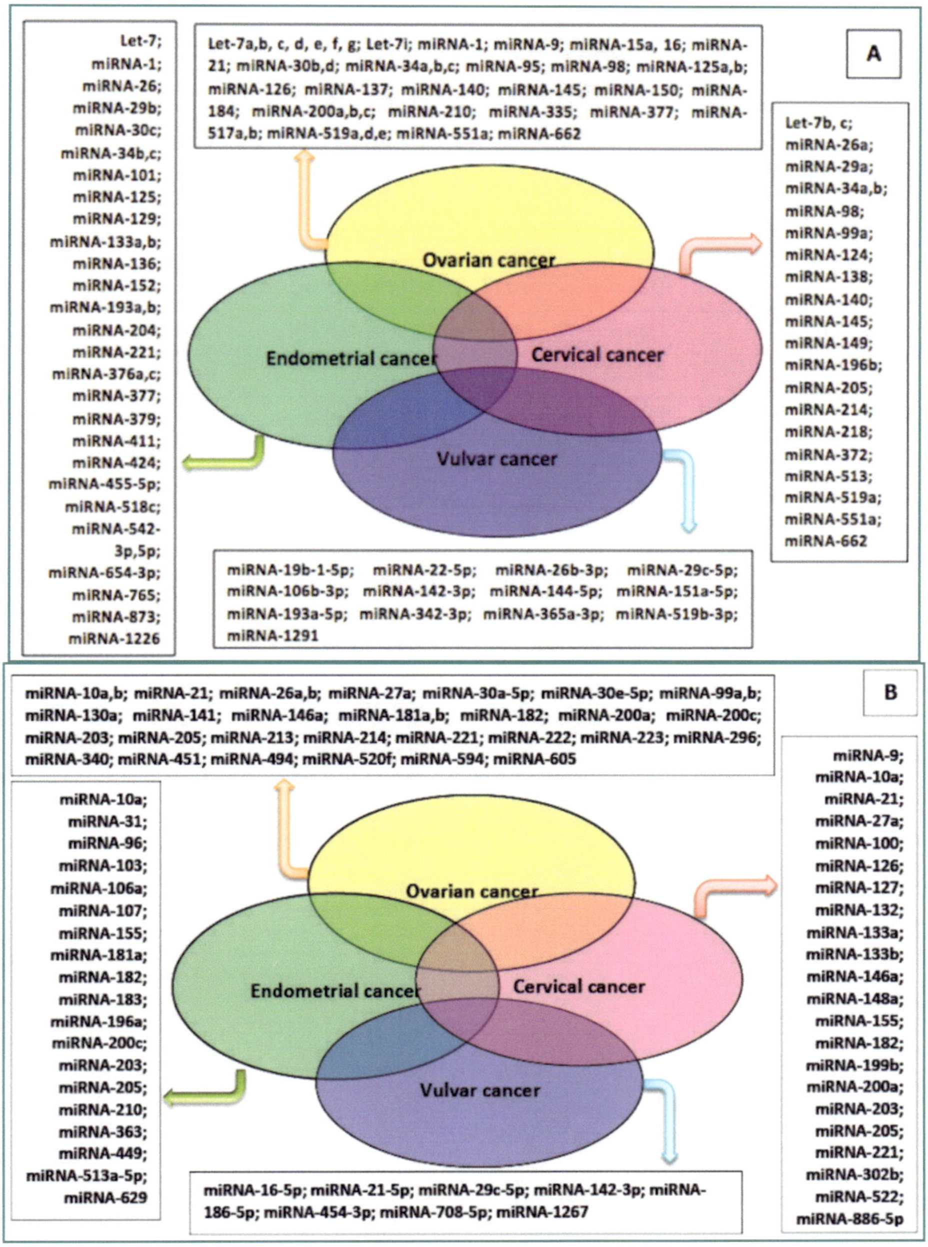

Figure 2. Venn diagram showing dysregulated miRNAs in gynecological cancers. (A) miRNAs downregulated, (B) miRNAs upregulated. Common miRNAs dysregulated signature between ovarian and other cancers are shown in red.

Specific miRNAs have effects on various molecular pathways, and specific miRNA expression signatures in gynecological cancers can be associated with diagnosis, prognosis, and therapy response. miRNAs can regulate a large number of target genes and Table 2 lists the estimated targets.

	miRNA(s)	Expression (Up/ downregulated)	Estimated target(s)	References
Ovarian cancer	Let-7a,b, c, d, e, f, g	Down	c-Myc, KRAS, HMGA2, IL-6, LIN28B, HIC2	217, 218
	Let-7i	Down	HMGA2, LIN28Bm TRIM71,IGF2BP1	219
	1	Down	FOXP1, HDAC4 c-Met, Pim1, HAND2	220
	9	Down	NF-kB, Bcl2, Bcl6, FGF, b-Raf	220, 221
	15a, 16	Down	BMI1	178
	21	Down	PTEN	222
	30b,d	Down	Unknown	223, 224
	34a,b,c	Down	SIRT1, MYC, NOTCH, BCL2, CCND1,WNT3	222, 223, 225
	95	Down	AIB1, GNAI2	226
	98	Down	HMGA2, LIN28B, HIC2	223
	125a, b	Down	ARID3B, LIN28b, Akt3, ETS1ARID3B, RBB2, ERBB3, TNFa, BMPR1B	223, 227, 228
	126	Down	SPRED1, PIK3R2, RGS4, RGS5, PI3K	229
	137	Down	CDK6, MITF, KLF12, PDLIM3	2
	140	Down	c-SRK, MMP13, FGF2	220,230
	145	Down	MAP3K3, MAP4K4, SOX2, OCT4, KLF4, c-myc	220, 230, 231
	150	Down	c-Myb, MAK9, Akt3, MAP2K4	230
	184	Down	TTK69, K10, Sax(A)	230
	200a,b,c	Down	ZEB1, ZEB2, FN1, PPM1E, EXOC5, GATA4, GATA6, TUBB3, TNC, TGF-b	219 ; 232, 233
	210	Down	E2F3, EFNA3, HoxA1, HoxA9	226, 234, 235, 236
	335	Down	P18SRP, HLF, CALU, MAX, HOXD8, SOX4, JAG1, TNC, c-Met, TNC	223, 228
	377	Down	REST, SOD1	230, 237
	517a, b	Down	CREAP-1, MAPKAPK5, NFKBIE, PTK2B	238
	519a, d,e	Down	FLJ31818, TGFBR2, HuR, EIF2C1, ARID4B, GATA2BD, SUV39H1	223,238, 239

miRNA(s)	Expression (Up/ downregulated)	Estimated target(s)	References
551a	Down	LPHN1, ERBB4, ZFP36	223
662	Down	NEGR1, MKX, CSF3	223
10a,b	Up	USF2, HOXA1, HOXD10, HOXB1, HOXB3, RB1CC1 and ribosomal proteins (enhances translation)	223,237,238, 240
21	Up	PDCD4, RPS7, NCAPG, TPM1, PTEN	222, 224, 228, 229, 238, 240
26a,b	Up	PTEN, IL6, KPNA6, CTDSPL, ITGA5, EZH2	230,237,238
27a	Up	ZBTB10, Myt-1, HMGB2, HOXA2, CYP1B1	226, 242
30a-5p, 30e-5p	Up	Unknown	223
99a,b	Up	SLC6A7, AIFM2, DNPEP, HS3ST2, DOHH	223, 229
130a	Up	MCSF, GAX, HOXA5	243, 244
141	Up	ZEB1, ZEB2	245
146a	Up	BRCA1, BRCA2	246
181a,b	Up	HOXA11, GATA6, NLK, CDX2, TBL1X, DPP6,KLF2	238, 247, 248
182	Up	FoxO3, FoxO1	238, 244, 249
200a	Up	ZEB1, ZEB2	245
200c	Up	TUBB3, ZEB1, ZEB2	245, 250
203	Up	p63, SOCS-3, ABL1, MCEF, ADAMTS6	220, 238
205	Up	ZEB1, ZEB2, E2F1, ERBB3, PKCe, SHIP2	220, 238,251
213	Up	APP, SATB2	252
214	Up	SLC2AB, KSR1, JMJD2B, EZH1, PLXNB3, NARG1, PTEN	226, 244
221	Up	CDKN1B (p27), CDKN1C (p57)	223, 235
222	Up	CDKN1B (p27), CDKN1C (p57)	253
223	Up	SEPT6, MMP9, USF2, KRAS, EGF	224,237, 254
296	Up	LYPLA2, IQSEC2, RNF44, HGS	223, 255
340	Up	PAM, RTN3, PPL, RNF34, ZNF513	252
451	Up	ZBTB10, Myt-1, HMGB2, HOXA2, CYP1B1	226, 242
494, 594	Up	Unknown	223
520f	Up	ZNF443, AK2, NFYA,TCERG1	247
605	Up	VGLL3, PHACTR2, SCAMP1, SEC24D	223, 256

	miRNA(s)	Expression (Up/ downregulated)	Estimated target(s)	References
Endometrial cancer	1	Down	c-Met, TIMP-3, TRIM2, ITGB3, ZNF264	257, 258
	Let-7	Down	KRAS, c-Myc, HMG2A, IL-6, HIC2	229
	26	Down	SMAD1, SOX2, Bcl6, SMAD4, BCL2,KLF4	229
	29b	Down	IGF1, Mcl-1	257
	30c	Down	MYH11, GPRASP2, DDR2, CKS2,C5	250
	34b,c	Down	NOTCH, BCL2, CCND1, WNT3, MYC, SIRT1	257, 259
	101	Down	COX2, EZH2	257
	125	Down	LIN28, ERBB2, ERBB3, Akt3 and ETS1	229
	129-2	Down	SOX4	192
	133a,b	Down	PKM2, Mcl-1,Bcl2l2	257
	136	Down	Rtl1	257
	152	Down	ENPP2, SNCAIP, LTBP4, MLH1,Bcl2l11	259, 260
	193a,b	Down	KIT, RAMP1, TSPYL5, ERBB4, ROBO4, UPA	250, 261
	204	Down	Ezrin, ESR1, CHD5, CAMTA1	261
	221	Down	LMOD, p27Kip1, p57Kip2, c-Kit	260
	376a,c	Down	PRPS1, BMPR2, KLF15,GRIK2	257, 262
	377	Down	ETS1, XIAP, RNF38	257
	379	Down	FOXP2, MTMR2, HLCS,CCNB1	257
	411	Down	MAP3K1, SP2, CDH2, FOXO1, SMAD4,SET	257
	424	Down	CCNE1, CCND1,NFI-A	257
	455-5p	Down	PP1R12A, KDR, SUZ12, FOXN3,PTPRJ	257, 263
	518c	Down	ID-1, HOXA3,HOXC8,RAP1B,ABCG2,HLA-G	245,257
	542-3p,5p	Down	COX-2, HSPG2, ZNF618, CREB5	257, 264
	654-3p	Down	KLF12, SORBS1, WDR26, RNF145, AP1S3	229, 265
	765	Down	KLK4, POU2F2, TIMP3, ADAM19, BCL6B	257
	873	Down	FOXK2, TBL1X, TMOD2, BMPR2, SFRS1	257
	1226	Down	MARCH9, PPFIBP1	257
	10a	Up	USF2, HOXA1, HOXD10, HOXB1, HOXB3, RB1CC1 and ribosomal proteins	250
	31	Up	FOXCP2, FOXP3	261
	96	Up	CHES1, FOXO1, FOXO3A	261, 266

	miRNA(s)	Expression (Up/ downregulated)	Estimated target(s)	References
	103	Up	GPD1, cdc5A, cdk6, cyclin D2, ENPP2, TIMP3	260, 268
	106a	Up	TGFB1I1, CNN1, OLFML2A, Rbp1-like, FOXA1, KIF1A, ZIC1	257, 260
	107	Up	ENPP2, CDK2, HIF1a	267
	142-5p	Up	E2F7, EGR3, IGF1, SOX11, SOX5, TGFBR2	257
	155	Up	UBE2J1, DCAF7, RAB34, SH3BP4	261
	181a	Up	GPRASP1, TBL1X, DPP6, KLF2, HOXA11, GATA6, NLK, CDX2	260, 268
	182, 183	Up	FOXO1, FOXO3, CASP3, CASP2, Fas	257, 260, 261, 266, 268
	196a	Up	ANXA1, HOXB8, HOXA7, HOXC8, HOXD8	269
	200c	Up	TUBB3	250
	203	Up	JPH4, ZIC1, CDK6, ABCE1, SMYD3, p63	257, 268
	205	Up	E2F1, ERBB3, JPH4, S100A2, ZEB1, ZEB2	257, 268
	210	Up	DCHS1, ENPP2, MYH11, KCNMB1, MNT, BDNF, PTPN1	257,260, 261, 268
	363	Up	CUL3, CXCL5, AGGF1, CIT, DUSP6, EPS8	261, 270
	449	Up	WISP2, MUC5B, EFNB1, VAMP2	261
	513a-5p	Up	CCRL1, MCHR2, CD274, RGS5, EPS8	257
	629	Up	LRP6, TCF4, SEPT1, ZNF436, SLC1A7	257
Cervical cancer	Let -7b, c	Down	Unknown	271
	29a	Down	Neurotrophin/TRK signaling	272, 273
	26a	Down	Unknown	274
	34a,b	Down	p18Ink4c, CDK4, CDK6, Cyclin E2, 2F1, E2F3, BCL2, BIRC3	199, 275
	99a	Down	IGF-1, BCL2L2, VEGFA CDK6	274
	124	Down	IGFBP7, CDK6	276
	138	Down	hTERT	277
	145	Down	IGF-1	274
	149,196b	Down	Unknown	271, 278
	205	Down	ZEB1, ZEB2, SIP1	279
	214	Down	MEK3, JNK1	175

	miRNA(s)	Expression (Up/ downregulated)	Estimated target(s)	References
	218	Down	LAMB3	280
	372	Down	CDK2, Cyclin A1	281
	513	Down	IGF-1, BCL2L2, VEGFA CDK6	274
	519a	Down	HuR	282
	9	Up	Unknown	283
	10a	Up	(HOX) genes	274
	21	Up	PTEN,TPM1, PDCD4	271, 284
	27a	Up	Unknown	285
	100	Up	PLK1	286
	126, 127	Up	Unknown	278, 287
	132	Up	(HOX) genes	274
	133a	Up	Unknown	278
	133b	Up	MST2,CDC42, RHOA,MAPK1,AKT1	288
	146a	Up	Unknown	285
	148a	Up	PTEN, P53INP1 and TP53INP2	274
	155	Up	Unknown	272, 278
	182, 199b	Up	Unknown	278, 280
	200a	Up	MYH10, ZEB1, DCP2, YWHAG, KIDINS220, ZEB2, TGFB2, RANBP5, EXOC5	283
	203	Up	p63	136
	205, 221	Up	Unknown	272, 285
	302b, 522	Up	Unknown	274
	886-5p	Up	BAX	289
Vulvar cancer	19b-1-5p; 22-5p; 26b-3p; 29c-5p; 106b-3p; 142-3p; 144-5p; 151a-5p; 193a-5p; 342-3p; 365a-3p; 519b-3p; 1291	Down	Unknown	72
	16-5p; 21-5p; 29c-5p; 142-3p; 186-5p; 454-3p; 708-5p; 1267	Up	Unknown	72

Table 2. Dysregulated miRNAs in gynecological cancer.

Specific biological functions affected by histone modifications in gynecological cancers are presented in Table 3.

	Genes	Functions	Expression Up/ downregulate	References
Ovarian cancer	EZH2	Lysine methyltransferase; Transcription regulator that acts in gene silencing and embryonic development;	Up	290
	SMYD2 (KMT3C)	Lysine methyltransferases; methylates both histones and nonhistone proteins, including p53/TP53 and RB1.	Up	291
	KDM4A	A demethylase that binds to androgen receptor and represses transcription; may play a role in regulation of cell cycle	Up	292
	EP300	Histone acetyltransferase that regulates transcription via chromatin remodeling	Down	293
	hMOF (KAT8)	Histone acetyltransferase which may be involved in transcriptional activation.	Down	294, 295
	CREBBP (KAT3A)	Plays critical roles in embryonic development, growth control, and homeostasis by coupling chromatin remodeling to transcription factor recognition.	Down	296
Endometrial cancer	HDAC1	Histone deacetylase 1, a transcriptional regulator that mediates histone deacetylation, antiapoptosis, synapse maturation, and hippocampus development	Up	297
	KDM4A	A demethylase that binds to androgen receptor and represses transcription; may play a role in regulation of cell cycle	Up	298
	EZH2	Transcription regulator that acts in gene silencing and embryonic development;	Up	299
Cervical cancer	KDM5B	Histone demethylase and transcription repressor that acts in regulation of Notch signaling, stem cell maintenance, and cell differentiation	Up	300
	EZH2	Transcription regulator that acts in gene silencing and embryonic development	Up	301
	KDM5C	A putative transcription regulator that may act in chromatin remodeling and brain development	Down	302
	KDM6A	Demethylates histone H3 lysine 27; induced expression by papillomavirus E7 oncoprotein results in epigenetic reprogramming	Up	303
	KDM6B	A transcription repressor that plays a role in gonad and lung development and defense response to Gram-positive	Up	303

Genes	Functions	Expression Up/ downregulate	References
	bacteria, regulates histone methylation, macrophage differentiation, and protein localization		
EP300	Histone acetyltransferase and regulates transcription via chromatin remodeling	Up	304
pCAF (KAT2B)	Histone acetyltransferase (HAT) to promote transcriptional activation	Up	305
HDAC1	Histone deacetylase 1; a transcriptional regulator that mediates histone deacetylation, antiapoptosis, synapse maturation, and hippocampus development	Up	306, 307
HDAC2	Histone deacetylase 2; a histone deacetylase and a transcriptional corepressor that acts in chromatin remodeling, inflammatory response, and regulation of translation	Up	307

Table 3. Histone modifications in gynecological cancer.

3. The roles of microenvironment-mediated epigenetic perturbations in the development of gynecological neoplasia

The complexity that governs the tumor phenotype cannot be explained only at the genetic level, as genetic abnormalities occur with low frequency. Therefore, major attention was focused on the study of the role of tumor microenvironment (TME) not only in tumor initiation but also in progression and metastasis. The hypothesis of cancer cell development and proliferation only in a conducive environment has been made by Paget since 1889 [308]. While Paget suggested that the microenvironment facilitates or inhibits metastasis through growth-promoting/ inhibiting factors, recent research sustains that the tumor is directed into one or several possible molecular evolution pathways by signals originating in native and/or modified microenvironmental factors [309]. The tumor microenvironment consists of epithelial cells, vascular endothelial cells, fibroblasts and myofibroblasts, macrophages, leukocytes, and the extracellular matrix (ECM). Together with the ECM, these nonmalignant cell types constitute the stromal tissue of the tumor that secretes ECM components, cytokines, and growth factors involved in tumor growth and invasion. All these components are dynamically interconnected around the tumor. In the tumorigenesis process, studies have shown the critical role of chronic inflammation by hyperexpression of the inflammatory mediators in the microenvironment. The inflammatory microenvironment is both the result of genetic alterations in cancer cells and of the tumor-infiltrating cells that produce inflammatory mediators [310].

While normal fibroblasts prevent tumor progression, cancer-associated fibroblasts (CAFs) that display a different secretory pattern generate an environment that favors tumor growth and invasiveness. Tumor formation is characterized by changes in cell behavior, like accelerated growth with loss of tissue architecture and epithelial dysfunction, angiogenesis, stromal activation, and migratory and invasive features. Therefore, dysfunction in the tumor microenvironment, in addition to epithelial dysfunction, is crucial for carcinogenesis as altering its components leads to impaired immune response. TME promotes tumorigenesis through new blood vessel formation. Although studies have suggested that some cells in TME contained mutations, recent data pointed, first, to the presence of mutations only in tumorigenic cells and second, to the contribution of these mutations to epigenetic changes in both nontumorigenic cells and TME. In turn, the cells in the microenvironment produce epigenetic changes in tumor cells reflected in their pattern of differentiation [311] and animal models demonstrate that the tumor microenvironment can induce epigenetic alterations and changes in gene expression in tumors [312].

It was suggested that the epigenome serves as the interface between the genome and the environment [313, 314]. The epigenetic role of TME in growth induction seems to be linked with transforming growth factor (TGF)-β and its receptor, whose expressions are regulated through chromatin remodeling [315], although no research on stromal fibroblasts was performed. TGFβ pathways are involved in the oncogenesis process, acting either as tumor suppressor or as tumor promotor, depending on TME crosstalk in the tumor microenvironment [316]. In malignant progression, epigenetic changes in the expression of 12 genes responsive to the TME stress suggest that coordinated transcriptional response of eukaryotic cells to microenvironment might be correlated with chemotherapy resistance of solid tumors [317]. Since tumor development is lead by physiological responses to an aberrant stromal environment, the interaction between the tumor and stromal cells determines tumoral progression [318]. In the chemokine network, epigenetic silencing of CXCR4 in SDF-1α/CXCR4 signaling of tumor microenvironment of cervical cancer cell lines and primary biopsy samples limited the cell response to the paracrine source of SDF-1α, which lead to loss of cell adhesion and disease progression [319]. Other authors reported miRNA's contribution to cancer progression and metastasis. While extracellular miRNAs are involved in cell–cell communication and stromal remodeling [320], specific intracellular ones lead to cell proliferation through cancer-associated fibroblast activation [321].

The acquisition of invasive properties in tumor cells seems to be partially linked to epithelial-mesenchymal transition by abrogation of homotypic cell–cell adhesion due to the absence of E-cadherin expression. Starting from the important role of transient E-cadherin expression in neoplasia, DesRoches and collaborators investigated its regulation by the microenvironment. Using 3D human tissue constructs, the authors suggested the role of epigenetic changes (DNA methylation, chromatin remodeling, and specific miRNA regulation) in the plasticity of E-cadherin-mediated adhesion in different tissue microenvironments during tumor cell invasion and metastasis [322]. The entry of the epithelial cells into the stroma is promoted through the E-cadherin intercellular junction disruption by MMP-3 and break down of the ECM collagen fibers by MMP-2 and MMP-9 [323]. MicroRNA suppression also influences the changes involved in epithelial–mesenchymal transition [324]. Reexpression of E-cadherin might reestablish cell–cell adhesion and may result in a mesenchymal–epithelial transition that might lead to proliferative growth of metastases.

Metastasis, as a multistage process (tumor cell migration from primary tumor, invasion of the surrounding tissues, intravasation into the circulation or the lymphatic system metastasis) involves communication with surrounding nonneoplastic cells [325] that can be epigenetically modulated to lead to ECM remodeling. Also, the epigenetic changes in the microenvironment have a significant impact on distant metastasis. In order to create a favorable local environment for cell proliferation in the metastatic sites, carcinoma cells induce epigenetic changes in both the stromal cells and bone marrow–derived cells [326]. The bone marrow cells are mobilized by the primary tumors to the metastatic sites before the actual metastasis creating a suitable microenvironment for metastasis [315, 327].

Due to their reversal character, epigenetic changes of TME might be targeted for controlling diseases and for therapeutic approach as drug resistance seems to also depend on TME. But, chemotherapeutic drug resistance depends at least partly on the TME rather than the tumor itself [328] and the combined treatment of both the tumor and the TME may be more efficient in the fight with cancer [315].

4. Molecular and epigenetic factors involved in drug resistance

Chemotherapy success is challenged by a multitude of intrinsic or acquired, molecular, genetic and epigenetic factors involved in drug transport, detoxification, signal transduction, gene expression, DNA repair, and programmed cell death. Drug resistance is a major challenge that chemotherapy should overcome. Even if the drug itself is efficient in destroying cancer cells, it is much more complicated to avoid triggering resistance than might appear at different levels of interaction between the drug and its cellular components.

The efflux mechanism is considered to be mainly responsible for the multiple drug resistance phenotypes in gynecologic cancers as well as in all types of cancers [329]. The process may be managed by cancer cells at the genetic and/or epigenetic level. While the genetic modifications of MDR1 and related multidrug resistance proteins were intensely explored over the past few decades, the contribution of epigenetic modification to the expression of MDR1 remains insufficiently explored in human gynecological cancers. It was observed that MDR1 was hypermethylated in 100% of ovarian cancer cell lines, and in 5 out of 13 (38%) primary ovarian cancers associated with loss of MDR1 mRNA expression in ovarian cancer cell lines, sustaining the importance role of epigenetic regulation in the expression of MDR1 and clinical treatment outcomes in human ovarian cancer [330]. However, in six ovarian cancer cell lines—W1MR, W1CR, W1DR, W1VR, W1TR, and W1PR that are respectively resistant to methotrexate, cisplatin, doxorubicin, vincristine, topotecan, and paclitaxel, P-gp is responsible for chemoresistance and, in the case of methotrexate, was found to have a relation between the MRP2 transcript level and drug resistance [331]. Among inhibitors of Pgp MDR, valspodar, an analog of cyclosporine A, showed no clinical benefit in a phase III trial with paclitaxel and carboplatin [332], because while these agents can block drug efflux at the cellular level, the effects are not tumor specific, requiring a reduction in dosage for minimizing the side effects but also the therapeutic advantage. On the other hand, miRNA was involved in resistance through the regulation of MDR proteins at a posttranscriptional level. The interaction of miRNAs with the targeted mRNA can downmodulate MDR proteins improving the response to anticancer drugs. It was described [329] that miR-223 can downregulate ABCB1 and mRNA levels. miR-124a and miR-506 significantly decreased the protein level of MRP4 (ABCC4), which is another efflux membrane transporter; however, these miRNAs did not change the gene transcription levels [333]. In addition, although there are many modalities acting on efflux proteins in order to circumvent drug resistance, their effective action can be compromised due to the diversity of signal transduction pathways involved in transporter-mediated MDR, such as MAPK, JNK, PI3K, among others; as well as some transcription factors, like NF-κB, TNF-α, and PTEN that could influence the levels of carrier proteins in different conditions [334].

Also, the signal transduction pathways can be involved in drug resistance. The Wnt signaling pathway, which is regulated by a multiprotein complex consisting of, among others, members of β-catenin, adenomatous polyposis coli APC, Axin, and GSK-3β [335], are involved in calcium-dependent cell adhesion due to the interaction between β-catenin and cadherin [336]. Different mutations in APC, promotes β-catenin proteolysis and reduces its transcriptional activity. PTEN, a lipid and protein phosphatase that is a negative regulator of phosphatidylinositol 3 (PI-3) kinase-dependent signaling interacts with the WNT pathway by impeding activation of integrin-linked kinase (ILK), which inhibits GSK-3β and thus causes accumulation of β-catenin [337]. The WNT signaling pathway is the most frequently altered pathway in the majority of cancers; therefore, individual components of the pathway are interesting targets for epigenetic inactivation. PI3K/Akt is another signaling pathway that is involved in acquired resistance of many cancers including gynecological ones. All of its isoforms (Akt1, Akt2, and Akt3) are activated (phosphorylated) by phosphatidylinositol 3-kinase (PI3-K) in response to growth factors and promote cell survival. It was demonstrated that the Akt pathway is directly related to the resistance of cancers against different drugs like sorafenib, trastuzumab, and erlotinib [329]. The epigenetic control of Akt and NF-κB is important for the establishment of drug resistance. RUNX3 suppresses Akt1 transcription by directly binding to the Akt1 promoter, and methylation of RUNX3 induces activation of the Akt signaling pathway [329].

Acquired resistance may develop additionally as blockage of apoptotic pathways or defective apoptotic signaling, often associated with loss of tumor suppressor protein p53, but also independent of p53, alteration of the control points of the cell cycle, increased ability to repair DNA, increased DNA damage tolerance, oncogene induction, and downmodulation of tumor suppressor genes. Eluding the normal process of programmed cell death is already known as a crucial strategy for cancer development and progression, but even more importantly, its participation in the intrinsic or acquired resistance of cancer cells to chemotherapy and radiation. Identification of the points of therapeutic intervention could potentially open up more efficient treatment opportunities. Epigenetic strategies might also be a feasible strategy to reactivate apoptosis or on the contrary to inactivate apoptosis-related genes that inhibit the process. However, it has now been demonstrated that inhibitors of DNA methylation and histone deacetylases can reactivate expression of tumor suppressor genes and induce histone hyperacetylation in the tumors of patients with cervical cancer after treatment with these agents. Preclinical studies have suggested a multitude of strategies to prevent or overcome resistance, but these approaches have not successfully translated to clinical practice yet [338].

5. Conclusions

This chapter underlined the importance of epigenetic events in gynecological cancer. Deciphering the relevant epigenetic changes associated with each step of tumor development might improve molecular diagnostic and cancer risk assessment. Advances in elucidating epigenetic regulation in cancer disease, as well as in the development of technology, lead to the identification of potential biomarkers for diagnostic screening. As epigenetic changes occur early in neoplastic process, epigenetic biomarkers seem to be more sensitive and specific in cancer detection and some have already been tested for several types of cancer, alone or in combination with traditional biomarkers. Unlike genetic changes, epigenetic alterations are essentially reversible and allow plasticity. These features are exploited and new therapeutic agents targeting epigenetic processes have been developed. The epigenetic changes of the transformed cells or TME can be modified by chemotherapeutic drugs and this epigenetic reversal therapy has potential in the future. In addition, miRNAs should be heavily explored as they might represent future alternatives for combined therapy of cancer. Many epigenetic targets are druggable and in order to overcome drug resistance, epigenetic therapy might also be a feasible strategy for induced cell death. Moreover, epigenetic patterns might be useful tools for therapy response prediction.

Author details

Coralia Bleotu[1*], Demetra Socolov[2], Mariana Anton[3], Anca Botezatu[1], Adriana Plesa[1], Iulia Virginia Iancu[1], Lorelei Irina Brasoveanu[1], Gabriela Anton[1] and Carmen Cristina Diaconu[1]

*Address all correspondence to: cbleotu@yahoo.com

1 Stefan S Nicolau Institute of Virology, Bucharest, Romania

2 University of Medicine and Pharmacy "Gr. T. Popa", Iassy, Romania

3 Carol Davila University of Medicine and Pharmacy, Bucharest, Romania

References

[1] Siedlecki P, Zielenkiewicz P. Mammalian DNA methyltransferases. Acta Biochim Pol. 2006;53(2):245–256.

[2] Bird AP. DNA methylation patterns and epigenetic memory. Genes Dev. 2002;16(1): 6–21.DOI: 10.1101/gad.947102.

[3] Takai D, Jones PA. Comprehensive analysis of CpG islands in human chromosomes 21 and 22. Proc Natl Acad Sci U S A. 2002;99:3740–3745. DOI: 10.1073/pnas. 052410099.

[4] Wang Y, Leung FC. An evaluation of new criteria for CpG islands in the human genome as gene markers. Bioinformatics. 2004;20:1170–1177. DOI: 10.1093/bioinformatics/bth059.

[5] Suzuki MM, Bird A. DNA methylation landscapes: provocative insights from epigenomics. Nat Rev Genet. 2008;9:465–476. DOI: 10.1038/nrg2341.

[6] Prendergast GC, Ziff EB. Methylation-sensitive sequence-specific DNA binding by the c-Myc basic region. Science. 1991;251:186–189.DOI: 10.1126/science.1987636.

[7] Watt F, Molloy PL. Cytosine methylation prevents binding to DNA of a HeLa cell transcription factor required for optimal expression of the adenovirus major late promoter. Genes Dev. 1988;2:1136–1143. DOI: 10.1101/gad.2.9.1136.

[8] Jones PL, Veenstra GJ, Wade PA, Vermaak D, Kass SU, *et al*. Methylated DNA and MeCP2 recruit histone deacetylase to repress transcription. Nat Genet. 1988;19:187–191. DOI: 10.1038/561.

[9] Nan X, Ng HH, Johnson CA, Laherty CD, Turner BM, *et al*. Transcriptional repression by the methyl-CpG binding protein MeCP2 involves a histone deacetylase complex. Nature. 1998;393:386–389. DOI:10.1038/30764.

[10] Bird AP, Taggart MH, Nicholls RD, Higgs DR, Non-methylated CpG-rich islands at the human alphaglobin locus: Implications for evolution of the alpha-globin pseudogene. The EMBO J. 1987;6(4):999–1004.

[11] Lan J, Hua S, He X, Zhang Y. DNA methyltransferases and methyl-binding proteins of mammals. Acta Biochim Biophys Sin. 2010;42(4):243–252. DOI: 10.1093/abbs/gmq015.

[12] Cuzick J, Bergeron C, von Knebel Doeberitz M, Gravitt P, *et al*. New technologies and procedures for cervical cancer screening. Vaccine. 2012;30S:F107–F116.

[13] Overmeer RM, Henken FE, Snijders PJ, Claassen-Kramer D, Berkhof J, *et al*. Association between dense CADM1 promoter methylation and reduced protein expression in high-grade CIN and cervical SCC. J Pathol. 2008;215(4):388–397.

[14] Jones PA, Baylin SB. The epigenomics of cancer. Cell. 2007;128:683–692.

[15] Yang HJ. Aberrant DNA methylation in cervical carcinogenesis. Chin J Cancer. 2013; 32:42–48.

[16] Esteller M, Corn PG, Baylin SB, *et al*. A gene hypermethylation profile of human cancer. Cancer Res. 2001;61:3225–3229.

[17] Esteller M. Epigenetics in cancer. N Engl J Med. 2008;358:1148–1159.

[18] Mulero Navarro S, Esteller M. Epigenetic biomarkers for human cancer: the time is now. Crit Rev Oncol Hematol. 2008;68:1–11.

[19] Qureshi SA, Bashir MU, Yaqinuddin A. Utility of DNA methylation markers for diagnosing cancer. Int J Surg. 2010;8:194–198.

[20] Kouzarides T. Chromatin modifications and their function. Cell. 2007;128:693–705:DOI: http://dx.doi.org/10.1016/j.cell.2007.02.005.

[21] Caterino TL, Hayes JJ. Chromatin structure depends on what's in the nucleosome's pocket. Nat Struct Mol Biol. 2007;14:1056–1058. DOI:10.1038/nsmb1107-1056.

[22] Shogren-Knaak M, Ishii H, Sun JM, Pazin MJ, Davie JR, *et al.* Histone H4-K16 acetylation controls chromatin structure and protein interactions. Science. 2006;311(5762): 844–847. DOI: 10.1126/science.1124000.

[23] Mikkelsen TS, Ku M, Jaffe DB, Issac B, Lieberman E, *et al.* Genome-wide maps of chromatin state in pluripotent and lineage-committed cells. Nature. 2007;448:553–560. DOI: 10.1038/nature06008.

[24] Ringrose L, Paro R. Polycomb/trithorax response elements and epigenetic memory of cell identity. Development. 2007;134:223–232. DOI: 10.1242/dev.02723.

[25] Kouzarides T. Histone methylation in transcriptional control. Curr Opin Genet Dev. 2002;12(2):198–209. DOI: 10.1016/S0959-437X(02)00287-3.

[26] Zardo G, Cimino G, Nervi C. Epigenetic plasticity of chromatin in embryonic and hematopoietic stem/progenitor cells: therapeutic potential of cell reprogramming. Leukemia. 2008;22(8):1503–1518. DOI: 10.1038/leu.2008.141.

[27] Schwartz YB, Pirrotta V. Polycomb silencing mechanisms and the management of genomic programmes. Nat Rev Genet. 2007;8(1):9–22.DOI: 10.1038/nrg1981.

[28] Simon JA, Kingston RE. Mechanisms of polycomb gene silencing: knowns and unknowns. Nat Rev Mol Cell Biol. 2009;10(10):697–708. DOI: 10.1038/nrm2763.

[29] Agger K, Cloos PA, Christensen J, Pasini D, Rose S, *et al.* UTX and JMJD3 are histone H3K27 demethylases involved in HOX gene regulation and development. Nature. 2007;449(7163):731–734. DOI: 10.1038/nature06145.

[30] De Santa F, Totaro MG, Prosperini E, Notarbartolo S, Testa G, *et al.* The histone H3 lysine-27 demethylase JMJD3 links inflammation to inhibition of polycombmediated gene silencing. Cell. 2007;130(6):1083–1094. DOI: http://dx.doi.org/10.1016/j.cell.2007.08.019.

[31] Lan F, Bayliss PE, Rinn JL, Whetstine JR, Wang JK, *et al.* A histone H3 lysine 27 demethylase regulates animal posterior development. Nature. 2007;449(7163):689–694. DOI: 10.1038/nature06192.

[32] Sharma S, Kelly TK, Jones PA. Epigenetics in cancer. Carcinogenesis. 2010;31(1):27–36. DOI: 10.1093/carcin/bgp220.

[33] Zhao XD, Han X, Chew JL, Liu J, Chiu KP, *et al.* Whole-genome mapping of histone H3 Lys4 and 27 trimethylations reveals distinct genomic compartments in human embryonic stem cells. Cell Stem Cell. 2007;1(3):286–298. DOI: 10.1016/j.stem.2007.08.004.

[34] Bernstein BE, Mikkelsen TS, Xie X, Kamal M, Huebert DJ, *et al.* A bivalent chromatin structure marks key developmental genes in embryonic stem cells. Cell. 2006;125(2):315–326. DOI: http://dx.doi.org/10.1016/j.cell.2006.02.041.

[35] Cedar H, Bergman Y. Linking DNA methylation and histone modification: patterns and paradigms. Nat Rev Genet. 2009;10:295–304. DOI: 10.1038/nrg2540.

[36] Tachibana M, Matsumura Y, Fukuda M, Kimura H, Shinkai Y. G9a/GLP complexes independently mediate H3K9 and DNA methylation to silence transcription. EMBO J. 2008;27:2681–2690. DOI: 10.1038/emboj.2008.192.

[37] Lehnertz B, Ueda Y, Derijck AA, Braunschweig U, Perez-Burgos L, *et al.* Suv39h-mediated histone H3 lysine 9 methylation directs DNA methylation to major satellite repeats at pericentric heterochromatin. Curr Biol. 2003;13:1192–1200. DOI: http://dx.doi.org/10.1016/S0960-9822(03)00432-9.

[38] Zhao Q, Rank G, Tan YT, Li H, Moritz RL, Simpson RJ, *et al.* PRMT5-mediated methylation of histone H4R3 recruits DNMT3A, coupling histone and DNA methylation in gene silencing. Nat Struct Mol Biol. 2009;16:304–311. DOI: 10.1038/nsmb.1568.

[39] Fuks F, Hurd PJ, Wolf D, Nan X, Bird AP, *et al.* The methyl-CpG-binding protein MeCP2 links DNA methylation to histone methylation. J. Biol. Chem. 2003;278:4035–4040. DOI: 10.1074/jbc.M210256200.

[40] Fraga MF, Ballestar E, Villar-Garea A, Boix-Chornet M, Espada J, *et al.* Loss of acetylation at Lys16 and trimethylation at Lys20 of histone H4 is a common hallmark of human cancer. Nat Genet. 2005;37:391–400. DOI: 10.1038/ng1531.

[41] Halkidou K, Gaughan L, Cook S, Leung HY, Neal DE, *et al.* Upregulation and nuclear recruitment of HDAC1 in hormone refractory prostate cancer. Prostate. 2004;59:177–189. DOI: 10.1002/pros.20022.

[42] Song J, Noh JH, Lee JH, Eun JW, Ahn YM, *et al.* Increased expression of histone deacetylase 2 is found in human gastric cancer. APMIS. 2005;113:264–268. DOI: 10.1111/j.1600-0463.2005.apm_04.x.

[43] Yang XJ. The diverse superfamily of lysine acetyltransferases and their roles in leukemia and other diseases. Nucleic Acids Res. 2004;32:959–976. DOI: 10.1093/nar/gkh252.

[44] Rougeulle C, Heard E. Antisense RNA in imprinting: spreading silence through air. Trends Genet. 2002;18:434–437. DOI: http://dx.doi.org/10.1016/S0168-9525(02)02749-X.

[45] Sleutels F, Zwart R, Barlow DP. The non-coding Air RNA is required for silencing autosomal imprinted genes. Nature. 2002;415:810–813. DOI:10.1038/415810a.

[46] Plath K, Mlynarczyk-Evans S, Nusinow DA, Panning B. Xist RNA and the mechanism of X chromosome inactivation. Annu. Rev. Genet. 2002;36:233–278. DOI: 10.1146/annurev.genet.36.042902.092433.

[47] Bartel DP. MicroRNAs: Genomics, biogenesis, mechanism, and function. Cell. 2004;116:281–297. DOI: http://dx.doi.org/10.1016/S0092-8674(04)00045-5.

[48] Lewis BP, Shih IH, Jones-Rhoades MW, Bartel DP, Burge CB. Prediction of mammalian microRNA targets. Cell. 2003;115:787–798. DOI: http://dx.doi.org/10.1016/S0092-8674(03)01018-3.

[49] Fabian MR, Sonenberg N. The mechanics of miRNA-mediated gene silencing: a look under the hood of miRISC. Nat Struct Mol Biol. 2012;19:586–593. DOI: 10.1038/nsmb.2296.

[50] Saj A, Lai EC. Control of microRNA biogenesis and transcription by cell signaling pathways. Curr Opin Genet Dev. 2011;21:504–551. DOI: 10.1016/j.gde.2011.04.010.

[51] Lagos-Quintana M, Rauhut R, Lendeckel W, Tuschl T. Identification of novel genes coding for small expressed RNAs. Science. 2001;294:853–858. DOI: 10.1126/science.1064921.

[52] Lau NC, Lim LP, Weinstein EG, Bartel DP. An abundant class of tiny RNAs with probable regulatory roles in *Caenorhabditis elegans*. Science. 2001;294:858–862. DOI: 10.1126/science.1065062.

[53] Lee RC, Ambros V. An extensive class of small RNAs in *Caenorhabditis elegans*. Science. 2001;294:862–864. DOI: 10.1126/science.1065329.

[54] Croce CM. Causes and consequences of microRNA dysregulation in cancer. Nat Rev Genet. 2009;10:704–714. DOI: 10.1038/nrg2634.

[55] Lu J, Getz G, Miska EA, Alvarez-Saavedra E, Lamb J, Peck D, *et al.* MicroRNA expression profiles classify human cancers. Nature 2005;435:834–838. DOI: 10.1038/nature03702.

[56] Munker R, Calin GA. MicroRNA profiling in cancer. Clin Sci (Lond). 2011;121:141–158. DOI: 10.1042/CS20110005.

[57] Volinia S, Calin GA, Liu CG, Ambs S, Cimmino A, *et al.* A microRNA expression signature of human solid tumors defines cancer gene targets. Proc Natl Acad Sci U S A. 2006;103:2257–2261. DOI: 10.1073/pnas.0510565103.

[58] Iorio MV, Croce CM. MicroRNA dysregulation in cancer: diagnostics, monitoring and therapeutics. A comprehensive review. EMBO Mol Med. 2012;4:143–159. DOI: 10.1002/emmm.201100209.

[59] Seo GJ, Fink LH, O'Hara B, Atwood WJ, Sullivan CS. Evolutionarily conserved function of a viral microRNA. J Virol. 2008 82(20), 9823–9828.

[60] Del Pino M, Rodriguez-Carunchio L, Ordi J. Pathways of vulvar intraepithelial neoplasia and squamous cell carcinoma. Histopathology 2013;62(1):161–175.

[61] Gadducci A, Tana R, Barsotti C, Guerrieri ME, Genazzani AR. Clinico-pathological and biological prognostic variables in squamous cell carcinoma of the vulva. Crit Rev Oncol Hematol 2012;83(1):71–83.

[62] van der Avoort IA, Shirango H, Hoevenaars BM, Grefte JM, de Hullu JA, *et al*. Vulvar squamous cell carcinoma is a multifactorial disease following two separate and independent pathways. Int J Gynecol Pathol. 2006;25(1):22–29.

[63] Schuurman MS, van den Einden LC, Massuger LF, Kiemeney LA, van der Aa MA, *et al*. Trends in incidence and survival of Dutch women with vulvar squamous cell carcinoma. Eur J Cancer. 2013;49(18):3872–3880.

[64] van de Nieuwenhof HP, Massuger LF, van der Avoort IA, Bekkers RL, Casparie M, *et al*. Vulvar squamous cell carcinoma development after diagnosis of VIN increases with age. Eur J Cancer 2009;45(5):851–856.

[65] McCluggage WG. Premalignant lesions of the lower female genital tract: cervix, vagina and vulva. Pathology 2013;45(3):214–328.

[66] Raspollini MR, Asirelli G, Moncini D, Taddei GL. A comparative analysis of lichen sclerosus of the vulva and lichen sclerosus that evolves to vulvar squamous cell carcinoma. Am J Obstet Gynecol. 2007;197(6):592–595.

[67] Sliutz G, Schmidt W, Tempfer C, Speiser P, Gitsch G, *et al*. Detection of p53 point mutations in primary human vulvar cancer by PCR and temperature gradient gel electrophoresis. Gynecol Oncol. 1997;64(1):93–98.

[68] Chulvis do Val IC, Almeida Filho GL, Valiante PM, Gondim C, Takiya CM, *et al*. Vulvar intraepithelial neoplasia p53 expression, p53 gene mutation and HPV in recurrent/progressive cases. J Reprod Med. 2004;49(11):868–874.

[69] Aulmann S, Schleibaum J, Penzel R, Schirmacher P, Gebauer G, *et al*. Gains of chromosome region 3q26 in intraepithelial neoplasia and invasive squamous cell carcinoma of the vulva are frequent and independent of HPV status. J Clin Pathol. 2008;61(9):1034–1037.

[70] Lavorato-Rocha AM, De Melo MB, Rodrigues IS, Stiepcich MMA, Baiocchi G, *et al*. Prognostication of vulvar cancer based on p14ARF status: molecular assessment of transcript and protein. Ann Surg Oncol. 2013; 20(1):31–39.

[71] Trietsch MD, Nooij LS, Gaarenstroom KN, van Poelgeest MIE. Genetic and epigenetic changes in vulvar squamous cell carcinoma and its precursor lesions: a review of the current literature. Gynecol Oncol. 2015; 136: 143–157.

[72] de Melo Maia B, Lavorato-Rocha AM, Rodrigues LS, Coutinho-Camillo CM, Baiocchi G, *et al.* microRNA portraits in human vulvar carcinoma. Cancer Prev Res (Phila). 2013;6(11):1231–1241. doi: 10.1158/1940-6207.CAPR-13-0121.

[73] de Martel C, Ferlay J, Franceschi S, Vignat J, Bray F, *et al.* Global burden of cancers attributable to infections in 2008: a review and synthetic analysis. Lancet Oncol. 2012;13:607–615.

[74] Rajaram S, Maheshwari A, Srivastava A. Staging for vaginal cancer. Best Pract Res Clin Obstet Gynaecol. 2015. http://dx.doi.org/10.1016/j.bpobgyn.2015.01.006.

[75] Grulich AE, van Leeuwen MT, Falster MO, Vajdic CM. Incidence of cancers in people with HIV/AIDS compared with immunosuppressed transplant recipients: a meta-analysis. Lancet 2007;370(9581):59–67.

[76] Hellman K, Silfverswärd C, Nilsson B, Hellström AC, Frankendal B, *et al.* Primary carcinoma of the vagina: factors influencing the age at diagnosis. The Radiumhemmet series 1956–96. Int J Gynecol Cancer. 2004;14(3):491–501.

[77] Daling JR, Madeleine MM, Schwartz SM, Shera KA, Carter JJ, *et al.* A population-based study of squamous cell vaginal cancer: HPV and cofactors. Gynecol Oncol 2002;84(2):263–270.

[78] Herbst AL, Ulfelder H, Poskanzer DC. Adenocarcinoma of the vagina. Association of maternal stilbestrol therapy with tumor appearance in young women. N Engl J Med 1971;284(15):878–881.

[79] Mittendorf R. Teratogen update: carcinogenesis and teratogenesis associated with exposure to diethylstilbestrol (DES) *in utero*. Teratology 1995;51(6):435–445.

[80] Treffers PE, Hanselaar AG, Helmerhorst TJ, Koster ME, van Leeuwen FE. Consequences of diethylstilbestrol during pregnancy; 50 years later still a significant problem. Ned Tijdschr Geneeskd. 2001;145(14):675–680.

[81] De Vuyst H, Clifford GM, Nascimento MC, Madeleine MM, Franceschi S. Prevalence and type distribution of human papillomavirus in carcinoma and intraepithelial neoplasia of the vulva, vagina and anus: a meta-analysis. Int J Cancer 2009;124(7):1626–1636.

[82] Alemany L, Saunier M, Tinoco L, Quirós B, Alvarado-Cabrero I, *et al.* HPV VVAP Study Group. Large contribution of human papillomavirus in vaginal neoplastic lesions: a worldwide study in 597 samples. Eur J Cancer. 2014; 50:2846–2854.

[83] Thierry F. Transcriptional regulation of the papillomavirus oncogenes by cellular and viral transcription factors in cervical carcinoma. Virology. 2009; 384:375–379.

[84] Thain A, Jenkins O, Clarke AR, Gaston K. CpG methylation directly inhibits binding of the human papillomavirus type 16 E2 protein to specific DNA sequences. J Virol 1996; 70: 7233–7235.

[85] Lillsunde Larsson G, Helenius G, Sorbe B, Karlsson MG. Viral load, integration and methylation of E2BS3 and 4 in human papilloma virus (HPV) 16-positive vaginal and vulvar carcinomas. PLoS ONE. 2014; 9(11): e112839. doi:10.1371/journal.pone.0112839.

[86] Palmer JR, Wise LA, Hatch EE, Troisi R, Titus-Ernstoff L, *et al.* Prenatal diethylstilbestrol exposure and risk of breast cancer. Cancer Epidemiol Biomarkers Prev. 2006; 15: 1509–1514.

[87] Hoover RN, Hyer M, Pfeiffer RM, Adam E, Bond B, *et al.* Adverse health outcomes in women exposed in utero to diethylstilbestrol. N Engl J Med. 2011; 365: 1304–1314. doi: 10.1056/NEJMoa1013961.

[88] Block K, Kardana A, Igarashi P, Taylor HS. In utero diethylstilbestrol (DES) exposure alters Hox gene expression in the developing mullerian system. FASEB J. 2000; 14:1101–1108.

[89] Newbold RR, Jefferson WN, Grissom SF, Padilla-Banks E, Snyder RJ, *et al.* Developmental exposure to diethylstilbestrol alters uterine gene expression that may be associated with uterine neoplasia later in life. Mol Carcinog. 2007; 46: 783–796.

[90] Vanhees K, Coort S, Ruijters EJ, Godschalk RW, van Schooten FJ, *et al.* Epigenetics: prenatal exposure to genistein leaves a permanent signature on the hematopoietic lineage. FASEB J. 2011; 25: 797–807. doi: 10.1096/fj.10-172155.

[91] Bromer JG, Wu J, Zhou Y, Taylor HS. Hypermethylation of homeobox A10 by *in utero* diethylstilbestrol exposure: an epigenetic mechanism for altered developmental programming. Endocrinology. 2009; 150: 3376–3382. doi: 10.1210/en.2009-0071.

[92] Li S, Washburn KA, Moore R, Uno T, Teng C, *et al.* Developmental exposure to diethylstilbestrol elicits demethylation of estrogen-responsive lactoferrin gene in mouse uterus. Cancer Res. 1997; 57: 4356–4359.

[93] Li S, Hursting SD, Davis BJ, McLachlan JA, Barrett JC. Environmental exposure, DNA methylation, and gene regulation: Lessons from diethylstilbesterol-induced cancers. Ann N Y Acad Sci. 2003; 983: 161–169.

[94] Harlid S, Xu Z, Panduri V, D'Aloisio AA, DeRoo LA, *et al.* In utero exposure to diethylstilbestrol and blood DNA methylation in women ages 40–59 years from the Sister Study. PLoS ONE. 2015; 10(3): e0118757. doi:10.1371/journal.pone.0118757.

[95] Dougan MM, Hankinson SE, Vivo I, Tworoger SS, Glynn RJ, *et al.* Prospective study of body size throughout the life-course and the incidence of endometrial cancer among premenopausal and postmenopausal women. Int J Cancer. 2015. doi: 10.1002/ijc.29427.

[96] Win AK, Reece JC, Ryan S. Family history and risk of endometrial cancer: a systematic review and meta-analysis. Obstet Gynecol. 2015;125(1):89–98. doi: 10.1097/AOG.0000000000000563.

[97] Yang HP, Cook LS, Weiderpass E, Adami HO, Anderson KE, *et al.* Infertility and incident endometrial cancer risk: a pooled analysis from the epidemiology of endometrial cancer consortium (E2C2). Br J Cancer. 2015;112(5):925–933.

[98] Graham JD, Clarke CL. Physiological action of progesterone in target tissues. Endocr Rev. 1997;18(4):502–519.

[99] Conneely OM, Lydon JP. Progesterone receptors in reproduction: functional impact of the A and B isoforms. Steroids. 2000;65(10–11):571–577.

[100] Yang S, Thiel KW, De Geest K, Leslie KK. Endometrial cancer: reviving progesterone therapy in the molecular age. Discov Med. 2011;12(64):205–212.

[101] Jones A, Teschendorff AE, Li Q, Hayward JD, Kannan A, *et al.* Role of DNA methylation and epigenetic silencing of HAND2 in endometrial cancer development. PLoS Med. 2013;10(11):e1001551. doi: 10.1371/journal.pmed.1001551.

[102] Srivastava D, Thomas T, Lin Q, Kirby ML, Brown D, *et al.* Regulation of cardiac mesodermal and neural crest development by the bHLH transcription factor, dHAND. Nat Genet. 1997;16: 154–160. doi:10.1038/ng0697-154.

[103] Li Q, Kannan A, DeMayo FJ, Lydon JP, Cooke PS, *et al.* The antiproliferative action of progesterone in uterine epithelium is mediated by Hand2. Science. 2011;331:912–916. doi:10.1126/science.1197454.

[104] Bagchi IC, Li Q, Cheon YP, Mantena SR, Kannan A, *et al.* Use of the progesterone receptor antagonist RU 486 to identify novel progesterone receptor-regulated pathways in implantation. Semin Reprod Med. 2005;23:38–45. doi:10.1055/s-2005-864032.

[105] Dassen H, Punyadeera C, Kamps R, Klomp J, Dunselman G, *et al.* Progesterone regulation of implantation-related genes: new insights into the role of oestrogen. Cell Mol Life Sci. 2007;64: 1009–1032. doi:10.1007/s00018-007-6553-9.

[106] Deacon JM, Evans CD, Yule R, *et al.* Sexual behaviour and smoking as determinants of cervical HPV infection and of CIN3 among those infected: a case–control study nested within the Manchester Cohort. Br J Cancer. 2000;83:1565–1572.

[107] Klumb EM, Araújo Jr ML, Jesus GR, *et al.* Is higher prevalence of cervical intraepithelial neoplasia in women with lupus due to immunosuppression? J Clin Rheumatol. 2010;16:153–157.

[108] Gadducci A, Barsotti C, Cosio S, Domenici L, Riccardo Genazzani A. Smoking habit, immune suppression, oral contraceptive use, and hormone replacement therapy use and cervical carcinogenesis: a review of the literature. Gynecol Endocrinol. 2011;27: 597–604.

[109] Lax S. Histopathology of cervical precursor lesions and cancer. Acta Dermatovenerol Alp Panonica Adriat. 2011;20:125–133.

[110] Kwasniewska A, Korobowicz E, Zdunek M, *et al*. Prevalence of *Chlamydia trachomatis* and herpes simplex virus 2 in cervical carcinoma associated with human papillomavirus detected in paraffin sectioned samples. Eur J Gynaecol Oncol. 2009;30:65–70.

[111] Chen CL, Liu SS, Ip SM, *et al*. E-cadherin expression is silenced by DNA methylation in cervical cancer cell lines and tumours. Eur J Cancer. 2003;39:517–523.

[112] Shivapurkar N, Sherman ME, Stastny V, *et al*. Evaluation of candidate methylation markers to detect cervical neoplasia. Gynecol Oncol. 2007;107:549–553.

[113] Kim JH, Choi YD, Lee JS, *et al*. Assessment of DNA methylation for the detection of cervical neoplasia in liquid based cytology specimens. Gynecol Oncol. 2010;116:99–104.

[114] Yang N, Nijhuis ER, Volders HH, *et al*. Gene promoter methylation patterns throughout the process of cervical carcinogenesis. Cell Oncol. 2010;32:131–143.

[115] Kitkumthorn N, Yanatatsanajit P, Kiatpongsan S, *et al*. Cyclin A1 promoter hypermethylation in human papillomavirus associated cervical cancer. BMC Cancer, 2006;6:55.

[116] Ki KD, Lee SK, Tong SY, *et al*. Role of 5'CpG island hypermethylation of the FHIT gene in cervical carcinoma. J Gynecol Oncol, 2008;19:117-122.

[117] Jha AK, Nikbakht M, Parashar G, *et al*. Reversal of hypermethylation and reactivation of the RARbeta2 gene by natural compounds in cervical cancer cell lines. Folia Biol (Praha). 2010;56:195–200.

[118] Hesson LB, Cooper WN, Latif F. The role of RASSF1A methylation in cancer. Dis Markers. 2007;23:73–87.

[119] Dong SM, Kim HS, Rha SH, *et al*. Promoter hypermethylation of multiple genes in carcinoma of the uterine cervix. Clin Cancer Res, 2001;7:1982-1986.

[120] Cheung TH, Lo KW, Yim SF, Chan LK, Heung MS, *et al*. Epigenetic and genetic alternation of PTEN in cervical neoplasm. Gynecol Oncol. 2004;93:621–627.

[121] Liu SS, Leung RC, Chan KY, *et al*. p73 expression is associated with the cellular radiosensitivity in cervical cancer after radiotherapy. Clin Cancer Res. 2004;10:3309–3316.

[122] Wentzensen N, Sherman ME, Schiffman M, *et al*. Utility of methylation markers in cervical cancer early detection: appraisal of the state of the science. Gynecol Oncol. 2009;112: 293–299.

[123] Lai HC, Lin YW, Huang RL, Chung MT, Wang HC, *et al*. Quantitative DNA methylation analysis detects cervical intraepithelial neoplasms type 3 and worse. Cancer. 2010;116(18):4266–4274.

[124] Eijsink JJ, Lendvai A, Deregowski V, Klip HG, Verpooten G, *et al.* A four gene methylation marker panel as triage test in hr-HPV positive patients. Int J Cancer. 2012;130(8):1861–1869.

[125] Hesselink AT, Heideman DA, Steenbergen RD, Coupé VM, Overmeer RM, Rijkaart D, *et al.* Combined promoter methylation analysis of CADM1 and MAL: an objective triage tool for high-risk human papillomavirus DNA-positive women. Clin Cancer Res. 2011;17(8): 2459–2465.

[126] Steenbergen RD, Kramer D, Braakhuis BJ, Stern PL, Verheijen RH, *et al.* TSLC1 gene silencing in cervical cancer cell lines and cervical neoplasia. J Natl Cancer Inst. 2004;96(4):294–305.

[127] Eijsink JJ, Yang N, Lendvai A, Klip HG, Volders HH, *et al.* Detection of cervical neoplasia by DNA methylation analysis in cervico-vaginal lavages, a feasibility study. Gynecol Oncol. 2011;120(2):280–283.

[128] Kalantari M, Calleja-Macias IE, Tewari D, Hagmar B, Lie K, *et al.* Conserved methylation patterns of human papillomavirus type 16 DNA in asymptomatic infection and cervical neoplasia. J Virol. 2004;78: 12762–12772.

[129] Turan T, Kalantari M, Calleja-Macias IE, Villa LL, Cubie HA, *et al.* Methylation of the human papillomavirus-18 L1 gene: A biomarker of neoplastic progression? Virology. 2006;349:175–183.

[130] Mirabello L, Sun C, Ghosh A, Rodriguez AC, Schiffman M, *et al.* Methylation of the HPV16 genome is associated with disease progression in a prospective population-based cohort. J Natl Cancer Inst. 2012;104(7):556–565.

[131] Mirabello L, Frimer M, Harari A, McAndrew T, Smith B, Chen Z, *et al.* HPV16 methyl-haplotypes determined by a novel next-generation sequencing method are associated with cervical precancer. Int J Cancer. 2015;136(4):E146-53. doi: 10.1002/ijc.29119.

[132] Zheng ZM, Wang X, Regulation of cellular miRNA expression by human papillomaviruses, Biochim Biophys Acta, 2011; 668–677.

[133] Skalsky RL, Cullen BR, Viruses, microRNAs, and host interactions. Annu Rev Microbiol. 2010;64:123–141.

[134] Wang X,Wang H-K, McCoy JP, *et al.* Oncogenic HPV infection interrupts the expression of tumor-suppressive miR-34a through viral oncoprotein E6. RNA. 2009;15:637–647.

[135] Wang X, Meyers C, Guo M, Zheng ZM. Upregulation of p18Ink4c expression by oncogenic HPV E6 via p53-miR-34a pathway. Int J Cancer. 2011;129:1362–1372.

[136] Melar-New M, Laimins LA. Human papillomaviruses modulate expression of microRNA 203 upon epithelial differentiation to control levels of p63 proteins. J Virol. 2010;84:5212–5221.

[137] Bo J, Yang G, Huo K, *et al*. microRNA-203 suppresses bladder cancer development by repressing bcl-w expression. FEBS J. 2011;278:786–792.

[138] Bian K, Fan J, Zhang X, *et al*. MicroRNA-203 leads to G1 phase cell cycle arrest in laryngeal carcinoma cells by directly targeting survivin. FEBS Lett. 2012;586:804–809.

[139] Takeshita N, Mori M, Kano M, *et al*. miR-203 inhibits the migration and invasion of esophageal squamous cell carcinoma by regulating LASP1. Int J Oncol. 2012;41:1653–1661.

[140] Ofir M, Hacohen D, Ginsberg D. MiR-15 and miR-16 are direct transcriptional targets of E2F1 that limit E2F-induced proliferation by targeting cyclin E. Mol Cancer Res. 2011;9:440–447.

[141] Myklebust M, Bruland O, Fluge O, Skarstein A, Balteskard L, *et al*. MicroRNA-15b is induced with E2F controlled genes in HPV-related cancer. Br J Cancer. 2011;105:1719–1725.

[142] Wang F, Fu X-D, Zhou Y, Zhang Y. Downregulation of the cyclin E1 oncogene expression by microRNA-16-1 induces cell cycle arrest in human cancer cells. BMB Rep. 2009;42:725–730.

[143] Chen J. Signaling pathways in HPV-associated cancers and therapeutic implications. Rev Med Virol. 2015;25 Suppl 1:24-53. doi: 10.1002/rmv.1823.

[144] Chudecka-Głaz, AM, ROMA, an algorithm for ovarian cancer. Clin Chim Acta. 2015;440:143–151.

[145] May T, Shoni M, Crum CP, Xian W, Vathipadiekal V, *et al*. Low-grade and high-grade serous Mullerian carcinoma: review and analysis of publicly available gene expression profiles. Gynecol Oncol. 2013;128(3):488-92. doi: 10.1016/j.ygyno.2012.12.009.

[146] Shih I, Kurman RJ. Ovarian tumorigenesis: a proposed model based on morphological and molecular genetic analysis. Am J Pathol 2004; 164:1511–1518.

[147] Wiegand KC, Shah SP, Al-Agha OM, *et al*. ARID1A mutations in endometriosis associated ovarian carcinomas. N Engl J Med. 2010;363:1532–1543.

[148] Kurman RJ, Shih I. Molecular pathogenesis and extraovarian origin of epithelial ovarian cancer—shifting the paradigm. Hum Pathol. 2011;42:918–931.

[149] Kurman RJ. Origin and molecular pathogenesis of ovarian high-grade serous carcinoma, Ann Oncol. 2013;24 (Supplement 10): x16–x21; doi:10.1093/annonc/mdt463.

[150] Przybycin CG, Kurman RJ, Ronnett BM, *et al*. Are all pelvic (nonuterine) serous carcinomas of tubal origin? Am J Surg Pathol. 2010;34:1407–1416.

[151] Tone AA, Begley H, Sharma M., *et al*. Gene expression profiles of luteal phase fallopian tube epithelium from BRCA mutation carriers resemble high-grade serous carcinoma. Clin Cancer Res. 2008;14:4067–4078.

[152] Kuhn E, Kurman RJ, Vang R., *et al*. TP53 mutations in serous tubal intraepithelial carcinoma and concurrent pelvic high-grade serous carcinoma—evidence supporting the clonal relationship of the two lesions. J Pathol. 2012;226:421–426.

[153] Cancer Genome Atlas Res Network. Integrated genomic analyses of ovarian carcinoma. Nature. 2011;474:609–615.

[154] Koukoura O, Spandidos DA, Daponte A, Sifakis S, DNA methylation profiles in ovarian cancer: implication in diagnosis and therapy (Review). Mol Med Rep. 2014;10:3–9.

[155] Baldwin RL, Nemeth E, Tran H, *et al*. BRCA1 promoter region hypermethylation in ovarian carcinoma: a population-based study. Cancer Res. 2000;60:5329–5333.

[156] Strathdee G, Appleton K, Illand M, *et al*. Primary ovarian carcinomas display multiple methylator phenotypes involving known tumor suppressor genes. Am J Pathol. 2001;158:1121–1127.

[157] Wang C, Horiuchi A, Imai T, *et al*. Expression of BRCA1 protein in benign, borderline, and malignant epithelial ovarian neoplasms and its relationship to methylation and allelic loss of the BRCA1 gene. J Pathol. 2004;202:215–223.

[158] Bol GM, Suijkerbuijk KP, Bart J, Vooijs M, van der Wall E, *et al*. Methylation profiles of hereditary and sporadic ovarian cancer. Histopathology. 2010;57:363–370.

[159] Rathi A, Virmani AK, Schorge JO, Elias KJ, Maruyama R et *al*. Methylation profiles of sporadic ovarian tumors and nonmalignant ovaries from high-risk women. Clin. Cancer Res. 2002;8(11):3324–3331.

[160] Yang HJ, Liu VW, Wang Y, Tsang PC, Ngan HY. Differential DNA methylation profiles in gynecological cancers and correlation with clinico-pathological data. BMC Cancer. 2006;6:212.

[161] Samuel S, Naora H. Homeobox gene expression in cancer: insights from developmental regulation and deregulation. Eur J Cancer. 2005;41:2428–2437.

[162] Kelly ZL, Michael A, Butler-Manuel S, Pandha HS, Morgan RG, HOX genes in ovarian cancer. J Ovarian Res. 2011;4:16.

[163] Montavon C, Gloss BS, Warton K, *et al*. Prognostic and diagnostic significance of DNA methylation patterns in high grade serous ovarian cancer. Gynecol Oncol. 2012;124:582–588.

[164] Widschwendter M, Apostolidou S, Jones AA, *et al*. HOXA methylation in normal endometrium from premenopausal women is associated with the presence of ovarian cancer: a proof of principle study. Int J Cancer. 2009;125: 2214–2218.

[165] Pattamadilok J, Huapai N, Rattanatanyong P, *et al*. LINE-1 hypomethylation level as a potential prognostic factor for epithelial ovarian cancer. Int J Gynecol Cancer. 2008;18:711–717.

[166] Woloszynska-Read A, James SR, Link PA, Yu J, Odunsi K, and Karpf AR. DNA methylation-dependent regulation of BORIS/CTCFL expression in ovarian cancer. Cancer Immun. 2007;7:21.

[167] Gupta A, Godwin AK, Vanderveer L, Lu A, Liu J. Hypomethylation of the synuclein gamma gene CpG island promotes its aberrant expression in breast carcinoma and ovarian carcinoma. Cancer Res. 2003;63:664–673.

[168] Chan KY, Ozçelik H, Cheung AN, Ngan HY, Khoo US. Epigenetic factors controlling the BRCA1 and BRCA2 genes in sporadic ovarian cancer. Cancer Res. 2002;62:4151–4156.

[169] Dann RB, DeLoia JA, Timms KM, Zorn KK, Potter J, *et al*. BRCA1/2 mutations andexpression:response to platinum chemotherapy in patients with advanced stage epithelial ovariancancer. Gynecol Oncol. 2012;125:677–82. DOI: 10.1016/j. ygyno. 2012.03.006.

[170] Kwon MJ, Kim SS, Choi YL, Jung HS, Balch C, *et al*. Derepression of CLDN3 and CLDN4 during ovarian tumorigenesisis associated with loss of repressive histone modifications. Carcinogenesis. 2010;31:974–983. DOI:10.1093/carcin/bgp336.

[171] Honda H, Pazin MJ, Ji H, Wernyj RP, Morin PJ. Crucial roles of Sp1 and epigenetic modifications in the regulation of the CLDN4 promoter in ovarian cancer cells. J Biol Chem. 2006;281:21433–21444. DOI:10.1074/jbc. M603767200.

[172] Honda H, Pazin MJ, D'Souza T, Ji H, Morin PJ. Regulation of the CLDN3 gene in ovarian cancer cells. Cancer Biol Ther. 2007;6:1733–1742. DOI:10.4161/cbt.6.11.4832.

[173] Cheng W, Jiang Y, Liu C, Shen O, Tang W, *et al*. Identification of aberrant promoter hypomethylation of HOXA10 in ovarian cancer. J Cancer Res Clin Oncol. 2010;136:1221–1227. doi:10.1007/s00432-010-0772-4.

[174] Fiegl H, Windbichler G, Mueller-Holzner E, Goebel G, Lechner M, *et al*. HOXA11 DNA methylation—a novel prognostic biomarker in ovarian cancer. Int J Cancer. 2008;123(3):725–729. DOI: 10.1002/ijc.23563.

[175] Frasco MA, Ayhan A, Zikan M, Cibula D, Iyibozkurt CA, Yavuz E, *et al*. HOXA methylation in normal endometrium from premenopausal women is associated with the presence of ovarian cancer: a proof of principle study. Int J Cancer. 2009;125(9): 2214–2218. DOI: 10.1002/ijc.24599.

[176] Lee PS, Teaberry VS, Bland AE, Huang Z, Whitaker RS, *et al*. Elevated MAL expression is accompanied by promoter hypomethylation and platinum resistance in epithelial ovarian cancer. Int J Cancer. 2010;126:1378–1389. DOI:10.1002/ijc.24797.

[177] Yang Z, Chen S, Luan X, Li Y, Liu M, *et al*. Micro RNA-214 is aberrantly expressed in cervical cancers and inhibits the growth of HeLa cells. IUBMB Life. 2009;61:1075–82. DOI:10.1002/iub.252.

[178] Bhattacharya R, Nicoloso M, Arvizo R, Wang E, Cortez A, *et al.* MiR-15a and MiR-16 control Bmi-1 expression in ovarian cancer. Cancer Res. 2009;69:9090–9095. DOI: 10.1158/0008-5472.CAN-09-2552.

[179] Izutsu N, Maesawa C, Shibazaki M, Oikawa H, Shoji T, *et al.* Epigenetic modification is involved inaberrant expression of class III beta-tubulin, TUBB3; in ovarian cancer cells. Int J Oncol. 2008;32:1227. DOI:10.3892/ijo_ 32_6_1227.

[180] Dahl KDC, Dahl R, Kruichak JN, Hudson LG. The epidermal growth factor receptor responsive miR25 are presses mesenchymal morphology in ovarian cancer cells. Neoplasia. 2009;11:1208. DOI:10.1593/neo.09942.

[181] GuanY, Yao H, Zheng Z, Qiu G, Sun K. MiR-125b targets BCL3 and suppresses ovarian cancer proliferation. Int J Cancer. 2011;128:2274–2283. DOI:10.1002/ijc.25575

[182] Ibanez de Caceres I, Battagli C, Esteller M, Herman JG, Dulaimi E, Edelson MI, *et al.* Tumor cell-specific BRCA1 and RASSF1A hypermethylation in serum, plasma, and peritoneal fluid from ovarian cancer patients. Cancer Res. 2004;64(18):6476–6481. DOI: 10.1158/0008-5472.CAN-04-1529.

[183] Makarla PB, Saboorian MH, Ashfaq R, Toyooka KO, Toyooka S, *et al.* Promoter hypermethylation profile of ovarian epithelial neoplasms. Clin. Cancer Res. 2005;11(15): 365–369. DOI: 10.1158/1078-0432.CCR-04-2455.

[184] Widschwendter M, Apostolidou S, Jones AA, Fourkala EO, Arora R, *et al.* Promoter hypermethylation contributes to frequent inactivation of a putative conditional tumor suppressor gene connective tissue growth factor in ovarian cancer. Cancer Res. 2007;67(15):7095–7105. DOI: 10.1158/0008-5472.CAN-06-4567.

[185] Barton CA, Gloss BS, Qu W, Statham AL, Hacker NF, *et al.* Collagen and calcium-binding EGF domains 1 is frequently inactivated in ovarian cancer by aberrant promoter hypermethylation and modulates cell migration and survival. Br J Cancer. 2010;102(1):87–96. DOI: 10.1038/sj.bjc.6605429.

[186] Gifford G, Paul J, Vasey PA, Kaye SB, Brown R. The acquisition of hMLH1 methylation in plasma DNA after chemotherapy predicts poor survival for ovarian cancer patients. Clin Cancer Res. 2004;10(13):4420–4426. DOI: 10.1158/1078-0432.CCR-03-0732.

[187] Hecht JL, Mutter GL. Molecular and pathologic aspects of endometrial carcinogenesis. J Clin Oncol. 2006;24(29):4783–4791. DOI 10.1200/JCO.2006.06.7173.

[188] Zhou XC, Dowdy SC, Podratz KC, Jiang SW. Epigenetic considerations for endometrial cancer prevention, diagnosis and treatment. Gynecol Oncol. 2007;107(1):143–153. DOI: http://dx.doi.org/10.1016/j.ygyno.2007.06.019.

[189] Barton CA, Hacker NF, Clark SJ, O'Brien PM. DNA methylation changes in ovarian cancer: implications for early diagnosis, prognosis and treatment. Gynecol Oncol. 2008;109(1):129–139. DOI 10.1016/j.ygyno.2007.12.017.

[190] Huang YW, Jansen RA, Fabbri E, Potter D, Liyanarachchi S, Chan MW, *et al*. Identification of candidate epigenetic biomarkers for ovarian cancer detection. Oncol Rep. 2009;22(4):853–861. DOI: 10.3892/or_00000509.

[191] Hsu YT, Gu F, Huang YW, Liu J, Ruan J, *et al*. Promoter hypomethylation of EpCAM regulated bone morphogenetic protein gene family in recurrent endometrial cancer. Clin Cancer Res. 2013;19:6272–6285. DOI:10.1158/1078-0432.CCR-13-1734.

[192] Huang YW, Liu JC, Deatherage DE, Luo J, Mutch DG, *et al*. Epigenetic repression of microRNA-129-2 leads to overexpression of SOX4 oncogene in endometrial cancer. Cancer Res. 2009;69:9038–9046. DOI:10.1158/ 0008-5472.CAN-09-1499.

[193] Muraki Y, Banno K, Yanokura M, Kobayashi Y, Kawaguchi M, *et al*. Epigenetic DNA hypermethylation: clinical applications in endometrial cancer. Oncol Rep. 2009;22:967–972. DOI: 10.3892/or_00000523.

[194] Banno K, Yanokura M, Iida M, Masuda K, Aoki D. Carcinogenic mechanisms of endometrial cancer:Involvement of genetics and epigenetics. J Obstet Gynaecol Res. 2014;40(8): 1957–1967. DOI:10.1111/jog.12442.

[195] Pallarés J, Velasco A, Eritja N, Santacana M, Dolcet X, Cuatrecasas M, *et al*. Promoter hypermethylation and reduced expression of RASSF1A are frequent molecular alterations of endometrial carcinoma. Mod Pathol. 2008;21: 691–699. DOI 0.1038/modpathol.2008.38.

[196] Jo H, Kim JW, Kang GH, Park NH, Song YS, *et al*. Association of promoter hypermethylation of the RASSF1A gene with prognostic parameters in endometrial cancer. Oncol Res. 2006;16(4):205–209. DOI: http://dx.doi.org/10.3727/000000006783981125.

[197] Kang S, Kim JW, Kang GH, Lee S, Park NH, *et al*. Comparison of DNA hypermethylation patterns in different types of uterine cancer: cervical squamous cell carcinoma, cervical adenocarcinoma and endometrial adenocarcinoma. Int J Cancer. 2006;118(9): 2168–2171. DOI: 10.1002/ijc.21609.

[198] Toyota M, Sasaki Y, Satoh A, Ogi K, Kikuchi T, *et al*. Epigenetic inactivation of CHFR in human tumors. Proc Natl Acad Sci U S A. 2003;100(13): 7818–7823. DOI: 10.1073/pnas.1337066100.

[199] Wang X, Yang Y, Xu C, Xiao L, Shen H, *et al.* CHFR suppression by hypermethylation sensitizes endometrial cancer cells to paclitaxel. Int J Gynecol Cancer. 2011;21(6): 996–1003. DOI: 10.1097/IGC.0b013e31821e05e8.

[200] Ignatov A, Bischoff J, Ignatov T, Schwarzenau C, Krebs T, *et al*. APC promoter hypermethylation is an early event in endometrial tumorigenesis. Cancer Sci. 2010;101:321–327. DOI 10.1111/j.1349-7006.2009.01397.x.

[201] Whitcomb BP, Mutch DG, Herzog TJ, Rader JS, Gibb RK, *et al.* Frequent HOXA11 and THBS2 promoter methylation, and a methylator phenotype in endometrial adenocarcinoma. Clin Cancer Res. 2003;9(6):2277–2287.

[202] Wong YF, Chung TK, Cheung TH, Nobori T, Yu AL, *et al.* Methylation of p16INK4A in primary gynecologic malignancy. Cancer Lett.1999;136(2):231–235. DOI: http://dx.doi.org/10.1016/S0304-3835(98)00327-9.

[203] Salvesen HB, MacDonald N, Ryan A, Jacobs IJ, Lynch ED, *et al.* PTEN methylation is associated with advanced stage and microsatellite instability in endometrial carcinoma. Int J Cancer. 2001;91(1):22–26. DOI: 10.1002/1097-0215(20010101)91:1<22::AID-IJC1002>3.0.CO;2-S.

[204] Yeh KT, Yang MY, Liu TC, Chen JC, Chan WL, *et al.* Abnormal expression of period 1 (PER1) in endometrial carcinoma. J Pathol. 2005;206(1):111–120. DOI: 10.1002/path.1756.

[205] Yamaguchi S, Asanoma K, Takao T, Kato K, Wake N. Homeobox gene HOPX is epigenetically silenced in human uterine endometrial cancer and suppresses estrogen-stimulated proliferation of cancer cells by inhibiting serum response factor. Int J Cancer. 2009;124(11):2577–2588. DOI: 10.1002/ijc.24217.

[206] Fiegl H, Gattringer C, Widschwendter A, Schneitter A, Ramoni A, *et al.* Methylated DNA collected by tampons—a new tool to detect endometrial cancer. Cancer Epidemiol Biomarkers Prev. 2004;13(5):882–888.

[207] Wu H, Chen Y, Liang J, Shi B, Wu G, *et al.* Hypomethylation-linked activation of PAX2 mediates tamoxifen-stimulated endometrial carcinogenesis. Nature. 2005;438(7070):981–987 (2005). DOI: 10.1038/nature04225.

[208] Soufir N, Queille S, Liboutet M, Thibaudeau O, Bachelier F, *et al.* Inactivation of the CDKN2A and the p53 tumour suppressor genes in external genital carcinomas and their precursors. Br J Dermatol. 2007;156(3):448–53. DOI: 10.1111/j.1365-2133.2006.07604.x.

[209] Oonk MH, Eijsink JJ, Volders HH, Hollema H, Wisman GB, *et al.* Identification of inguinofemoral lymph node metastases by methylation markers in vulvar cancer. Gynecol Oncol. 2012;125(2):352–357. DOI: 10.1016/j.ygyno.2012.01.013.

[210] Guerrero D, Guarch R, Ojer A, Casas JM, Méndez-Meca C, *et al.* Differential hypermethylation of genes in vulvar cancer and lichen sclerosus coexisting or not with vulvar cancer. Int J Cancer. 2011;128(12):2853–2864. DOI: 10.1002/ijc.25629.

[211] Stephen JK, Chen KM, Raitanen M, Grénman S, Worsham MJ. DNA hypermethylation profiles in squamous cell carcinoma of the vulva. Int J Gynecol Pathol. 2009;28(1):63–75. doi: 10.1097/PGP.0b013e31817d9c61.

[212] Guerrero-Setas D, Perez-Janices N, Ojer A, Blanco-Fernandez L, Guarch-Troyas C, *et al.* Differential gene hypermethylation in genital lichen sclerosus and cancer: a comparative study. Histopathology. 2013;63(5):659–669.

[213] Lee TS, Kim JW, Kang GH, Park NH, Song YS, *et al*. DNA hypomethylation of CAGE promoters in squamous cell carcinoma of uterine cervix. Ann N Y Acad Sci. 2006;1091:218–224. DOI:10.1196/annals.1378.068.

[214] Huang F, Lin C, Shi YH, Kuerban G. Micro RNA-101 inhibits cell proliferation, invasion, and promotes apoptosis by regulating cyclooxygenase-2 in Hela cervical carcinoma cells. Asian Pac J Cancer Prev. 2013;14:5915–5920. DOI:10.7314/APJCP.2013.14.10.5915.

[215] Yamamoto N, Kinoshita T, Nohata N, Yoshino H, Itesako T, *et al*. Tumor-suppressive microRNA-29a inhibits cancer cell migration and invasion via targeting HSP47in cervical squamous cell carcinoma. Int J Oncol. 2013;43:1855–1863. DOI:10.3892/ijo.2013.2145.

[216] Zhu X, Er K, Mao C, Yan Q, Xu H, *et al*. miR-203 suppresses tumor growth and angiogenesis by targeting VEGFA in cervical cancer. Cell Physiol Biochem. 2013;32:64–73. DOI:10.1159/000350125.

[217] Shell S, Park SM, Radjabi AR, Schickel R, Kistner EO, *et al*. Let-7 expression defines two differentiation stages of cancer. Proc Natl Acad Sci U S A. 2007;104(27):11400–11405. DOI: 10.1073/pnas.0704372104.

[218] Poleshko A, Einarson MB, Shalginskikh N, Zhang R, Adams PD, *et al*. Identification of a functional network of human epigenetic silencing factors. J Biol Chem. 2010;285(1):422–433. DOI: 10.1074/jbc.M109.064667.

[219] Yang N, Kaur S, Volinia S, Greshock J, Lassus H, *et al*. MicroRNA microarray identifies Let-7i as a novel biomarker and therapeutic target in human epithelial ovarian cancer. Cancer Res. 2008;68(24):10307-14. DOI: 10.1158/0008-5472.CAN-08-1954.

[220] Iorio MV, Visone R, Di Leva G, Donati V, Petrocca F, Casalini P, *et al*. MicroRNA signatures in human ovarian cancer. Cancer Res. 2007;67(18):8699–8707. DOI: 10.1158/0008-5472.CAN-07-1936.

[221] Guo LM, Pu Y, Han Z, Liu T, Li YX, *et al*. MicroRNA-9 inhibits ovarian cancer cell growth through regulation of NF-kappaB1. FEBS J. 2009;276(19):5537–5546. DOI: 10.1111/j.1742-4658.2009.07237.x.

[222] Nam EJ, Yoon H, Kim SW, Kim H, Kim YT, *et al*. MicroRNA expression profiles in serous ovarian carcinoma. Clin Cancer Res. 2008;14(9):2690–2695. DOI: 10.1158/1078-0432.CCR-07-1731.

[223] Dahiya N, Sherman-Baust CA, Wang TL, Davidson B, Shih IeM, *et al*. MicroRNA expression and identification of putative miRNA targets in ovarian cancer. PLoS ONE. 2008;3(6):e2436. DOI: 10.1371/journal.pone.0002436.

[224] Laios A, O'Toole S, Flavin R, Martin C, Kelly L, Ring M, *et al*. Potential role of miR-9 and miR-223 in recurrent ovarian cancer. Mol Cancer. 2008;7:35. DOI 10.1186/1476-4598-7-35.

[225] Corney DC, Flesken-Nikitin A, Godwin AK, Wang W, Nikitin AY. MicroRNA-34b and microRNA-34c are targets of p53 and cooperate in control of cell proliferation and adhesion-independent growth. Cancer Res. 2007;67(18):8433–8438. DOI: 10.1158/0008-5472.CAN-07-1585.

[226] Zhang L, Huang J, Yang N, Greshock J, Megraw MS, *et al.* microRNAs exhibit high frequency genomic alterations in human cancer. Proc Natl Acad Sci U S A. 2006;103(24),9136–9141. DOI: 10.1073/pnas.0508889103.

[227] Cowden Dahl KD, Dahl R, Kruichak JN, Hudson LG. The epidermal growth factor receptor responsive miR-125a represses mesenchymal morphology in ovarian cancer cells. Neoplasia. 2009;11(11):1208–1215. DOI 10.1593/neo.09942.

[228] Sorrentino A, Liu CG, Addario A, Peschle C, Scambia G, *et al.* Role of microRNAs in drug-resistant ovarian cancer cells. Gynecol Oncol. 2008;111(3):478–486. DOI: 10.1016/j.ygyno.2008.08.017.

[229] Resnick KE, Alder H, Hagan JP, Richardson DL, Croce CM, *et al.* The detection of differentially expressed microRNAs from the serum of ovarian cancer patients using a novel real-time PCR platform. Gynecol Oncol. 2009;112(1):55–59. DOI: 10.1016/j.ygyno.2008.08.036.

[230] Zhang L, Volinia S, Bonome T, Calin GA, Greshock J, *et al.*Genomic and epigenetic alterations deregulate microRNA expression in human epithelial ovarian cancer. Proc Natl Acad Sci U S A. 2008;105(19):7004–7009. DOI: 10.1073/pnas.0801615105.

[231] Papagiannakopoulos T, Pan G, Thomson JA, Kosik KS. MicroRNA-145 regulates OCT4; SOX2; and KLF4 and represses pluripotency in human embryonic stem cells. Cell. 2009;137(4):647–658. DOI: 10.1016/j.cell.2009.02.038.

[232] Hu X, Macdonald DM, Huettner PC, Feng Z, *et al.* miR-200 microRNA cluster as prognostic marker in advanced ovarian cancer. Gynecol Oncol. 2009;114(3):457–464. DOI 10.1016/j.ygyno.2009.05.022.

[233] Shimono Y, Zabala M, Cho RW, Lobo N, Dalerba P, Qian D, *et al.* Downregulation of miRNA-200c links breast cancer stem cells with normal stem cells. Cell. 2009;138(3): 592–603. DOI: 10.1016/j.cell.2009.07.011.

[234] Choi YL, Kim J, Kwon MJ, Choi JS, Kim TJ, Bae DS, *et al.* Expression profile of tight junction protein claudin 3 and claudin 4 in ovarian serous adenocarcinoma with prognostic correlation. Histol Histopathol. 2007;22(11):1185–1195. DOI: http://www.hh.um.es.

[235] Fasanaro P, Greco S, Lorenzi M, Pescatori M, Brioschi M, *et al.* An integrated approach for experimental target identification of hypoxia-induced miR-210. J Biol Chem. 2009;284(50):35134–35143. DOI: 10.1074/jbc.M109.052779.

[236] Giannakakis A, Sandaltzopoulos R, Greshock J, Liang S, Huang J, Hasegawa K, *et al.* miR-210 links hypoxia with cell cycle regulation and is deleted in human epithelial ovarian cancer. Cancer Biol Ther. 2008;7(2):255–264. DOI: 10.4161/cbt.7.2.5297.

[237] Wyman SK, Parkin RK, Mitchell PS, Fritz BR, O'Briant K, Godwin AK, *et al.* Repertoire of microRNAs in epithelial ovarian cancer as determined by next generation sequencing of small RNA cDNA libraries. PLoS One. 2009;4(4): E5311. DOI: 10.1371/journal.pone.0005311.

[238] Lee CH, Subramanian S, Beck AH, Espinosa I, Senz J, *et al.* MicroRNA profiling of BRCA1/2 mutation-carrying and non-mutation-carrying high-grade serous carcinomas of ovary. PLoS One. 2009;4(10):E7314. DOI: 10.1371/journal.pone.0007314.

[239] Abdelmohsen K, Srikantan S, Kuwano Y, Gorospe M. miR-519 reduces cell proliferation by lowering RNA-binding protein HuR levels. Proc Natl Acad Sci U S A. 2008;105(51):20297–20302. DOI: 10.1073/pnas.0809376106.

[240] Bearfoot JL, Choong DY, Gorringe KL, Campbell IG. Genetic analysis of cancer-implicated microRNA in ovarian cancer. Clin. Cancer Res. 2008;14(22):7246–7250. DOI: 10.1158/1078-0432.CCR-08-1348.

[241] Yang Y, Chaerkady R, Beer MA, Mendell JT, Pandey A. Identification of miR-21 targets in breast cancer cells using a quantitative proteomic approach. Proteomics. 2009;9(5):1374–1384. DOI: 10.1002/pmic.200800551.

[242] Shibata D, Mori Y, Cai K, Zhang L, Yin J, *et al.* RAB32 hypermethylation and microsatellite instability in gastric and endometrial adenocarcinomas. Int J Cancer. 2006;119(4), 801–806. DOI: 10.1002/ijc.21912.

[243] Eitan R, Kushnir M, Lithwick-Yanai G, David MB, Hoshen M, Glezerman M, *et al.* Tumor microRNA expression patterns associated with resistance to platinum based chemotherapy and survival in ovarian cancer patients. Gynecol Oncol. 2009;114(2): 253–259. DOI: 10.1016/j.ygyno.2009.04.024.

[244] Taylor DD, Gercel-Taylor C. MicroRNA signatures of tumor-derived exosomes as diagnostic biomarkers of ovarian cancer. Gynecol Oncol. 2008;110(1):13–21. DOI: 10.1016/j.ygyno.2008.04.033.

[245] Bendoraite A, Knouf EC, Garg KS, Parkin RK, Kroh EM, *et al.* Regulation of miR-200 family microRNAs and ZEB transcription factors in ovarian cancer: evidence supporting a mesothelial-to-epithelial transition. Gynecol Oncol. 2010;116(1):117–125. DOI: 10.1016/j.ygyno.2009.08.009.

[246] Shen J, Ambrosone CB, DiCioccio RA, Odunsi K, Lele SB, Zhao H. A functional polymorphism in the miR-146a gene and age of familial breast/ovarian cancer diagnosis. Carcinogenesis. 2008;29(10):1963–1966. DOI: 10.1093/carcin/bgn172.

[247] Risinger JI, Maxwell GL, Chandramouli GV, Aprelikova O, Litzi T, *et al.* Gene expression profiling of microsatellite unstable and microsatellite stable endometrial cancers

indicates distinct pathways of aberrant signaling. Cancer Res. 2005;65(12):5031–5037. DOI: 10.1158/0008-5472.CAN-04-0850.

[248] Ji J, Yamashita T, Budhu A, Forgues M, Jia HL, *et al.* Identification of microRNA-181 by genome-wide screening as a critical player in EpCAM-positive hepatic cancer stem cells. Hepatology. 2009;50(2):472–480. DOI: 10.1002/hep.22989.

[249] Zhu H, Wu H, Liu X, Evans BR, Medina DJ, *et al.* Role of microRNA miR-27a and miR-451 in the regulation of MDR1/P-glycoprotein expression in human cancer cells. Biochem Pharmacol. 2008;76(5):582–588. DOI: 10.1016/j.bcp.2008.06.007.

[250] Cochrane DR, Spoelstra NS, Howe EN, Nordeen SK, Richer JK. MicroRNA-200c mitigates invasiveness and restores sensitivity to microtubule-targeting chemotherapeutic agents. Mol Cancer Ther. 2009;8(5):1055–1066. DOI: 10.1158/1535-7163.MCT-08-1046.

[251] Yu J, Ryan DG, Getsios S, Oliveira-Fernandes M, Fatima A, Lavker RM. MicroRNA-184 antagonizes microRNA-205 to maintain SHIP2 levels in epithelia. Proc Natl Acad Sci U S A. 2008;105(49):19300–19305. DOI: 10.1073/pnas.0803992105.

[252] Boren T, Xiong Y, Hakam A, Wenham R, Apte S, Chan G, *et al.* MicroRNAs and their target messenger RNAs associated with ovarian cancer response to chemotherapy. Gynecol Oncol. 2009;113(2):249–255. DOI: 10.1016/j.ygyno.2009.01.014.

[253] Wurz K, Garcia RL, Goff BA, Mitchell PS, Lee JH, *et al.* MiR-221 and MiR-222 alterations in sporadic ovarian carcinoma: relationship to CDKN1B, CDKNIC and overall survival. Genes Chromosomes Cancer. 2010;49(7):577–584. DOI: 10.1002/gcc.20768.

[254] Fukao T, Fukuda Y, Kiga K, Sharif J, Hino K, *et al.* An evolutionarily conserved mechanism for microRNA-223 expression revealed by microRNA gene profiling. Cell. 2007;129(3):617–631. DOI: http://dx.doi.org/10.1016/j.cell.2007.02.048.

[255] Würdinger T, Tannous BA, Saydam O, Skog J, Grau S, Soutschek J, *et al.* miR-296 regulates growth factor receptor overexpression in angiogenic endothelial cells. Cancer Cell. 2008;14(5):382–393. DOI: 10.1016/j.ccr.2008.10.005.

[256] Yang WT, Lewis MT, Hess K, Wong H, Tsimelzon A, Karadag N, *et al.* Decreased TGFb signaling and increased COX2 expression in high risk women with increased mammographic breast density. Breast Cancer Res Treat. 2010;119(2):305–314. DOI: 10.1007/s10549-009-0350-0.

[257] Hiroki E, Akahira J, Suzuki F, Nagase S, Ito K, *et al.* Changes in microRNA expression levels correlate with clinicopathological features and prognoses in endometrial serous adenocarcinomas. Cancer Sci. 2009;101(1):241–249. DOI: 10.1111/j.1349-7006.2009.01385.x.

[258] Dalmay T, Edwards DR. MicroRNAs and the hallmarks of cancer. Oncogene. 2006;25(46):6170–6175. DOI: 10.1038/sj.onc.1209911.

[259] Lujambio A, Calin GA, Villanueva A, Ropero S, Sánchez-Céspedes M, *et al.* A microRNA DNA methylation signature for human cancer metastasis. Proc Natl Acad Sci U S A. 2008;105(36):13556–13561. DOI: 10.1073/pnas.0803055105.

[260] Boren T, Xiong Y, Hakam A, Wenham R, Apte S, *et al.* MicroRNAs and their target messenger RNAs associated with endometrial carcinogenesis. Gynecol Oncol. 2008;110(2):206–215. DOI: 10.1016/j.ygyno.2008.03.023.

[261] Wu W, Lin Z, Zhuang Z, Liang X. Expression profile of mammalian microRNAs in endometrioid adenocarcinoma. Eur J Cancer Prev. 2009;18(1):50–55. DOI: 10.1097/CEJ.0b013e328305a07a.

[262] Kawahara Y, Zinshteyn B, Sethupathy P, Iizasa H, Hatzigeorgiou AG, Nishikura K. Redirection of silencing targets by adenosine-to-inosine editing of miRNAs. Science. 2007;315(5815):1137–1140. DOI: 10.1126/science.1138050.

[263] Mayr D, Kanitz V, Anderegg B, Luthardt B, Engel J, *et al.* Analysis of gene amplification and prognostic markers in ovarian cancer using comparative genomic hybridization for microarrays and immunohistochemical analysis for tissue microarrays. Am J Clin Pathol. 2006;126(1):101–109. DOI: 10.1309/N6X5MB24BP42KP20.

[264] Toloubeydokhti T, Pan Q, Luo X, Bukulmez O, Chegini N. The expression and ovarian steroid regulation of endometrial micro-RNAs. Reprod Sci. 2008;15(10):993–1001. DOI: 10.1177/1933719108324132.

[265] Kim JY, Tavare S, Shibata D. Counting human somatic cell replications: methylation mirrors endometrial stem cell divisions. Proc Natl Acad Sci U S A. 2005;102(49): 17739–17744. DOI: 10.1073/pnas.0503976102.

[266] Myatt SS, Wang J, Monteiro LJ, Christian M, Ho KK, *et al.* Definition of microRNAs that repress expression of the tumor suppressor gene FOXO1 in endometrial cancer. Cancer Res. 2010;70:367–377. DOI: 10.1158/0008-5472.CAN-09-1891.

[267] Orom UA, Nielsen FC, Lund AH. MicroRNA-10a binds the 5′UTR of ribosomal protein mRNAs and enhances their translation. Mol Cell. 2008;30(4):460–471. DOI: 10.1016/j.molcel.2008.05.001.

[268] Chung TK, Cheung TH, Huen NY, Wong KW, Lo KW, Yim SF, *et al.* Dysregulated microRNAs and their predicted targets associated with endometrioid endometrial adenocarcinoma in Hong Kong women. Int J Cancer. 2009;124(6):1358–1365. DOI: 10.1002/ijc.24071.

[269] Luthra R, Singh RR, Luthra MG, Li YX, Hannah C, *et al.* MicroRNA-196a targets annexin A1: a microRNA-mediated mechanism of annexin A1 downregulation in cancers. Oncogene. 2008;27(52):6667–6678. DOI: 10.1038/onc.2008.256.

[270] Kim YK, Yu J, Han TS, Park SY, Namkoong B, Kim DH, Hur K, Yoo MW, Lee HJ, Yang HK, Kim VN. Functional links between clustered microRNAs: suppression of

cell-cycle inhibitors by microRNA clusters in gastric cancer. Nucleic Acids Res. 2009;37(5):1672–1681. DOI: 10.1093/nar/gkp002.

[271] Lui WO, Pourmand N, Patterson BK, Fire A. Patterns of known and novel small RNAs in human cervical cancer. Cancer Res. 2007;67(13):6031–6043. DOI: 10.1158/0008-5472.CAN-06-0561.

[272] Wang X, Tang S, Le SY, Lu R, Rader JS, *et al.* Aberrant expression of oncogenic and tumor-suppressive microRNAs in cervical cancer is required for cancer cell growth. PLoS ONE. 2008;3(7):e2557. DOI: 10.1371/journal.pone.0002557.

[273] Torres A, Torres K, Maciejewski R, Harvey WH. Micro-RNAs and their role in gynecological tumors. Med Res Rev. 2011;31(6):895–923. DOI: 10.1002/med.20205.

[274] Pereira PM, Marques JP, Soares AR, Carreto L, Santos MA. MicroRNA expression variability in human cervical tissues. PLoS One. 2010;5(7):e11780. DOI: 10.1371/journal.pone.0011780.

[275] Botezatu A, Goia-Rusanu CD, Iancu IV, Huica I, Plesa A, *et al.* Quantitative analysis of the relationship between microRNA-124a, -34b and -203 gene methylation and cervical oncogenesis. Mol Med Rep. 2011;4(1):121–128. DOI: 10.3892/mmr.2010.394.

[276] Wilting SM, van Boerdonk RA, Henken FE, Meijer CJ, Diosdado B, Meijer GA, *et al.* Methylation-mediated silencing and tumour suppressive function of hsa-miR-124 in cervical cancer. Mol Cancer. 2010;9:167–181. DOI: 10.1186/1476-4598-9-167.

[277] Chakrabarti M, Banik NL, Ray SK. miR-138 overexpression is more than hTERT knockdown to potentiate apigenin for apoptosis in neuroblastoma in vitro and *in vivo*. Expl Cell Res. 2013;319(10);1575–1585. DOI: 10.1016/j.yexcr.2013.02.025.

[278] Lee JW, Choi CH, Choi JJ, Park YA, Kim SJ, *et al.* Altered MicroRNA expression in cervical carcinomas. Clin Cancer Res. 2008;14: 2535–2542. DOI: 10.1158/1078-0432.CCR-07-1231.

[279] Gregory PA, Bracken CP, Bert AG, Goodall GJ. MicroRNAs as regulators of epithelial–mesenchymal transition. Cell Cycle. 2008;7(20):3112-8. DOI:10.4161/cc.7.20.6851.

[280] Martinez I, Gardiner AS, Board KF, Monzon FA, Edwards RP, Khan SA. Human papillomavirus type 16 reduces the expression of microRNA-218 in cervical carcinoma cells. Oncogene. 2008;27(18):2575–2582. DOI:10.1038/sj.onc.1210919.

[281] Tian RQ, Wang XH, Hou LJ, Jia WH, Yang Q, *et al.* MicroRNA-372 is down-regulated and targets cyclin-dependent kinase 2 (CDK2) and cyclin A1 in human cervical cancer, which may contribute to tumorigenesis. J Biol Chem. 2011;286(29):25556–25563. DOI: 10.1074/jbc.M111.221564.

[282] Abdelmohsen K, Kim MM, Srikantan S, Mercken EM, Brennan SE, *et al.* miR-519 suppresses tumor growth by reducing HuR levels. Cell Cycle. 2010;9(7):1354–1359. DOI: 10.4161/cc.9.7.11164.

[283] Hu X, Schwarz JK, Lewis JS Jr, Huettner PC, Rader JS, *et al.* A microRNA expression signature for cervical cancer prognosis. Cancer Res. 2010;70(4):1441–1448. DOI: 10.1158/0008-5472.CAN-09-3289.

[284] Yao Q, Xu H, Zhang QQ, Zhou H, Qu LH. MicroRNA-21 promotes cell proliferation and down-regulates the expression of programmed cell death 4 (PDCD4) in HeLa cervical carcinoma cells. Biochem Biophys Res Commun. 2009;388(3):539-42. DOI: 10.1016/j.bbrc.2009.08.044.

[285] Gocze K, Gombos K, Juhasz K, Kovacs K, Kajtar B, *et al.* Unique microRNA expression profiles in cervical cancer. Anticancer Res 2013;33(6):2561–2567.

[286] Li BH, Zhou JS, Ye F, Cheng XD, Zhou CY, *et al.* Reduced miR-100 expression in cervical cancer and precursors and its carcinogenic effect through targeting PLK1 protein. Eur J Cancer. 2011;47(14):2166–2174. DOI: 10.1016/j.ejca.2011.04.037.

[287] Gilad S, Meiri E, Yogev Y, Benjamin S, Lebanony D, Yerushalmi N, *et al.* Serum microRNAs are promising novel biomarkers, PLoS One. 2008;3(9):e3148. DOI: 10.1371/journal.pone.0003148.

[288] Qin W, Dong P, Ma C, Mitchelson K, Deng T, Zhang L, *et al.* MicroRNA-133b is a key promoter of cervical carcinoma development through the activation of the ERK and AKT1 pathways. Oncogene. 2011;31(36):4067–4075. DOI: 10.1038/onc.2011.561.

[289] Li JH, Xiao X, Zhang YN, Wang YM, Feng LM, *et al.* MicroRNA miR-886-5p inhibits apoptosis by down-regulating Bax expression in human cervical carcinoma cells. Gynecol Oncol. 2011;120(1):145–151. doi:10.1016/j.ygyno.2010.09.009.

[290] Li H, Zhang R. Role of EZH2 in epithelial ovarian cancer: from biological insights to therapeutic target. FrontOncol. 2013; 3:47. DOI:10.3389/fonc.2013.00047.

[291] Scoumanne A, Chen X. Protein methylation: a new mechanism of p53 tumor suppressor regulation. Histol Histopathol. 2008; 23: 1143–1149.

[292] Black JC, Manning AL, Van Rechem C, Kim J, Ladd B, *et al.* KDM4A lysine demethylase induces site-specific copy gain and rereplication of regions amplified in tumors. Cell. 2013;154:541–555. DOI: 10.1016/j.cell.2013.06.051.

[293] Bryan EJ, Jokubaitis VJ, Chamberlain NL, Baxter SW, Dawson E, *et al.* Mutation analysis of EP300 in colon, breast and ovarian carcinomas. Int J Cancer. 2002;102:137–141. DOI: 10.1002/ijc.10682.

[294] Cai M, Hu Z, Liu J, Gao J, Tan M, *et al.* Expression of hMOF in different ovarian tissues and its effects on ovarian cancer prognosis. Oncol Rep. 2015;33(2):685–692. DOI: 10.3892/or.2014.3649.

[295] Liu N, Zhang R, Zhao X, Su J, Bian X, *et al.* A potential diagnostic marker for ovarian cancer: involvement of the histone acetyltransferase, human males absent on the first. Oncol Lett. 2013;2:393–400. DOI:10.3892/ol.2013.1380.

[296] Ward R, Johnson M, Shridhar V, van Deursen J, Couch FJ. CBP truncating mutations in ovarian cancer. J Med Genet. 2005;42:514–518. DOI: 10.1136/jmg.2004.025080.

[297] Weichert W, Denkert C, Noske A, Darb-Esfahani S, Dietel M, *et al*. Expression of class I histone deacetylases indicates poor prognosis in endometrioid subtypes of ovarian and endometrial carcinomas. Neoplasia. 2008;10(9):1021–1027. DOI: 0.1593/neo.08474

[298] Wang HL, Liu MM, Ma X, Fang L, Zhang ZF, *et al*. Expression and effects of JMJD2A histone demethylase in endometrial carcinoma. Asian Pac J Cancer Prev. 2014;15:3051–3056.

[299] Bachmann IM, Halvorsen OJ, Collett K, Stefansson IM, Straume O, *et al*. EZH2 expression is associated with high proliferation rate and aggressive tumor subgroups in cutaneous melanoma and cancers of the endometrium, prostate,and breast. J Clin Oncol. 2006;24:268–273. DOI: 10.1200/JCO.2005.01.5180.

[300] Hayami S, Yoshimatsu M, Veerakumarasivam A, Unoki M, Iwai Y, Tsunoda T, *et al*. Overexpression of the JmjC histone demethylase KDM5B in human carcinogenesis: involvement in the proliferation of cancer cells through the E2F/RB pathway. Mol Cancer. 2010;9:59. DOI: 10.1186/1476-4598-9-59.

[301] Hyland PL, McDade SS, McCloskey R, Dickson GJ, Arthur K, *et al*. Evidence for alteration of EZH2; BMI1; and KDM6A and epigenetic reprogramming in human papillomavirus type 16 E6/E7-expressing keratinocytes. J Virol. 2011;85(21):10999–11006. DOI: 10.1128/JVI.00160-11.

[302] Smith JA, White EA, Sowa ME, Powell ML, Ottinger M, *et al*. Genome-wide siRNA screen identifies SMCX, EP400; and Brd4 as E2-dependent regulators of human papillomavirus oncogene expression. Proc Natl Acad Sci U S A. 2010;107(8):3752-7.DOI: 10.1073/pnas.0914818107.

[303] McLaughlin-Drubin ME, Crum CP, Münger K. Human papillomavirus E7 oncoprotein induces KDM6A and KDM6B histone demethylase expression and causes epigenetic reprogramming. Proc Natl Acad Sci U S A. 2011;108(5):2130–2135. DOI: 10.1073/pnas.1009933108.

[304] Bernat A, Avvakumov N, Mymryk JS, Banks L. Interaction between the HPV E7 oncoprotein and the transcriptional coactivator p300. Oncogene. 2003;22:7871–7881. DOI: 10.1038/sj.onc.1206896.

[305] Avvakumov N, Torchia J, Mymryk JS. Interaction of the HPV E7 proteins with the pCAF acetyltransferase. Oncogene. 2003;22:3833–3841. DOI: 10.1038/sj.onc.1206562.

[306] Longworth MS, Laimins LA. The binding of histone deacetylases and the integrity of zinc finger-like motifs of the E7 protein are essential for the life cycle of human papillomavirus type 31. J Virol. 2004;78:3533–3541. DOI: 10.1128/JVI.78.7.3533-3541.2004.

[307] Brehm A, Nielsen SJ, Miska EA, McCance DJ, Reid JL, *et al*. The E7 oncoprotein associates with Mi2 and histone deacetylase activity to promote cell growth. EMBO J. 1999;18:2449–2458. DOI: 10.1093/emboj/18.9.2449.

[308] Westhoff MA, Brühl O, Debatin KM. Cancer therapy: know your enemy? Mol Cell Pediatr. 2014; 1:10. http://www.molcellped.com/content/1/1/10.

[309] Witz IP, The tumor microenvironment: the making of a paradigm. Cancer Microenviron. 2009;S1:9–17. doi: 10.1007/s12307-009-0025-8.

[310] Tsai MJ, Chang WA, Huang MS, Kuo PL. Tumor microenvironment: a new treatment target for cancer. ISRN Biochem. 2014. http://dx.doi.org/10.1155/2014/351959.

[311] Ma XJ, Dahiya S, Richardson E, Erlander M, Sgroi DC. Gene expression profiling of the tumor microenvironment during breast cancer progression. Breast Cancer Res. 2009;11(1):R7.

[312] Hamm CA, Stevens JW, Xie H, Vanin EF, Morcuende JA, *et al*. Microenvironment alters epigenetic and gene expression profiles in Swarm rat chondrosarcoma tumors. BMC Cancer. 2010;10:471.

[313] Feil R, Fraga MF. Epigenetics and the environment: emerging patterns and implications. Nat Rev Genet. 2011;13:97–109. doi: 10.1038/nrg3142.

[314] Jirtle RL, Skinner MK. Environmental epigenomics and disease susceptibility. Nat Rev Genet. 2007;8: 253–262.

[315] Dey P. Epigenetics meets the tumor microenvironment. Med Epigenet. 2013; 31–36. DOI: 10.1159/000354283.

[316] Bierie B, Moses HL. Tumour microenvironment: TGFβ: the molecular Jekyll and Hyde of cancers. Nat Rev Cancer 2006; 6:506–520. doi:10.1038/nrc1926.

[317] Denko N, Schindler C, Koong A, Laderoute K, Green C, *et al*. Epigenetic regulation of gene expression in cervical cancer cells by the tumor microenvironment. Clin Cancer Res. 2000;6(2): 480–487.

[318] Kiaris H, Trimis G, Papavassiliou AG. Regulation of tumor-stromal fibroblast interactions: implications in anticancer therapy. Curr Med Chem. 2008;15:3062–3067.

[319] Yadav SS, Prasad SB, Das M, Kumari S, Pandey LK, *et al*. Epigenetic silencing of CXCR4 promotes loss of cell adhesion in cervical cancer. BioMed Res Int. 2014; doi.org/10.1155/2014/581403.

[320] Rusek AM, Abba M, Eljaszewicz A, Moniuszko M, Niklinski J, *et al*. MicroRNA modulators of epigenetic regulation, the tumor microenvironment and the immune system in lung cancer. Mol Cancer. 2015; 14:34. DOI 10.1186/s12943-015-0302-8.

[321] Mitra AK, Zillhardt M, Hua Y, Tiwari P, Murmann AE, *et al.* MicroRNAs reprogram normal fibroblasts into cancer-associated fibroblasts in ovarian cancer. Cancer Discov. 2012;2:1100–1108.

[322] DesRochers TM, Shamis Y, Alt-Holland A, Kudo Y, Takata T, *et al.* The 3D tissue microenvironment modulates DNA methylation and E-cadherin expression in squamous cell carcinoma. Epigenetics. 2012;7(1): 34–46.

[323] Li JR, Li MQ, Bao JT, Li JZ: Correlation between expression of metastasis-associated gene 1 and matrix metalloproteinase 9 and invasion and metastasis of breast cancer. Zhonghua Yi Xue Za Zhi. 2008;88:2278–2280.

[324] Talbot LJ, Bhattacharya SD, Kuo PC. Epithelial–mesenchymal transition, the tumor microenvironment, and metastatic behavior of epithelial malignancies. Int J Biochem Mol Biol. 2012;3(2):117–136.

[325] Ungefroren H, Sebens S, Seidl D, Lehnert H, Hass R. Interaction of tumor cells with the microenvironment. Cell Commun Signal. 2011;9:18. http://www.biosignaling.com/content/9/1/18.

[326] Kaplan RN, Rafii S, Lyden D. Preparing the 'soil': the premetastatic niche. Cancer Res. 2006; 66: 11089–11093.

[327] Schedin P, Elias A. Multistep tumorigenesis and the microenvironment. Breast Cancer Res. 2004; 6: 93–101.

[328] Farmer P, Bonnefoi H, Anderle P, Cameron D, Wirapati P, *et al.* A stroma related gene signature predicts resistance to neoadjuvant chemotherapy in breast cancer. Nat Med. 2009; 15: 68–74.

[329] Niero EL, Rocha-Sales B, Lauand C, Cortez BA, Medina de Souza M, *et al.* The multiple facets of drug resistance: one history, different approaches. J Exp Clin Cancer Res. 2014; 33:37. doi:10.1186/1756-9966-33-37.

[330] Kawakami Y, Miyamoto K, Takehara K, Kumagai M, Samura O, *et al.* Down-regulation of MDR1 by epigenetic alteration in human epithelial ovarian cancer cells. J Clin Oncol. 27; 2009 (suppl; abstr e16556).

[331] Januchowski R, Wojtowicz K, Sujka-Kordowska P, Andrzejewska M, Zabel M. MDR gene expression analysis of six drug-resistant ovarian cancer cell lines. Biomed Res Int. 2013;2013:241763. doi: 10.1155/2013/241763.

[332] Lhomme´ C, Joly F, Walker JL *et al.* Phase III study of valspodar (PSC 833) combined with paclitaxel and carboplatin compared with paclitaxel and carboplatin alone in patients with stage IV or suboptimally debulked stage III epithelial ovarian cancer or primary peritoneal cancer. J Clin Oncol. 2008;26:2674–2682.

[333] Markova SM, Kroetz DL. ABCC4 is regulated by microRNA-124a and microRNA-506. Biochem Pharmacol. 2014;87:515–522.

[334] Sui H, Fan Z-Z, Li Q. Signal transduction pathways and transcriptional mechanisms of ABCB1/Pgp-mediated multiple drug resistance in human cancer cells. J Int Med Res 2012; 40:426–435.

[335] Uthoff SM, Eichenberger MR, McAuliffe TL, Hamilton CJ, Galandiuk S. Wingless-type frizzled protein receptor signaling and its putative role in human colon cancer. Mol Carcinogen. 2001;31:56–62.

[336] Hajra KM, Fearon ER. Cadherin and catenin alterations in human cancer. Genes Chromosomes Cancer 2002; 34:255–268.

[337] Persad S, Troussard AA, McPhee TR, Mulholland DJ, Dedhar S. Tumor suppressor PTEN inhibits nuclear accumulation of beta-catenin and T cell/lymphoid enhancer factor 1-mediated transcriptional activation. J Cell Biol. 2001;153:1161–1174.

[338] Bookman MA. The addition of new drugs to standard therapy in the first-line treatment of ovarian cancer. Ann Oncol. 2010;21(Supplement 7): vii211–vii217. doi: 10.1093/annonc/mdq368.

Chapter 3

Antiangiogenic Therapy in Epithelial Ovarian Cancer

M.A. Alonso Bermejo, L. Rey Iglesias ,
M.E. Pérez López, A. Fernández Montes and
J. García Mata

Additional information is available at the end of the chapter

http://dx.doi.org/10.5772/60822

Abstract

Approximately 75% of women with ovarian cancer are diagnosed at advanced stages (FIGO stage III/IV), with 15-23 months median global survival and 20% 5-year survival. Angiogenesis plays an important role in tumour development and proliferation. Increased angiogenesis is associated with worse clinical outcome in ovarian cancer. Here we review the play of bevacizumab in the treatment of ovarian cancer and also other antiangiogenic drugs. In total, to date there are no promising results for most of the reviewed antiangiogenic agents, except those already known for bevacizumab, trebananib, pazopanib, cediranib and nintedanib. Ongoing research will shed more light on this fascinating tumour process and its control.

Keywords: angiogenesis, ovarian cancer

1. Introduction

Approximately 75% of women with ovarian cancer are diagnosed at advanced stages (FIGO stage III/IV), with 15–23 months median global survival and 20% 5-year survival [1].

Although approximately 80% of patients respond to first-line chemotherapy, more than 70% relapse and develop resistance to chemotherapy [2]. This requires the development of more effective treatments to improve survival in advanced disease. This was not achieved by adding a third cytotoxic agent to the standard treatment [3–7], and so the latest research is focused on new molecular targets.

Angiogenesis plays an important role in tumor development and proliferation. Increased angiogenesis is associated with worse clinical outcome in ovarian cancer.

The vascular endothelial growth factor (VEGF) family comprises VEGF-A (known as VEGF), VEGF-B, VEGF-C, VEGF-D, placental growth factor (PGF), VEGF-E, and VEGF-F (Figure 1).

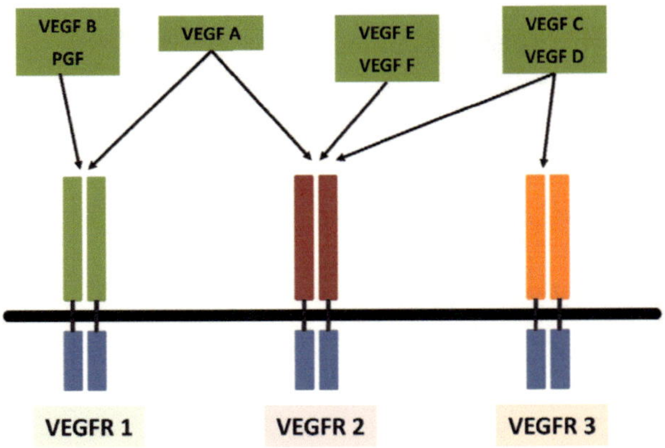

Figure 1. VEGF-A, VEGF-B, VEGF-C, VEGF-D, VEGF-E, VEGF-F, and PGF bind differentially to receptors VEGFR-1, VEGFR-2, and VEGFR-3.

The relationship between VEGF overexpression, increased angiogenesis, and ovarian cancer development is well established, as well as in peritoneal dissemination and malignant ascites development [8]. Ovarian tumors overexpress several proangiogenic factors such as vascular endothelial growth factor (VEGF), angiopoietin, fibroblast growth factors, platelet-derived growth factors (PDGFs), and proangiogenic cytokines [9].

The most investigated is VEGF, which promotes endothelial cell proliferation and migration for the formation of new blood vessels and increases the permeability of existing blood vessels [10].

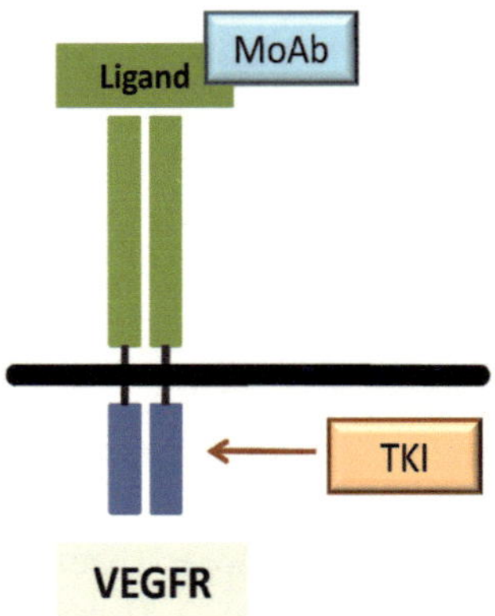

Figure 2. Monoclonal antibodies (MoAb) inhibit VEGF ligand, and TKI inhibits the VEGFR.

http://dx.doi.org/10.5772/60822

The angiogenesis pathway can be inhibited by two strategies (Figure 2): inhibition of the VEGF ligand with antibodies or soluble receptors and inhibition of the VEGF receptor with tyrosine kinase inhibitors (TKI). Several antiangiogenic drugs have been studied in ovarian cancer in different settings, and we will review them in this chapter.

2. Bevacizumab

Bevacizumab is a recombinant humanized monoclonal antibody that binds to all VEGF isoforms [11]. It has shown its efficacy in different neoplasms, such as colorectal cancer, breast cancer, or kidney cancer.

To date, bevacizumab is the antiangiogenic agent that has shown the best results in the treatment of ovarian cancer.

The first-line efficacy data come from two phase III clinical trials: ICON7 and GOG 218.

The ICON7 clinical trial [12] randomized 1528 women to receive carboplatin (AUC 5 or 6) and paclitaxel (175 mg/m^2) every 3 weeks for 6 cycles, or the same regimen plus bevacizumab (7.5 mg/kg) every 3 weeks during chemotherapy, followed by 12 cycles or until unacceptable toxicity or disease progression. The study included patients with initial (FIGO I/IIA), high-risk (G3 or clear cells), or advanced (FIGO IIB–IV) cancer stage. The primary objective was progression-free survival (PFS) measured by RECIST criteria, and the secondary objectives included overall survival (OS), response to treatment, toxicity, and quality of life. Most of the patients (94%) had good performance status (ECOG Performance Status 0–1). A total of 70% patients were diagnosed at FIGO stage IIIC/IV.

With a median follow-up of 19.4 months, PFS was greater in the group with bevacizumab, and the difference was statistically significant (19.0 months vs. 17.3 months; HR = 0.81 (95% CI = 0.70–0.94); $p = 0.0041$). This difference in PFS was greater in the high-risk-of-progression group (stage IIIC with suboptimal surgery and IV), 15.9 vs. 10.5 months; HR = 0.68 (95% CI = 0.55–0.85); $p < 0.001$).

In the final analysis, with a median follow-up of 49 months, the increase in PFS is maintained in the high-risk-of-progression group, with an increase of 5.5 months (16.0 vs. 10.5 months; HR = 0.73 (95% CI = 0.61–0.88); $p = 0.001$), and there is an increase of 9.4 months in OS in the high-risk-of-progression group (39.7 vs. 30.3 months; HR = 0.78 (95% CI = 0.63–0.97); $p = 0.03$).

The treatment with bevacizumab was associated with an increase in bleeding (especially grade 1 mucocutaneous bleeding), grade 2 (G2) or greater acute hypertension (18% vs. 2%), grade 3 (G3) or higher thromboembolic events (7% vs. 3%), and gastrointestinal perforation (10 cases vs. 3 cases). The quality of life scores measured by the EORTC QLQ-C30 and QLQ-OV28 questionnaires show that continuation of treatment with bevacizumab appears to be associated with a small but clinically significant decline in quality of life compared to standard chemotherapy, so PFS and quality of life over the period of time in question have to be considered when treatment decisions are made [13].

The GOG 218 clinical trial [14] randomized 1873 women with stage III (incompletely resected) or stage IV epithelial ovarian cancer after cytoreduction surgery in three groups. In the three groups, the patients received carboplatin AUC 6 and paclitaxel 175 mg/m^2 every 3 weeks for 6 cycles and the study treatment. In the first arm (placebo arm), patients received placebo every 3 weeks from cycle 2 to cycle 22; in the second arm (bevacizumab initiation), patients received bevacizumab 15 mg/kg every 21 days from cycle 2 to cycle 6 followed by placebo from cycle 7 to cycle 22; in the third arm (bevacizumab throughout), patients received bevacizumab at the same dose from cycle 2 to cycle 22. The primary objective was PFS according to RECIST, CA-125, or clinical criteria. The secondary objectives included OS, safety, and quality of life. Once again, most of the patients (93%) maintained an ECOG PS 0-1. The group had a relatively poor prognosis, as 40% had stage III disease with residual disease greater than 1 cm and 26% had stage IV disease.

With a median follow-up of 17.4 months, the arm with bevacizumab (bevacizumab throughout) compared with the standard chemotherapy arm (placebo arm) showed a statistically significant increase in PFS (14.1 vs. 10.3 months; HR = 0.717 (95% CI = 0.625–0.824); $p = 0.0001$). In the bevacizumab initiation group, there was no increase in PFS (11.2 vs. 10.3 months; HR = 0.908 (95% CI = 0.759–1.040); $p = 0.080$). OS was similar in the three groups: 39.3, 38.7, and 39.7 months for the placebo arm, bevacizumab initiation group, and bevacizumab-throughout group, respectively, with no statistically significant differences.

G2 or higher hypertension was the only toxicity that was more common in a statistically significant manner in the bevacizumab groups than in the placebo arm (22.9% in bevacizumab throughout vs. 7.2% in the placebo arm). There were no differences in other toxicities such as gastrointestinal perforation or fistula, G3 or higher proteinuria, G4 neutropenia, febrile neutropenia, or venous or arterial thrombosis.

The main open questions left by these two trials are dosage and duration of treatment with bevacizumab. The dosage recommendation is to use the 15 mg/kg dose, which is in the summary of product characteristics, although benefit with bevacizumab is shown in a 7.5–15 mg/kg dose range [14]. As for treatment duration, both studies show that the widest separation of the PFS curves is found at 12 months in ICON7 and 15 months in GOG 218, which is at the termination of the bevacizumab. Thus, it is advisable to maintain bevacizumab treatment up to 15 months and to consider extending this period.

Two phase II studies showed the activity of bevacizumab in patients pretreated with chemotherapy. Those studies included platinum-sensitive and platinum-resistant patients.

A first study conducted by the GOG, GOG 170D, evaluated the efficacy of bevacizumab at 15 mg/kg every 3 weeks in 62 patients with advanced ovarian cancer after having received one or more treatment lines for advanced disease and found a 21% response rate and 10.3 months median response duration, with no intestinal perforation [15].

A second study in 70 patients evaluated the addition of cyclophosphamide (50 mg orally per day) to bevacizumab (10 mg/kg every 2 weeks) in patients who had received one to three previous chemotherapy lines and found a 24% response rate, 56% of patients relapse-free at 6 months, and 5.7% suffering intestinal perforations [16].

Subsequently, the OCEANS trial was initiated as a phase II study; after a safety review focused on intestinal perforations, it was converted to a phase III trial. Then 484 patients with platinum-sensitive recurrent ovarian cancer were randomized to receive carboplatin/gemcitabine for 6–10 cycles with bevacizumab (15 mg/m^2 every 3 weeks) or placebo until disease progression or unacceptable toxicity. Progression was documented by radiological (RECIST 1.0) or clinical criteria but not by CA-12.5 elevations. The primary objective was PFS determined by the investigators. The secondary objectives included response rate and OS. It also included an analysis of the primary objective by an independent committee.

The addition of bevacizumab to carboplatin/gemcitabine showed a median increase in PFS of 12.4 months versus 8.4 months (HR = 0.484, 95% CI = 0.388–0.605). These figures were repeated when evaluated by an independent committee (12.3 months vs. 8.6 months, $p = 0.0001$). This increase benefited all subgroups irrespective of age, ECOG, presence of cytoreduction surgery, time since last recurrence, and CA-12.5 levels. The secondary objectives also showed a 21.1% increase in response rate in the bevacizumab arm (response rate 78.5% vs. 57.4%, $p = 0.0001$). At cutoff date with a small number of events, there were not statistically significant differences in median survival, 35.2 months in the placebo arm and 33.3 months in the bevacizumab arm.

The most relevant G3 toxicities in the bevacizumab arm were proteinuria (0.9% vs. 8.5%) and hypertension (0.4% vs. 17.4%). No gastrointestinal perforation was documented during the study [17].

This study is the first randomized trial to describe the role of bevacizumab in platinum-sensitive disease. In this context, there is an ongoing study, GOG 213, which is evaluating the addition of bevacizumab to carboplatin and paclitaxel in platinum-sensitive relapse, with OS as its primary objective [18].

Two more studies are also evaluating bevacizumab in this context. The MITO-16/Mango OV-2BBP study is evaluating the addition of bevacizumab versus placebo to a carboplatin regimen with gemcitabine or pegylated liposomal adriamycin or paclitaxel in platinum-sensitive disease. Its primary objective is PFS, and OS is one of its secondary objectives [19]. The AGO/OVAR 2.21 study aims to show superiority in PFS for the carboplatin regimen with pegylated liposomal adriamycin and bevacizumab versus carboplatin with gemcitabine and bevacizumab [20].

There is a single phase II study in platinum-resistant disease; 44 patients who had received two or three previous treatment lines that included topotecan or liposomal anthracyclines were treated with bevacizumab, finding a 15.9% response rate and 27.8% of patients disease-free at 6 months. Perforations were found in a large percentage of patients, 11.4%, leading to its premature closure [21].

The AURELIA trial tested the addition of an antiangiogenic drug to chemotherapy in platinum-resistant disease. In this trial, 361 women with platinum-resistant ovarian cancer were randomized to receive single-agent chemotherapy (paclitaxel, pegylated liposomal doxorubicin, or topotecan) or the same chemotherapy with bevacizumab (10 mg/kg every 2 weeks or 15 mg/kg every 3 weeks in the regimen that included topotecan every 3 weeks). The therapeutic regimen was to be decided by the investigators, permitting any of those mentioned above. On the basis of the high rate of gastrointestinal perforations found in the aforementioned phase II study, the inclusion of both platinum-resistant patients who had received at least two lines of chemotherapy and platinum-refractory patients (progression while being treated with platinum) was ruled out, as well as patients with a history of intestinal obstruction (including subocclusive cases), intestinal perforation, abdominal fistula, intra-abdominal abscess, rectum or sigmoid colon affected by the disease, intestinal affectation by CT, or radiotherapy on the abdomen or pelvis. Its primary objective was PFS evaluated by the investigator. The secondary objectives included radiological response rate according to RECIST 1.0 criteria and CA-12.5, OS, safety, tolerability, and quality of life.

PFS was greater in the bevacizumab arm, with 6.7 months versus 3.4 months (HR = 0.42, $p < 0.001$), showing its efficacy in all the subgroups analyzed. There was also a greater response rate (27.3% in the bevacizumab arm vs. 11.8% in the placebo arm, $p = 0.001$) according to radiologic criteria and also a greater CA-12.5 serologic response rate, 11.6% in the placebo arm and 31.8% in the bevacizumab arm. There were no differences in OS (HR = 0.85; 95% CI = 0.66–1.08; $p = 0.174$). This finding can possibly be explained by the crossover in 40% of the patients assigned to the chemotherapy arm.

Toxicity in the bevacizumab arm included greater proteinuria and G3 hypertension. There was also a 2.2% incidence of gastrointestinal perforations. Overall, this is the first study to evaluate that the addition of an antiangiogenic to chemotherapy has an impact on PFS [22].

Another question to be investigated is the combination of bevacizumab with other strategies that have shown good results in the first-line treatment of ovarian cancer, such as intense doses of chemotherapy or intraperitoneal chemotherapy.

The combination of bevacizumab with intense-dose chemotherapy was studied in the OCTAVIA phase II clinical trial [23]. The primary objective was PFS according to RECIST criteria; the secondary objectives included the overall response rate, response duration in responder patients, OS, progression defined by CA-125, safety, and tolerability. The study included 189 patients diagnosed with stage I/IIA (grade 3/clear cells) or stages IIB–IV (any grade) ovarian cancer who underwent surgery. The patients received 6–8 cycles of bevacizumab (7.5 mg/kg, day 1 every 3 weeks) with weekly paclitaxel (80 mg/m^2, days 1, 8, and 15 every 3 weeks) and carboplatin (AUC 6, day 1 every 3 weeks); bevacizumab continued at the same dose as a single agent every 3 weeks up to a total of 17 cycles (1 year). A PFS of more than 18 months was considered to be clinically significant. Most of the patients were stage IIIC/IV (74%). With a median follow-up of 26.3 months, PFS was 23.7 months (95% CI = 19.8–26.4). PFS in the patients with stage III disease and >1.0 cm of residual disease after debulking surgery, or with stage IV disease, was 18.1 months. The response rate by RECIST in the 91 patients with measurable disease was 84.6% (95%CI = 75.5–91.3%), with 30.8% (95% CI = 21.5–41.3%) of complete responses. OS at 1 and 2 years was 97.8% and 92.1%, respectively. The most common grade ≥3 undesirable effects related to bevacizumab were hypertension (4.2%) and thromboembolic events (6.3%). In the study update [24], the limited number of events (17% of patients) for the planned final study analysis means that the OS results would be premature.

The combination of bevacizumab and chemotherapy at intense doses was also studied in the phase III GOG 262 clinical trial, which compared the standard chemotherapy regimen with carboplatin and paclitaxel every 3 weeks versus carboplatin every 3 weeks and paclitaxel weekly. The patients could also receive bevacizumab at the investigator's discretion [25].

The combination of bevacizumab and intraperitoneal chemotherapy is being studied in the GOG 252 phase III clinical trial [26].

3. Trebananib

Angiopoietins 1 and 2 (Ang1 and Ang2) are ligands of the Tie2 receptor, which is expressed in endothelial and some hematopoietic and lymph cells, mediating in vascular remodeling; it has a different signaling pathway from VEGF.

Trebananib (AMG 386) is a peptibody that inhibits angiopoietin 1 and 2, preventing interaction with the Tie2 receptor; it shows antiangiogenic effects in preclinical ovarian cancer models.

Having shown its safety and efficacy when administered intravenously in monotherapy at a maximum dose of 30 mg/kg weekly in phase I studies [27], and increasing PFS in phase II studies that used a dose of 10 mg/kg [28], it can be inferred that this benefit will be even greater using higher doses (such as 15 mg/kg), as doses of up to 30 mg/kg are tolerated without an increased toxicity.

The phase III study (TRINOVA-1) [29] examines the addition of trebananib to weekly paclitaxel versus weekly paclitaxel, showing a significant increase in PFS. It is a randomized, double-blind, placebo-controlled study. The inclusion criteria are as follows: woman over 18 years of age with histological diagnosis of epithelial ovarian cancer; primary peritoneal cancer or Fallopian tube cancer; having previously received chemotherapy based on a platinum regimen and progressed to 2 treatment lines; performance status 0–1; correct hematological, hepatic, and renal function; correct blood pressure figures (accepting appropriate control by taking antihypertensive treatment); and life expectancy of 3 months or more. Platinum-sensitive patients (platinum-free interval of more than 12 months) and platinum-refractory patients (disease recurrence or progression in the first 6 months or less after starting first-line platinum-based chemotherapy) were excluded and were also excluded in other histologies such as borderline, mucous and clear-cell tumors, patients who had presented a thromboembolic or hemorrhagic event in the last 12 months, unhealed wound, ulcer, fracture or infection, metastasis in the central nervous system, presence of grade 1 or higher neuropathy, presence of hepatitis B or C virus, and HIV infection. A total of 912 patients were randomized to receive in a 1:1 proportion of placebo and paclitaxel weekly or trebananib and paclitaxel weekly. The patients were stratified by platinum-free interval (0–6 months, or more than 6 months but less than 12), geographic region, and presence of radiologically measurable disease or not.

Patients received 80 mg/m^2 of paclitaxel IV (3 weeks on and 1 week off) and placebo or 15 mg/kg i.v. trebananib weekly, until progression according to RECIST 1.1 criteria, toxicity, or withdrawal of consent. A reduction in the dose of paclitaxel was allowed, but not of the placebo or trebananib. If necessary due to toxicity (e.g., edema), the drug was suspended until the toxicity was resolved, and it was definitively suspended if the delay due to toxic effects lasted more than 28 days. The patients were reassessed every 8 weeks by computerized tomography (CT) of the chest, abdomen, and pelvis. The tumor marker (specific cancer antigen (CA-125)) did not contribute to the assessment of disease response and progression. The primary objective was PFS, and the secondary objectives are survival and response rate.

The groups comprised 458 patients in the control arm (paclitaxel–placebo) and 461 in the experimental arm (paclitaxel–trebananib); median patient follow-up was 10.1 months.

Median PFS was greater in the group that received trebananib (5.4 vs. 7.2 months, HR = 0.6, 95% CI = 0.57–0.77), $p < 0.0001$, with all patient subgroups benefiting. The response rate by RECIST was greater in the experimental group (30% vs. 38%), and this difference was greater according to CA-125 levels, with a significant reduction of this (49% vs. 56%, $p = 0.03$). The interim overall OS analysis showed no differences between the groups (17.3 months vs. 19 months, HR = 0.86, 95% CI = 0.69–1.08, $p = 0.19$). Grade 3 or more side effects were described in 28% of the control subjects (paclitaxel–placebo) and 34% of the experimental group (paclitaxel–trebananib). The most common adverse reaction to the study drug was edema, which even became a cause of suspension of the treatment. Cases of hypertension, bleeding, pulmonary and arterial thromboembolism, proteinuria, and gastrointestinal perforations were also described. Trebananib added to paclitaxel for the treatment of recurring ovarian cancer significantly increases PFS versus placebo.

There are 2 phase III studies in which trebananib is added to pegylated liposomal doxorubicin (TRINOVA-2) [30] and trebananib in the first line associated to carboplatin–paclitaxel (TRINOVA-3) [31], although no conclusions have yet been reached.

4. Pazopanib

Pazopanib is an orally administered multikinase inhibitor of vascular endothelial growth factor receptor (VEGFR)-1/-2/-3 and of platelet-derived growth factor receptor (PDGFR)-α/-β and of c-Kit.

This drug has been approved for the treatment of metastatic renal cancer and soft tissue sarcomas.

Its role in several combinations has been analyzed, initially in a phase I/II study in combination with carboplatin and paclitaxel, after surgery, in order to increase the disease-free interval. This open-label phase I/II study was conducted to evaluate the safety and efficacy of paclitaxel 175 mg/m^2 plus carboplatin (AUC 5 (group A) or AUC 6 (group B)) once every 3 weeks for up to six cycles, with either 800 or 400 mg per day of pazopanib. Dose-limiting toxicities (DLT) were detected in two of the first six patients included in the pazopanib 800 mg plus paclitaxel 175 mg/m^2 plus carboplatin AUC 5 arm. There was also DLT in 2 of these first 6 patients at the lowest dosage level (pazopanib 400 mg plus paclitaxel 175 mg/m^2 plus carboplatin AUC 5).

Two of the 4 DLTs were gastrointestinal perforations, and severe myelotoxicity was reported in 6 of the 12 patients, leading to suspension of the study [32].

Subsequently, its use in monotherapy was investigated in a multicenter, nonrandomized, phase II study (VEG104450; NCT00281632) in patients with recurrence of epithelial ovarian or Fallopian tube cancer or primary peritoneal carcinoma who had presented complete response of CA-125 levels with platinum-based chemotherapy regimens. At relapse, patients with CA-12 levels reaching ≥42 U/mL (>2 × ULN) were treated with pazopanib 800 mg/day until progression or toxicity. Inclusion criteria were ECOG 0–1 and good hepatic and renal function. The primary objective was the response rate (determined by normalization of CA-125 levels or not), and the secondary objectives were overall response (measured as biochemical, radiological, and physical response) and PFS. Eleven out of 36 patients (31%) presented CA-125 response with a mean duration of 113 days; the overall response rate in patients with measurable disease was 18%. The most common adverse events leading to suspension of the treatment were transaminase elevation, with only 1 case of grade 4 edema [33].

This led to the study of the role of pazopanib as maintenance therapy in ovarian cancer patients who had not progressed during first-line chemotherapy. A total of 940 patients were included, with epithelial ovarian, Fallopian tube, or primary peritoneal cancer; FIGO stages II–IV, with no evidence of progression after surgery; and 6 cycles of platinum plus taxane chemotherapy. They were randomized 1:1 to receive pazopanib 800 mg once daily or placebo for 24 months. The primary objective was PFS by RECIST 1.0 criteria. It was shown that maintenance therapy with pazopanib increased PFS compared with placebo: 17.9 vs. 12.3 months, HR = 0.77; 95% CI = 0.64–0.91; $p = 0.0021$. Grades 3 and 4 adverse events were hypertension (30.8%), neutropenia (9.9%), transaminase elevation (9.4%), diarrhea (8.2%), fatigue (2.7%), thrombocytopenia (2.5%), and palmoplantar erythrodysesthesia (1.9%) in the pazopanib arm. Suspension of the treatment was significantly greater in the pazopanib arm (33.3%) versus placebo (5.6%) [34].

Maintenance therapy with pazopanib leads to an improvement in the median PFS of 5.6 months (HR = 0.77), with a 23% risk reduction for 2 years in women with FIGO stages II–IV who had not progressed to the first line of treatment. An increase in OS has not yet been shown, so the use of pazopanib is not currently recommended for this clinical situation.

5. Nintedanib

Nintedanib (BIBF 1120) is a powerful triple angiokinase inhibitor. It inhibits VEGFR-1, VEGFR-2, and VEGFR-3; PDGFR α and β; and FGFR-1, FGFR-2, and FGFR-3. The first data, obtained in a phase I study, in combination with carboplatin and paclitaxel administered twice a day, with doses of 100–250 mg, in 22 patients with locally advanced or recurring metastatic ovarian cancer, indicated that the maximum tolerated dose was 200 mg/12 h. Higher doses were related to higher significant gastrointestinal toxicity in the form of diarrhea, alanine aminotrnasferase (ALT) and aspartate aminotransferase (AST) elevation, and hematological toxicity, basically in white blood cells [35].

Nintedanib 250 mg/12 h was studied in a phase II randomized trial versus placebo in 83 women with recurring (in second or subsequent lines) ovarian cancer who had responded to chemotherapy but presented high risk of relapse. The primary objectives were PFS, OS, and toxicity. The patients received at least 9 cycles of the treatment or placebo, continuing until disease progression (unless the patient withdrew from the study). PFS at 36 weeks was 16.3% versus 5%, with HR = 0.65, 95% CI = 0.42–1.02, and $p = 0.06$. The reported G3/4 adverse events were similar in both arms (34.9% vs. 27.5%, respectively, $p = 0.49$), but in the nintedanib group, there was greater gastrointestinal toxicity in the form of diarrhea, nausea, and vomiting ($p < 0.001$) versus placebo. Likewise, there was greater G3/4 hepatotoxicity with nintedanib versus placebo (51.2% vs. 7.5%, $p < 0.001$ [36]).

There is currently an ongoing phase III, randomized, double-blind trial (AGO-OVAR 12/LUME) in first-line treatment of locally advanced or metastatic ovarian cancer (stages IIB–IV) that compares the combination of carboplatin, paclitaxel, and nintedanib 200 mg/12 h and maintenance with nintedanib for 120 weeks versus the same chemotherapy regimen with placebo and maintenance with placebo, also for 120 weeks. A total of 1366 patients have been included, and to date, it has reported an advantage in PFS in favor of the arm with the combination of nintedanib with chemotherapy and subsequent maintenance (17.3 months vs. 16.6 months), HR = 0.84 and 95% CI (0.72–0.98), $p = 0.0239$, versus placebo [37].

Another phase II trial is being conducted with this drug in recurrent or persistent disease or disease already treated with bevacizumab [38].

6. Cediranib

Cediranib (AZD 2171) is a tyrosine kinase agent with antiangiogenic activity, blocking the VEGF receptor (VEGFR 1, VEGFR2 and VEGFR3) and c-Kit.

Although women were included in the phase I study of the drug, they did not have ovarian cancer. It was found that the dose was tolerable up to 45 mg/24 h [39]. The phase II studies used both this and lower doses.

At the 2008 ASCO meeting, Hirte et al. presented data from 60 patients with relapse of ovarian or Fallopian tube carcinoma or peritoneal carcinomatosis treated with cediranib, showing that the 30 mg/24 h dose was well tolerated and active in this patient group [40].

In 2009, the results of a phase II study were published, including 46 patients with platinum-sensitive and platinum-resistant relapse of ovarian carcinoma, Fallopian tube carcinoma, or peritoneal carcinomatosis. The patients received cediranib 45 mg/24 h until progression, intolerable toxicity, or withdrawal of consent. After the toxicity seen in 11 patients, the dose was reduced to 30 mg/24 h. More than 20% of the patients presented G3 adverse events, the most common being hypertension (46%), fatigue (24%), and diarrhea (13%); 8.7% of them presented G4 adverse events [41].

The randomized, double-blind ICON 6 study compares a platinum-based chemotherapy arm with cediranib (concurrent), another similar arm (concurrent) plus continuation (for 18 months or until progression) of maintenance cediranib, and the same chemotherapy regimen with placebo in relapse of platinum-sensitive disease. The preliminary data (60 women enrolled) show benefit with the combination of cediranib and its maintenance versus the arm in which placebo was added, both in PFS (11.4 vs. 9.4 months, HR = 0.68, $p = 0.0022$) and in OS (20.3 vs. 17.6 months, HR = 0.70, $p = 0.049$). The dose of cediranib had to be reduced during the study to 20 mg/24 h due to toxicity and reduced adherence to treatment [42]. The results update at the 2013 ESMO congress show greater benefit in PFS (12.5 vs. 9.4 months, HR = 0.57, $p = 0.00001$) and a benefit of 2.7 months in OS in the cediranib maintenance group. It is the first oral antiangiogenic agent to date to show benefit in terms of OS. The most common adverse events were diarrhea, nausea, and fatigue [43].

Cediranib was combined with olaparib in a randomized phase II study versus olaparib in monotherapy in women presenting platinum-sensitive relapse of ovarian cancer associated with BRCA mutation. The patients received olaparib 200 mg/24 h and cediranib 30 mg/24h in the combination arm and olaparib 400 mg/24 h in the monotherapy arm. PFS was 17.7 months with the combination and 9 months with olaparib in monotherapy, HR = 2.9 and 95% CI (1.5–5.6), $p = 0.001$. There were 2 complete and 21 partial responses, 56% objective responses with the monotherapy, and 3 complete, 33 partial, and 84% objective responses in the experimental group. The incidence of G3/4 adverse events was 70% with the combination and only 7% with olaparib; the most common were fatigue, diarrhea, and hypertension [44].

7. Aflibercept

Aflibercept is a recombinant fusion protein, also called VEFG-Trap, that binds to and neutralizes all forms of VEGF-A and VEGF-B and inhibits placental growth factor (PGF) activation. In several preclinical models, it was seen to inhibit tumor growth and metastasis formation, and another study showed evident reduction in ascites and tumor size in murine models that developed human ovarian tumors [45].

Various phase II studies have tested the activity of this drug in ovarian cancer. In the first of these, aflibercept is combined with docetaxel in 49 patients with platinum-resistant relapse with a maximum of two previous chemotherapy regimens. It was administered at a dose of 6 mg/kg until progression or intolerable toxicity. There was a 54% response rate; 10 cases presented complete response, and relapse was not detected in 4 of them at 1-year posttreatment (range 5–22 months). Median PFS was 6.2 months, and OS was 24.3 months [46].

Gotlieb et al. published a multicenter, randomized, double-blind phase II study that included 55 patients with relapse of platinum-resistant ovarian cancer, who had received a median of at least 4 previous lines (range 2–12) that compared aflibercept 4 mg/kg every 14 days versus placebo. The patients were stratified according to the need for paracentesis in 2 periods, ≤2 weeks and >2 weeks. The primary objective was time to new paracentesis. Time to paracentesis from randomization was significantly greater in the aflibercept arm (55.1 vs. 23.3 days), and in two patients, new paracentesis was not required until 6 months later. There was more toxicity in the form of dyspnea (20% vs. 8%) in the aflibercept arm and also intestinal perforation (3 patients vs. 1). However, there was more fatigue or asthenia (13% vs. 44%) and more dehydration (10% vs. 12%) with placebo [47].

Similar to the previous study, and with the same doses, another multicenter group tried to answer the same question in another phase II study: the utility of aflibercept in control of gynecologic tumor ascites. They included 16 platinum-resistant and very pretreated patients, with similar results obtained [48].

These last two studies show the activity and effect of the drug in reducing the need for paracentesis, although a small risk of intestinal perforation in peritoneal carcinomatosis cannot be ruled out. It should only be used after thoroughly evaluating the risk/benefit ratio in each specific case.

8. Sorafenib

Sorafenib is a multikinase inhibitor with activity on different tyrosine kinase receptors, including VEGFR-2 and VEGFR-3, PDGFR-β, c-Kit, and Flt-3 receptor and the v-raf oncogene.

Limited activity of this drug has been shown in 71 women who presented ovarian tumor relapse within 12 months of completing platinum treatment (after one or two previous regimens). The primary objectives were PFS at 6 months and safety; the secondary objectives were percentage response and duration of PFS and OS. The dose used was 400 mg/12 h. Efficacy was evaluated only in the 59 patients with measurable disease: 14 women (24%) presented PFS of at least 6 months. Partial response was obtained in 2 women, stabilization in 20, while 30 patients presented progression; response could not be measured in 7 patients. The most common G3/4 adverse events were as expected (rash, hand/foot syndrome, gastrointestinal, and metabolic and, to a lesser extent, cardiovascular and pulmonary toxicity) [49].

A Canadian group from the Princess Margaret Hospital studied sorafenib, at the same doses, in combination with gemcitabine weekly in a phase II trial in 43 pretreated patients with platinum-resistant relapse; 2 of them presented partial response, and the disease remained stable for at least 6 months in 10 of them. However, the proportion of responses was only 4.7%. The most common G3/4 events were hematological (28% lymphocytopenia and 26% neutropenia), leading to significant delays in the administration of the therapeutic regimen [50].

German investigators tested the addition of the drug to the carboplatin–paclitaxel combination in the neoadjuvant context in patients with large disease volume and ascites. This phase II trial included only 4 patients, as it was stopped due to severe G3/4 toxicity, largely cardiovascular [51].

The combination with topotecan in platinum-resistant patients was also evaluated. There was important hematologic toxicity and G3/4 toxicity in the form of transaminase elevation [52].

The possibility of continuation or maintenance treatment was evaluated in women after they completed the first-line treatment with carboplatin and paclitaxel and had presented complete response. Two hundred and forty-six patients were included and randomized to receive

Sorafenib 400 mg/12 h or placebo until progression, intolerable toxicity, or withdrawal of consent. The patient was withdrawn from the study if there was more than a 30-day delay in the administration of the treatment or if more than two dose reductions were required. The primary objectives were to evaluate the efficacy and safety of this approach. There were no differences between the two groups in PFS, with a trend toward better results in the placebo arm, and there were clearly more adverse events with sorafenib, with a toxicity profile similar to that found in previous studies. The conclusions of the study were that maintenance therapy with this drug could not be recommended [53].

The combination of paclitaxel, carboplatin, and sorafenib was investigated in first-line treatment for metastatic disease in women with stages III and IV. After two treatment cycles, the patients with stabilization or partial response continued the chemotherapy for six cycles, and sorafenib was maintained for 52 weeks; 85 patients were included. Efficacy was similar in proportion of responses, PFS, and 2-year survival. The addition of sorafenib clearly increased toxicity: EPP, mucositis, and HT, and so its use was not recommended [54].

9. Sunitinib

Sunitinib is also another multikinase inhibitor that binds to VEGF, PDGF, c-Kit, and Ftl-3. As with sorafenib, the response rates of therapy with this drug are low.

In a phase II trial that included 30 women with platinum-sensitive (73%) and platinum-resistant (27%) relapse who had received one or two previous lines, treated with the standard 50 mg/day dose for 4 weeks and 2 weeks of rest, there was one partial response and 16 stabilizations [55].

In another phase II study with 73 platinum-resistant patients who had received three or more previous lines, they were randomized to receive sunitinib at standard dose or 37.5 mg/day continually. There were differences in median PFS in favor of the standard administration (4.8 vs. 2.9 months) but not in OS (13.6 vs. 13.7 months). The pattern and the frequency of adverse events were similar in the two groups and as expected: fatigue, cardiovascular and gastrointestinal toxicity, hematological alterations, and hepatic function disorders [56].

The continuous administration of 37.5 mg/day was also evaluated in another Dana–Farber phase II study in 18 platinum-resistant patients, continuing to find a response (partial and complete) rate of around 8% and median PFS of just 10 weeks. There was also considerable toxicity in the form of hypertension and gastrointestinal events [57].

10. Imatinib mesylate

Imatinib belongs to the tyrosine kinase inhibitor family; it prevents PDGF from binding to its receptor and prevents the triggering of the AKT intracellular signaling cascade responsible for tumor growth and metastatic dissemination.

Its possible therapeutic effect on platinum-resistant ovarian tumors after progression to other treatments has also been studied. Most studies treated patients at the standard dose of 600 mg/day after selecting them according to immunohistochemical c-Kit expression. They included a small number of patients, and the drug was tested in monotherapy [58, 59] and in combination with docetaxel [60] or paclitaxel [61]. Few responses were obtained (0–2%), primarily obtaining stabilizations, with repeated dose reductions required due to toxicity in the form of edemas, gastrointestinal, or hematological adverse events.

More recently, Anderson's work found that there was no correlation between responses in platinum-refractory patients who had progressed to taxanes and expression of the aforementioned biomarkers. The efficacy and toxicity results were similar to those of previous studies, concluding that it was not an active treatment in this group of patients [62].

11. Vandetanib

Vandetanib (ZD6474) also belongs to the oral tyrosine kinase inhibitor family and inhibits VEGFR-2 and VEGFR-3, EGFR, and RET.

In a phase I/II study in combination with pegylated liposomal doxorubicin (50 mg/m^2, day 1/28 days), at a dose of 100 mg/24 h in platinum-resistant patients, 14 patients were included and few responses (around 10%) were found, with close to 40% stabilizations, but significant toxicity led to discontinuation of the treatment in nearly 30% of patients [63].

Combined with concomitant docetaxel, the SWOG S0904 study compared it to docetaxel in monotherapy. A total of 131 patients were included and randomized to one of the arms; no benefit was found from the addition of vandetanib in PFS; there was G4 hematological toxicity in nearly 30% of the included women [64].

12. Ramucirumab

Ramucirumab, or IMC-1121B, is an Ig G1 humanized monoclonal antibody that has affinity for the extracellular domain of VEGFR-2 and prevents VEGF from binding to its ligands, thus inhibiting endothelial cell proliferation and migration and new vessel formation.

A multicenter study with 70 women with platinum-resistant relapse in 75% of them only obtained 5% partial responses, nearly 60% stabilizations, and 25% 6-month PFS (both primary end points); ramucirumab was not found to be particularly active in this context [65].

13. Zibotentan

Zibotentan or ZD4054 is an oral ET-A receptor antagonist that is involved in activation of endothelin growth, and thus in cell proliferation and tumor invasion and migration.

In a multicenter study that combines the drug (at a dose of 10 mg/24 h) with carboplatin and paclitaxel versus the same chemotherapy and placebo, no benefit was found in PFS, percentage of responses, or reduction of CA-125 in women with platinum-sensitive disease. The toxicities most commonly found with the drug were anemia and neutropenia, alopecia, nausea, and headache in nearly 50% of patients [66].

In total, to date there are no promising results for most of the reviewed antiangiogenic agents, except those already known for bevacizumab, trebananib, pazopanib, cediranib, and nintedanib. Ongoing research will shed more light on this fascinating tumor process and its control.

Author details

M.A. Alonso Bermejo, L. Rey Iglesias , M.E. Pérez López, A. Fernández Montes* and J. García Mata

*Address all correspondence to: afm1003@hotmail.com

Medical Oncology Service at the University Hospital Ourense, Ourense, Spain

References

[1] Colombo N, Peiretti M, Parma G, et al. Newly diagnosed and relapsed epitelial ovarian carcinoma: ESMO Clinical Practice Guidelines for diagnosis, treatment and follow-up. Ann Oncol 2010; 21 (Suppl 5): v23–v30.

[2] Monk BJ, Coleman RL. Changing the paradigm in the treatment of platinum-sensitive recurrent ovarian cancer: from platinum doublets to nonplatinum doublets and adding antiangiogenesis compounds. Int J Gynecol Cancer 2009; 19 (Suppl 2): s63–s67.

[3] Bookman MA, Brady MF, McGuire WP, et al. Evaluation of new platinum-based treatment regimens in advanced-stage ovarian cancer: a Phase III Trial of the Gynecologic Cancer Intergroup. J Clin Oncol 2009; 27 (9): 1419–1425.

[4] du Bois A, Herrstedt J, Hardy-Bessard AC, et al. Phase III trial of carboplatin plus paclitaxel with or without gemcitabine in first-line treatment of epithelial ovarian cancer. J Clin Oncol 2010; 28: 4162–4169.

[5] du Bois A, Weber B, Rochon J, et al. Addition of epirubicin as a third drug to carboplatin-paclitaxel in first-line treatment of advanced ovarian cancer: a prospectively randomized gynecologic cancer intergroup trial by the Arbeitsgemeinschaft Gynaekologische Onkologie Ovarian Cancer Study Group and the Groupe d'Investigateurs Nationaux pour l'Etude des Cancers Ovariens. J Clin Oncol 2006; 24: 1127–1135.

[6] Bolis G, Scarfone G, Raspagliesi F, et al. Paclitaxel/carboplatin versus topotecan/paclitaxel/carboplatin in patients with FIGO suboptimally resected stage III–IV epithelial ovarian cancer: a multicenter, randomized study. Eur J Cancer 2010; 46: 2905–2912.

[7] Pfisterer J, Weber B, Reuss A, et al. Randomized phase III trial of topotecan following carboplatin and paclitaxel in first-line treatment of advanced ovarian cancer: a gynecologic cancer intergroup trial of the AGO-OVAR and GINECO. J Natl Cancer Inst 2006; 98: 1036–1045.

[8] Aravantinos G, Pectasides D. Bevacizumab in combination with chemotherapy for the treatment of advanced ovarian cancer: a systematic review. J Ovarian Res 2014; 7: 57.

[9] Martin L, Schilder R. Novel approaches in advancing the treatment of epithelial ovarian cancer: the role of angiogenesis inhibition. J Clin Oncol 2007; 25 (20): 2894–2901.

[10] Nagy JA, Dvorak AM, Dvorak HF. VEGF-A and the induction of pathological angiogenesis. Annu Rev Pathol 2007; 2: 251–275.

[11] Ferrara N, Hillan KJ, Novotny W. Bevacizumab (Avastin), a humanized anti-VEGF monoclonal antibody for cancer therapy. Biochem Biophys Res Commun 2005; 333: 328–335.

[12] Perren TJ, Swart AM, Pfisterer J, et al. A phase 3 trial of bevacizumab in ovarian cancer. N Engl J Med 2011; 365: 2484–2496.

[13] Stark D, Nankivell M, Pujade-Lauraine E, et al. Standard chemotherapy with or without bevacizumab in advanced ovarian cancer: quality-of-life outcomes from the International Collaboration on Ovarian Neoplasm (ICON 7) phase 3 randomised trial. Lancet Oncol 2013; 14: 236–243.

[14] Burger RA, Brady MF, Bookman MA, et al. Incorporation of bevacizumab in the primary treatment of ovarian cancer. N Engl J Med 2011; 365: 2473–2483.

[15] Burger RA, Sill MW, Monk BJ, et al. Phase II trial of bevacizumab in persistent or recurrent epithelial ovarian cancer or primary peritoneal cancer: a Gynecologic Oncology Group Study. J Clin Oncol 2007;25: 5165–5171.

[16] Garcia AA, Hirte H, Fleming G, et al. Phase II clinical trial of bevacizumab and low-dose metronomic oral cyclophosphamide in recurrent ovarian cancer: a trial of the California, Chicago and Princess Margaret Hospital phase II consortia. J Clin Oncol 2008;26: 76–82.

[17] Aghajanian C, Blank SV, Goff BA, et al. OCEANS: a randomized, double-blind, placebo-controlled phase III trial of chemotherapy with or without bevacizumab in patients with platinum-sensitive recurrent epithelial ovarian, primary peritoneal, or fallopian tube cancer. J Clin Oncol 2012; 30: 2039–2045.

[18] A Phase III Randomized Controlled Clinical Trial of Carboplatin and Paclitaxel (or Gemcitabine) Alone or in Combination with Bevacizumab (NSC #704865) Followed by Bevacizumab and Secondary Cytoreductive Surgery in Platinum-Sensitive, Recurrent Ovarian, Peritoneal Primary and Fallopian Tube Cancer. National Library of Medicine. http://www.clinicaltrials.gov/show/NCT00565851

[19] Study of Clinical and Biological Prognostic Factors in Patients with Ovarian Cancer Receiving Carboplatin +Paclitaxel With Bevacizumab (MITO16/MANGO-2). http://www.clinicaltrials.gov/show/NCT01706120

[20] Evaluation of Optimal Treatment with Bevacizumab in Patients with Platinum-Sensitive Recurrent Ovarian Cancer. AGO-OVAR 2.21/ENGOT ov-18. http://www.clinicaltrials.gov/show/NCT01837251

[21] Cannistra SA, Matulonis UA, Penson RT, et al. Phase II study of bevacizumab in patients with platinum-resistant ovarian cancer or peritoneal serous cancer. J Clin Oncol 2007; 25: 5180–5186.

[22] [22]. Pujade-Lauraine E, Hilpert F, Weber B, et al. Bevacizumab combined with chemotherapy for platinum-resistant recurrent ovarian cancer: the AURELIA open-label randomized phase III trial. J Clin Oncol 2014; 32: 1302–1308.

[23] Gonzalez-Martin A, Gladieff L, Tholander B, et al. Efficacy and safety results from OCTAVIA, a single-arm phase II study evaluating front-line bevacizumab, carboplatin and weekly paclitaxel for ovarian cancer. Eur J Cancer 2013; 49: 3831–3838.

[24] Gonzalez-Martin A, Gladieff L, Tholander B, et al. Updated results from OCTAVIA (front-line Bevacizumab, carboplatin and weekly paclitaxel therapy for ovarian cancer). Eur J Cancer 2014; 50: 862–863.

[25] Paclitaxel and Carboplatin with or without Bevacizumab in Treating Patients with Stage II, Stage III, or Stage IV Ovarian Epithelial Cancer, Primary Peritoneal Cancer, or Fallopian Tube Cancer. http://www.clinicaltirals.gov/ct2/show/NCT01167712

[26] Bevacizumab and Intravenous or Intraperitoneal Chemotherapy in Treating Patients with Stage II–III Ovarian Epithelial Cancer, Fallopian Tube Cancer, or Primary Peritoneal Cancer. http://www.clinicaltrials.gov/ct2/show/NCT00951496

[27] Herbst RS, Hong d, Chap L., et al. Safety, pharmacokinetics, and antitumor activity of AMG 386, a selective angiopoietin inhibitor, in adult patients with advanced solid tumors. J Clin Oncol 2009;27: 3557–3565.

[28] Karlan BY, Oza AM, Richardson GE, et al. Randomized, double-blind, placebo-controlled phase II study of AMG 386 combined with weekly paclitaxel in patients with recurrent ovarian cancer. J Clin Oncol 2012; 30: 362–371.

[29] Monk BJ, Poveda A, Vergote I, et al. Anti-angiopoietin therapy with trebananib for recurrent ovarian cancer (TRINOVA-1): a randomised, multicentre, double-blind, placebo-controlled phase 3 trial. Lancet Oncol 2014; 15: 799–808.

[30] Amgen: TRINOVA-2: Trebananib in Ovarian Cancer-2. http://www.clinicaltrials.gov/show/NCT01281254

[31] Amgen: TRINOVA-3: A Study of AMG 386 Placebo in Combination with Paclitaxel and Carboplatin to Treat Ovarian Cancer. http://www.clinicaltrials.gov/show/NCT01493505

[32] du Bois A, Vergote I, Wimberger P, et al. Open-label feasibility study of pazopanib, carboplatin, and paclitaxel in women with newly diagnosed, untreated, gynaecologic tumours: a phase I/II trial of the AGO study group. Br J Cancer 2012; 106: 629–632.

[33] Friedlander M, Hancock KC, Rischin D, et al. A phase II, open-label study evaluating pazopanib in patients with recurrent ovarian cancer. Gynecol Oncol 2010; 119: 32–37.

[34] du Bois A, Floquet A, Kim JW, et al. Incorporation of pazopanib in maintenance therapy of ovarian cancer. J Clin Oncol 2014; 32: 3314–3382.

[35] Du Bois A, Huober J, Stopfer P, et al. A phase I open-label dose-escalation study of oral BIBF 1120 combined con standard paclitaxel and carboplatin in patients with advanced gynecological malignancies. Ann Oncol 2010; 21: 370–375.

[36] Lederman JA, Hackshaw A, Kaye S, et al. Randomized phase II placebo-controlled trial of maintenance therapy using the oral triple angiokinase inhibitor BIBF 1120 after chemotherapy for relapsed ovarian cancer. J Clin Oncol 2011; 29: 3798–3804.

[37] Du Bois A, Kristensen G, Ray-Coquard I, et al. AGO-OVAR 12: a randomized placebo-controlled GCIG/ENGOT-intergroup phase III trial of standard frontline chemotherapy +/– nintedanib for advanced ovarian cancer [abstract]. Int J Gynecol 2013; 23(Suppl 1):LBA1.

[38] Boehringer Ingelheim: BIBF1120 in bevacizumab resistant, persistent or recurrent epithelial ovarian cancer. National of Library of Medicine. http://www.clinicaltrials.gov/show/NCT01669798

[39] Drevs J, Siegert P, Medinger M, et al. Phase I clinical study of AZD2171, an oral vascular endothelial growth factor signaling inhibitor, in patients with advanced solid tumors. J Clin Oncol 2007; 25: 3045–3054.

[40] Hirte HW, Vidal L, Fleming GF, et al. A phase II study of cediranib (AZD2171) in recurrent or persistent ovarian, peritoneal or fallopian tube cancer: final results of a PMH, Chicago and California consortia trial. J Clin Oncol 2008; 26: Abstract 5521.

[41] Matulonis UA, Berlin S, Ivy P, et al. Cediranib, an oral inhibitor of vascular endothelial growth factor receptor kinases, is an active drug in recurrent epithelial ovarian, fallopian tube, and peritoneal cancer. J Clin Oncol 2009; 27: 5601–5606.

[42] Raja FA, Griffin CL, Qian W, et al. Initial toxicity assessment of ICON6: a randomised trial of cediranib plus chemotherapy in platinum-sensitive relapsed ovarian cancer. B J Cancer 2011; 105: 884–889.

[43] Ledermann J, Perren TJ, Raja FA, et al. Randomised double-blind phase III trial of cediranib (AZD 2171) in relapsed platinum sensitive ovarian cancer: results of the ICON6 trial. E J Cancer 2013, 49: LBA: 10.

[44] Liu J, Barry WT, Birrer MJ, et al. Combination cediranib and olaparib versus olaparib alone for women with recurrent platinum-sensitive ovarian cancer: a randomised phase 2 study. Lancet Oncol 2014; 15: 1207–1214.

[45] Byrne AT, Ross L, Holash J, et al. Vascular endothelial growth factor-trap decreases tumor burden, inhibits ascites, and causes dramatic vascular remodeling in an ovarian cancer model. Clin Cancer Res 2003; 9: 5721–5728.

[46] Coleman RL, Duska LR, Ramirez PT, et al. Phase II multi-institutional study of docetaxel plus aflibercept (AVE0005, NSC# 724700) in patients with recurrent ovarian, primary peritoneal and fallopian tube cancer. J Clin Oncol 2011; 20: Abstract 5017.

[47] Gotlieb WH, Amant F, Advani S, et al. Intravenous aflibercept for treatment of recurrent symptomatic malignant ascites in patients with advanced ovarian cancer: a phase 2, randomised, double-blind, placebo controlled study. Lancet Oncol 2012; 13: 154–162.

[48] Colombo N, Mangili G, Mammoliti S, et al. A phase II study of aflibercept in patients with advanced epithelial ovarian cancer and symptomatic malignant ascites. Gynecol Oncol 2012; 125: 42–47.

[49] Matei D, Sill MW, Lankes HA, et al. Activity of sorafenib in recurrent ovarian cancer and primary peritoneal carcinomatosis: a Gynecologic Oncology Group trial. J Clin Oncol 2010; 29: 69–75.

[50] Welch SA, Hirte HW, Elit L, et al. Sorafenib in combination with gemcitabine in recurrent epithelial ovarian cancer: a study of the Princess Margaret Hospital Phase II Consortium. Int J Gynecol Cancer 2010; 20: 787–793.

[51] Polcher M, Eckhardt M, Coch C, et al. 2010. Sorafenib in combination with carboplatin and paclitaxel as neoadjuvant chemotherapy in patients with advanced ovarian cancer. Cancer Chemother Pharmacol 2010; 66: 203–207.

[52] Chekerov R, Mahner S, Lorenz R, et al. NOGGO-AGO Intergroup Study: efficacy and safety of sorafenib added to topotecan in patients with platinum-resistant recurrent ovarian cancer: A NOGGO-AGO intergroup run-in-study (TRIAS). Int J Gynecol Cancer 2011; 21: S597.

[53] Herzog TJ, Scambia G, Kim BG, et al. A randomized phase II trial of maintenance therapy with sorafenib in front-line ovarian carcinoma. Gynecol Oncol 2013; 130: 25–30.

[54] Hainsworth JD, Thompson DS, Bismayer JA. Paclitaxel/carboplatin with or without sorafenib in the first-line treatment of patients with stage III/IV epithelial ovarian

cancer: a randomized phase II study of the Sarah Cannon Research Institute. Cancer Med 2014 Dec 31. doi: 10.1002/cam4.376. [Epub ahead of print]

[55] Biagi JJ, Oza AM, Chalchal HI, Grimshaw R, Ellard SL, Lee U, et al. A phase II study of sunitinib in patients with recurrent epithelial ovarian and primary peritoneal carcinoma: an NCIC Clinical Trials Group Study. Ann Oncol 2011; 22: 335–340.

[56] Baumann KH, du Bois A, Meier W, et al. A phase II trial (AGO 2.11) in platinum-resistant ovarian cancer: a randomized multicenter trial with sunitinib (SU11248) to evaluate dosage, schedule, tolerability, toxicity and effectiveness of a multitargeted receptor tyrosine kinase inhibitor monotherapy. Ann Oncol 2012; 23: 2265–2271.

[57] Campos SM, Penson RT, Matulonis U, et al. A phase II trial of Sunitinib malate in recurrent and refractory ovarian, fallopian tube and peritoneal carcinoma. Gynecol Oncol 2013; 128: 215–220.

[58] Alberts DS, Liu PY, Wilczynski SP, et al. Phase II trial of imatinib mesylate in recurrent, biomarker positive, ovarian cancer (SWOG S0211). Int J Gynecol Cancer 2007; 17(4): 784–788.

[59] Juretzka M, Hensley ML, Tew W, et al. A phase 2 trial of oral imatinib in patients with epithelial ovarian, fallopian tube, or peritoneal carcinoma in second or greater remission. Eur J Gynaecol Oncol 2008; 29: 568–572.

[60] Matei D, Emerson RE, Schilder J, et al. Imatinib mesylate in combination with docetaxel for the treatment of patients with advanced, platinum-resistant ovarian cancer and primary peritoneal carcinomatosis. Cancer 2008; 113: 723–732.

[61] Safra T, Andreopoulou E, Levinson B, et al. Weekly paclitaxel with intermittent imatinib mesylate (Gleevec): tolerance and activity in recurrent epithelial ovarian cancer. Anticancer Res 2010; 30: 3243–3247.

[62] Noguera IR, Sun CC, Broaddus RR, et al. Phase II trial of imatinib mesylate in patients with recurrent platinum- and taxane-resistant low-grade serous carcinoma of the ovary, peritoneum, or fallopian tube. Gynecol Oncol 2012; 125: 640–645.

[63] Harter P, Sehouli J, Kimmig R, et al. Addition of vandetanib to pegylated liposomal doxorubicin (PLD) in patients with recurrent ovarian cancer. A randomized phase I/II study of the AGO Study Group (AGO-OVAR 2.13). Invest New Drugs 2013; 31: 1499–1504.

[64] Coleman RL, Moon J, Sood AK, et al. Randomised phase II study of docetaxel plus vandetanib versus docetaxel followed by vandetanib in patients with persistent or recurrent epithelial ovarian, fallopian tube or primary peritoneal carcinoma: SWOG S0904. E J Cancer 2014; 50: 1638–1648.

[65] Penson RT, Moore KM, Fleming GF, et al. A phase II study of ramucirumab (IMC-1121B) in the treatment of persistent or recurrent epithelial ovarian, fallopian tube or primary peritoneal carcinoma. Gynecol Oncol 2014; 134: 478–485.

[66] Cognetti F, Bagnato A, Colombo N, et al. A phase II, randomized, double-blind study of zibotentan (ZD4054) in combination with carboplatin/paclitaxel versus placebo in combination with carboplatin/paclitaxel in patients with advanced ovarian cancer sensitive to platinum-based chemotherapy (AGO-OVAR 2.14). Gynecol Oncol 2013; 103: 31–37.

Chapter 4

Peritonectomy Procedures and HIPEC for Peritoneal Metastasis from Ovarian Cancer

Angelo Di Giorgio, Daniele Biacchi, Antonio Ciardi, Alessio Impagnatiello, Maurizio Cardi, Simone Sibio, Bianca Sollazzo, Joseph Maher Fouad Atta, Giuseppe Naso, Fabio Accarpio and Paolo Sammartino

Additional information is available at the end of the chapter

http://dx.doi.org/10.5772/60844

Abstract

Peritoneal carcinomatosis (PC) is the most impressive and frequent evidence of loco-regional spread of epithelial ovarian cancer (EOC). For most of its natural history, PC remains confined to the peritoneal district, thus representing a target for various combinations of surgery and systemic or loco-regional chemotherapy. PC is observed both in primary settings, i.e. in patients first treated for locally advanced EOC, and in recurrent, previously treated, EOC patients at any FIGO stage. Since 2000s, the use of hyperthermic intraperitoneal chemotherapy (HIPEC) combined with maximum cytoreduction (peritonectomy) has gradually spread in the treatment of PC from ovarian cancer, as well as for gastrointestinal carcinomatosis and primary tumours of the peritoneum. Use of combined peritonectomy + HIPEC in the treatment of ovarian carcinomatosis is the most discussed issue among those concerning peritoneal surface malignancy (PSM). The main criticism concerns the use of HIPEC, since the need for maximal cytoreduction is consolidated and does not raise any doubts. Communities of surgeon and oncologic gynaecologists who believes in the role of HIPEC have started controlled clinical trials aimed at clarifying the role of HIPEC associated to peritonectomy, but these studies are difficult to conduct and time-consuming. At present and pending the results of future prospective trials, the role and limits of application of the procedure are drawn from experiences from three basic study groups: collective reviews, multicentre studies, monocentric case studies produced by high-volume HIPEC centers. A comprehensive literature review and an in-depth analysis of our personal experience, based on the largest monocentric case series (130 cases), have helped to provide an assessment on the role of peritonectomy + HIPEC in about 2000 patients treated for initial and recurrent PC from ovarian cancer. Comparison of the overall results drawn from these studies, indicates that peritonectomy + HIPEC is able to guarantee in these patients better overall survival (OS) and higher progression-free survival (PFS) rates than those derived from traditional treatments, with acceptable morbidity and mortality. Notwithstanding, some specific aspects, including the role of chemoresistance and neoadjuvant and adjuvant treatments, should be clarified by further experience and the results of on-going trials.

Keywords: Epithelial Ovarian Cancer, Peritoneal Carcinomatosis, Peritonectomy, HIPEC

---

1. Introduction

Peritoneal metastasis is the most common type of diffusion and the most frequent cause of death from EOC.

Intra-abdominal and pelvic parietal and visceral peritoneal metastases, often associated with ascites, resectable hepatic metastasis, deep bowel wall infiltration up to mucosa, identify stage III or IV ovarian cancer with diffuse PC [1,2]. Treatment of these conditions is traditionally based on cytoreductive surgery (CRS) combined with systemic carbotaxol-based chemotherapy at first line. Despite high rates of chemosensitivity, relapses are detected in up to 50% of cases in the first two years and in almost 100% in the first 5 years post-treatment. [3]

For most of its natural history, EOC is confined to the abdominal cavity, developing further peritoneal tumour implants and producing pelvic and lumbar lymph node metastases without extra-abdominal diffusion.

For this reason, new integrate therapeutic strategies have emphasized the role of local aggressive treatments, represented by maximal cytoreductive surgery (peritonectomy) combined with loco-regional HIPEC.

Peritonectomy (PRT) associated with HIPEC has been used since the second half of the 90's in the treatment of ovarian PC, as well as in other primary and metastatic peritoneal surface malignancies.

PC is observed both in primary settings, i.e. in patients first treated for locally advanced EOC, and as a recurrence in patients previously treated for ovarian cancer at any stage.

2. Initial and recurrent ovarian carcinomatosis

About 75% of ovarian cancers are diagnosed and treated in primary settings as FIGO Stage IIIc/IV, meaning that they are confined to the abdominal and pelvic cavity and characterised by diffuse visceral and parietal PC [4]. PC is frequently associated with lymphnode metastases and less commonly with haematogenous hepatic metastases.

Such a high percentage of PC at first presentation is mainly caused by the relevant delay in diagnosing EOC at early stages, due to the lack of symptoms and to the low sensitivity and specificity of diagnostic tools. Only 20% to 30% of EOC in developed countries are diagnosed at FIGO Stage I and II and the diagnosis is usually accidental: either via sonography, computerised tomography (CT scanning) or during laparoscopic investigations [5,6].

The pathogenesis of late PC in patients already treated for EOC at any stage is more complex.

At FIGO stages I and II it may be related to a number of factors:

1. Limited and incorrect application of standard surgical procedures;

2. Inherent limitations to the procedures established by international guidelines;

3. Chemoresistance.

Point 1 of the above is sometimes dictated by special clinical situations, which require conservative treatment. Young patients with small ovarian tumours can be treated with simple unilateral oophorectomy, in order to preserve their reproduction function. The results of this strategy are not uniform and tend to show an unjustifiable risk of surgical relapse. Rupture of the ovarian tumour during open surgery, or more often during laparoscopic surgery, is one of the most frequent cause of peritoneal recurrence [7].

Omission of appendectomy or total omentectomy is also not a rare cause of peritoneal recurrence or persistence of the disease (Fig. 1).

As to point 2, despite international guidelines advice for infra-colic limited resection of the greater omentum and for not total omentectomy, the presence of histologically-proven tumour implants in the latter tissue is associated to elevated rates of peritoneal and omental recurrence.

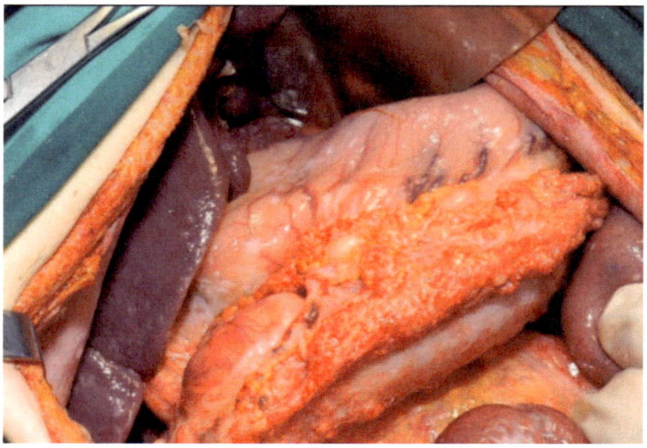

Figure 1. Residual greater omentum involved in recurrent peritoneal carcinomatosis.

On the other hand, the anatomical structure of the omentum is unitary and limited resection is, therefore, not plausible. It should be reminded that the omentum often harbours EOC deposits by virtue of its peculiar anatomy and function. It contains milky spots, which are responsible for the concentration and reabsorption of intraperitoneal fluid, including malignant ascites. It is through the milky spots that the tumour cells take root into the omentum. This phenomenon facilitates the formation of carcinomatous nodules of various sizes, in some cases involving the complete replacement of the omental tissue with tumour tissue ("omental cake").

Omission of lymphadenectomy in early stage EOC is frequent and correlates significantly with subsequent loco-regional lymph-node metastases and PC (over 50% in our series of recurrent EOC patients).

Finally, chemoresistance to first-line adjuvant treatments with carbotaxol is detectable in 20% of cases and is a further cause of relapse after treatment for stage I and II EOC [8].

Peritoneal recurrences after treatments for FIGO stages III or IV intraperitoneal EOC, can be mainly attributed to the lack of aggressiveness of the standard treatments. The current standard therapy, i.e. CRS combined with systemic chemotherapy, shows limited efficacy in high stage EOC, and is followed in most cases by abdomino-pelvic loco-regional recurrence.

Most often relapses occur as PC, associated with ascites in 60% of cases.

Further attempts to treat ovarian cancer at stage III — aimed at curbing the incidence of peritoneal recurrence — involve the use of intra-peritoneal normothermic chemotherapy (IP CHT).

Several randomized trials have demonstrated the effectiveness of this method, especially after optimal CRS; nevertheless it is still rarely used mainly due to catheter-related complications which significantly reduce its applicability. [9,10]

In conclusion, PC is the most frequent and characteristic manifestation of EOC, whether identified early at first assessment or later as persistent or recurrent disease following standard treatments. These include surgical debulking and systemic chemotherapy, are characterised by high recurrence rates and cannot guarantee long-term survival and improvement in the quality of life.

3. Epidemiology

EOC affects over 200.000 women and causes 125.000 deaths annually worldwide, with a deaths/new cases ratio of 62,5 % [11]. These data demonstrate that standard treatments are not able to deal effectively with this disease, and success rates are distant from other common types of cancer, such as colorectal cancer, for which the deaths/new cases ratio was 45.9% over the same period. The low impact of standard treatments is also corroborated by the analysis of the causes of death for EOC patients. Our National Institute of Statistics (ISTAT) data referred to 2013-2014 showed that 80% of deaths in EOC patients is exclusively due to peritoneal recurrence, 10% to peritoneal recurrence associated with extra-peritoneal metastasis, and only 10% exclusively to extra-peritoneal metastases. Therefore, alternative therapeutic strategies are needed, also considering that distant metastases are a late occurrence in EOC patients, mainly due to the little effectiveness of standard treatments.

4. Macroscopy and microscopy

Traditionally the origin of carcinomas of the ovary is identified in the Ovarian Surface Epithelium (OSE). Growing evidence indicates that the majority of EOC have an extraovarian source. [12]

The new paradigm that increasingly fits with the extraovarian origin of EOC establishes common characteristics for ovarian, tubal and primitive peritoneal tumours that unite these malignancies in a common family, divided into two broad groups: type I and type II ovarian cancers.

Molecular profiling contributes to better distinguish the two types of ovarian cancer (high grade vs. low grade) as well as identifying various subtypes, i.e., serous, mucinous, endometrioid and clear cell cancer.

The application of these new classifications will be invaluable in identifying "ovarian" tumours with different prognosis and targets for specific therapeutic strategies. [10]

Major studies on ovarian PC include ovarian, tubal and primitive peritoneal carcinomas grouped together due to their histological and pathological similarities and the treatment options which are identical for all three forms.

Macroscopically the ovarian carcinomatosis is similar to other forms of PSM. It can be present as nodules varying in size from less than 1 mm to various centimetres, isolated or conglomerated in the form of solid or cystic masses or plaques of varying sizes and thicknesses.

The serous or mucinous content of carcinomatous implants and their degree of invasiveness of the peritoneum and of the underlying structures is extremely variable.

Previous treatments with chemotherapy can influence the appearance of ovarian carcinomatosis. After neoadjuvant or adjuvant chemotherapies, the peritoneum can show evident signs of carcinomatosis regression on its surface, ranging from significant reduction to complete disappearance; in each case the signs of previous disease are still evident.

In particular, the increase in thickness of the parietal and visceral peritoneal membrane, its opacification, and the presence of blurs and reddish spots indicate the location and extent of previous carcinomatosis.

Histological and immunohistochemical studies of biopsies of these tissues often show the presence of microscopic foci of disease in the context of thick, fibrotic areas.

These macroscopic and microscopic features are potential justifications for relapse after neoadjuvant or adjuvant chemotherapy in patients subjected to an apparently negative

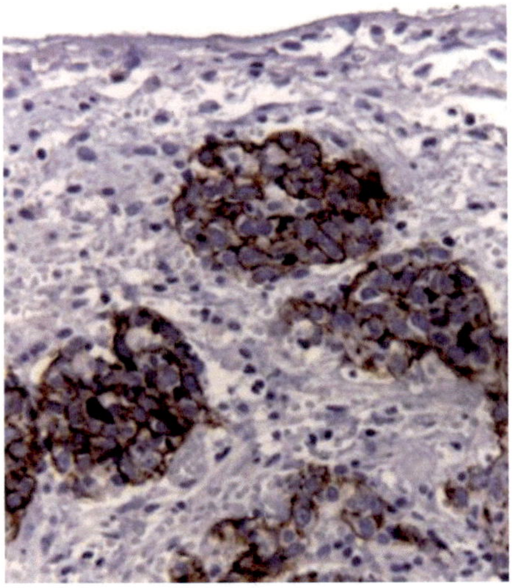

Figure 2. Microfocus of neoplastic cells inside fibrous desmoplastic tissue- CA-125 immunohistochemistry.

second-look. Indeed, fibrosis encapsulating foci of neoplastic cells may preserve them from effects of further systemic or locoregional therapies.

Furthermore, total chemical cytoreduction runs the risk of both surgical and chemotherapic undertreatment, especially if obtained after effective neoadjuvant treatments.

PC may involve any anatomic site and bowel segment or parenchyma in high percentages (parietal and visceral peritoneum 90%; omentum 60%; diaphragm 40%; liver and spleen capsule 15%). Lymphatic and haematogenous metastases in the liver may also be detected contemporaneously (respectively 50-60% and 5%). Ascites is present in about 60%.

5. Diagnosis and staging of peritoneal carcinomatosis

The ovarian carcinomatosis is paucisymptomatic until it assumes a considerable size or is associated with ascites or occlusion. Therefore diagnosis is often delayed and more than 70% of ovarian cancer patients are diagnosed at FIGO stages IIIC/IV.

Clinical examination with vaginal and rectal exploration plays a critical role in assessing the pelvic spread of the disease.

Diagnosis is based on a set of efficient morphological investigations (CT, MRI, PET). CA 125, in association or not to CA 19.9, and currently to HE-4, are the most sensitive tumour markers for specific diagnosis of ovarian cancer. Laparoscopy plays an important role in doubtful cases, allowing the direct visualization and biopsy of suspected lesions.

The intraoperative staging of PC from ovarian cancer, as in other forms of PSM, relies mainly on PCI classification proposed by Sugarbaker [13], although other classifications have been proposed.

The correct staging of PC is important to assess resectability, prognosis and risk of complications. For this reason, much effort is made to adopt the PCI classification also prior to surgery by applying it to data from morphological imaging (CT, MR, PET) or laparoscopy investigations.

Being able to determine reliably in the preoperative phase the peritoneal spread of the disease and the involvement of sensitive anatomical areas, PCI could avoid unnecessary surgical approaches and improve the overall strategy as well as identify cases to be submitted to neoadjuvant chemotherapy (NACT).

However results are still unsatisfactory both due the complexity of PCI classification and the difficulty in its preoperative application; recently a new and simpler method to stage peritoneal carcinomatosis via laparoscopy has been proposed [14].

If the above described set of diagnostic procedures increases the percentage of successful diagnosis of PC, including the identification of the primary tumour and the eventual presence of extra-peritoneal disease, the reliability of the current standard diagnostic tools used in staging intraperitoneal spread must be considered as unsatisfactory. Many authors emphasize the role of laparoscopy in staging intraperitoneal spread of carcinomatosis, but the obvious limits of feasibility in pervasive forms of recurrence restrict the use and significance of this method [14-17]. Moreover risk of contamination of port site access by tumor cells at laparoscopy should be considered [18-20].

6. Evaluation of residual disease after cytoreductive surgery

Evaluation of tumor residues after cytoreductive surgery is of relevant importance because of residual disease volume is the major prognostic factor in the treatment of EOC.[21-30]

The degree of cytoreduction can be assessed with various classification systems, the most used of them is the Sugarbaker scoring classification [Completeness of Cytoreduction score (CC)] [31]. This system provides four values from 0 to 3, where 0 indicates complete cytoreduction of peritoneal carcinomatosis with total absence of macroscopic residual disease at the end of the surgical phase. The maximum therapeutic efficacy of the integrated procedure is carried out in cases where an "optimal" cytoreduction (CC0 - CC1) is achieved.

7. Peritonectomy and HIPEC

The limits of success of standard treatments of PC from ovarian cancer have led to test new therapeutic possibilities, borrowing from the experiences made in other forms of peritoneal carcinomatosis a therapeutic strategy based on the association of maximal cytoreduction (Peritonectomy) with Hyperthermic Intraperitoneal Chemotherapy (HIPEC).

Peritonectomy is aimed to complete removal of macroscopic disease; HIPEC is aimed to treat microscopic or millimetric tumor residues after surgical cytoreductive phase.

7.1. Rationale

The association between PRT and HIPEC is based on a complex rationale that takes into account the mechanism of intraperitoneal spread of free cancer cells, Gompertzian tumor growth kinetics, Goldie&Coldman mathematical model about drug resistance, pharmacokinetic and pharmacodynamic events related to intraperitoneal chemotherapy associated with hyperthermia. [32]

Maximal cytoreduction reducing drastically tumor volume, induces the remaining cells to enter the fast proliferating phase of the cell cycle becoming more responsive to chemotherapic drugs. Moreover microscopic or millimetric residual tumor volumes include a minor rate of chemoresistant clones and can be totally permeated by drugs delivered by intraperitoneal chemotherapy [33-36].

The association of HIPEC is based on a series of advantages related by a part to the fact that the chemotherapy is carried out at the end of the surgical stage directly into abdominal cavity and by the other part to the fact that drugs used are brought to a constant temperature of 42-43° for the entire treatment period of infusion (usually 60 minutes).

The benefits of loco-regional chemotherapy consist of:

- direct exposure of whole anatomical region to chemotherapy being absent adhesions
- possibility of using high concentrations of chemotherapics
- possibility of allowing a prolonged exposure time
- low systemic toxicity

The combination of hyperthermia provides additional benefits:

- hyperthermia damages cancer cells
- increases the effectiveness of some chemotherapics (CDDP, MMC, DOX, gemcitabine)
- does not involve increased toxicity
- promotes tissue penetration of chemotherapeutic drugs

In particular, hyperthermia favours drug penetration into the tissues to a depth of 5 mm, a value significantly greater than what occurs in isothermal conditions (2 mm). Therefore the more the peritonectomy is effective achieving "optimal" cytoreduction (CC0 - CC1), i.e. up to allow the total removal of the disease or leaving residues of minimum size (up to 2.5mm), the more associated chemo-hyperthermia will be able to successfully attack microscopic or minimum size tumor residues.

http://dx.doi.org/10.5772/60844

8. Peritonectomy

The term of peritonectomy identifies precisely the meaning of the surgical procedure: removal of parietal and visceral peritoneum affected by the neoplastic pathology.

Peritonectomy procedures comprise:

- exeresis of parietal peritoneum
- exeresis of visceral peritoneum by visceral and parenchymal resection
- excision/in situ destruction of single implants
- resection of abdominal wall, muscle implants and laparoscopic trocar sites
- lymphadenectomy

At parietal level the procedure entails complete or partial removal of the peritoneum lining the abdominal wall, the diaphragms and the pelvis according to disease extension. General consensus is in removing parietal peritoneum limited to involved areas, sparing a unaffected zones.

If healthy areas are limited, large parietal peritonectomies should be performed up to complete parietal peritonectomy.

In principle, the resection of the parietal and pelvic peritoneum below the transverse umbilical line should be performed in all cases of peritoneal carcinomatosis from ovarian cancer.

Parietal peritonectomy includes greater and lesser omentectomy, resection of round and falciform ligaments, stripping of omental bursa peritoneum.

When PC spreads deeply beyond peritoneal membrane trough abdominal wall, full or partial thickness parietal resection is performed.

Laparoscopic trocar sites are removed by full thickness cylindrical parietal resection when involved by carcinomatosis or when suspected to be contaminated by tumor cells. Umbilicus, regardless its previous use as trocar sites, should be removed on principle in recurrent cases being a frequent site of metastasis.

Visceral peritoneum cannot be separated from underlying visceral tissue and removed separately as with the peritoneum lying the abdominal walls and diaphragms. Therefore visceral peritonectomy involves exeresis of endoperitoneal viscera or organs deeply infiltrated by PC. Rarely and only in special anatomical situations is possible the removal of visceral peritoneum only as when PC does not deeply infiltrate the visceral wall or when it concerned the Glisson's capsule.

Bowel resection is the most frequent peritonectomy procedure in treating peritoneal carcinomatosis from ovarian cancer.

Contemporaneous involvement of multiple viscera induces to multivisceral resections for what en bloc resection should be preferred (Fig 3-4).

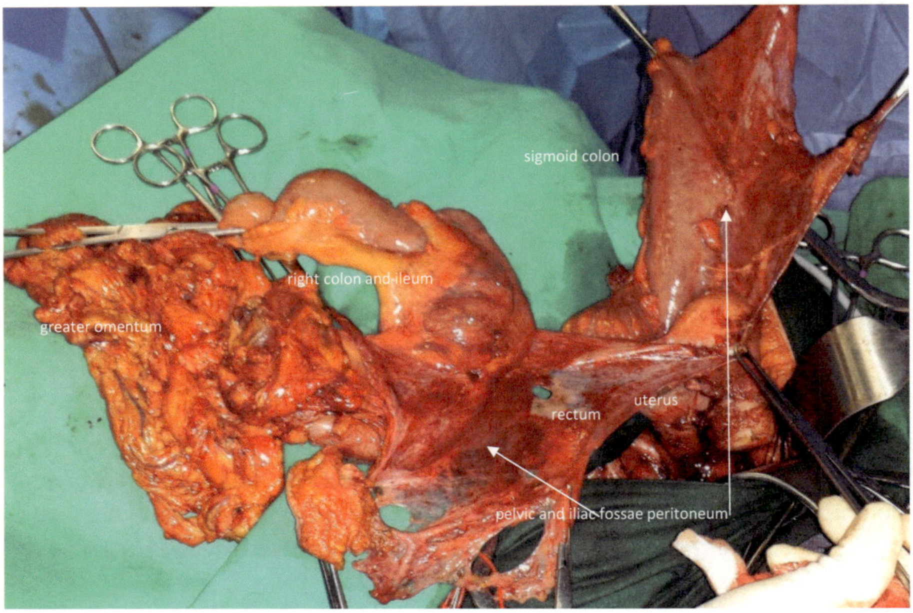

Figure 3. Pelvic peritonectomy: the moment of rectal resection as final step to remove en-bloc the surgical specimen.

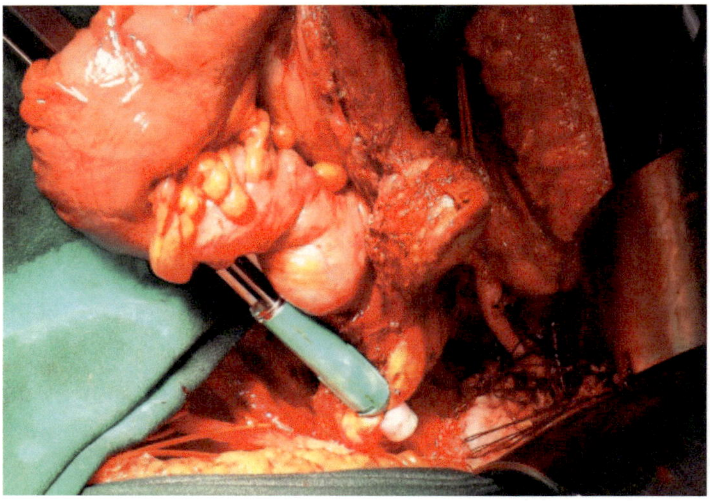

Figure 4. Pelvic peritonectomy: en bloc resection of uterus, adnexa, rectosigmoid colon, pelvic and iliac fossae peritoneum, right colon and greater omentum.

Small and large bowel resections are the most frequent surgical procedures because of deep parietal involvement by tumor implants. Thickness of the gastric wall is such as to allow prevailingly a conservative cleaning of the tumor implants without the need to perform major gastric resections.

Among large bowel resections, which may include all types of colon resection, left colorectal exeresis is the most frequent. Widespread pelvic involvement by primary tumor and peritoneal metastases with infiltration of the pouch and colorectal wall, provides colorectal resection. Such exeresis should include mesorectal resection and section of mesenteric vessel at their origin to achieve the same radicality requested for primary colorectal cancer treatment. Same radicality criteria should be followed resecting other large bowel sectors. This policy allows to remove both a large amount of mesocolon, frequently infiltrated by implants, and loco-regional lymph nodes which are metastasized in over 50% of cases. [37]

Lymphadenectomy plays a relevant role in strategy of peritonectomy for ovarian carcinomatosis and its prognostic role is highly significant: the only performing the procedure involves a significant increase in survival regardless metastastic involvement of lymph nodes[38-40].

The incidence of loco-regional lymph node metastasis is high exceeding 50% of cases and should induce a policy of radicalization of surgery in lymph nodes as well as in peritoneum.

Iliac-obturator and lumbar lymphadenectomy must be performed routinely in primary forms. In secondary forms lymphadenectomy should be performed if it was not done in previous surgery, or if it has been made necessary by evident nodal relapse in the seats already treated.

Additional forms of lymphadenectomy, at the level of hepatic pedicle, splenic hilum, mesentery or lesser omentum should be performed in the presence of lymphadenopathy macroscopically evident.

9. Removal / "in situ" destruction of implants

The treatment of peritoneal implants does not absolutely require the exeresis of wide portions of peritoneum or the mandatory sacrifice of wide tracts of gut or other structures involved in the disease. In relation to quality, quantity, and macroscopic and microscopic (histology) characteristics of carcinomatous implants, the exeresis should respond to general criteria of saving structures and avoiding useless tissue and visceral sacrifices, when local removal or in situ destruction with an appropriate technology allow a radical result.

A conservative approach is achievable when implants are superficial, few infiltrating the underlying structures, and when are prevailingly mucinous. In these conditions, it is possible to spare wide visceral resection especially when small or large intestine are involved. Local excision or local destruction can be assured effectively with curved scissors, electric scalpels with various tips, radiofrequency (Tissue Link), argon beam laser.

In patients undergone neoadjuvant treatments an additional contribution to HIPEC efficacy is given by argon or electric scalpels use over peritoneal areas where an apparent response to chemotherapy was achieved.

These areas are identified by the presence of specific morphological changes, including opacification, thickening, fibrosis of serous peritoneal membrane and presence of red spots.

Extensive treatment on such areas with argon or ball tip electro-surgery permits diffuse local damage and partial destruction of fibrosis.

The loss of structural continuity will permit a deeper tissue penetration of chemotherapics and a better contact with eventual encapsulated microscopic residuals in post-chemotherapy fibrosis.

10. HIPEC

HIPEC is performed at the end of surgical phase by using a 2.5-4.5 litres solution of chemotherapy drugs. Chemotherapy drugs, HIPEC techniques and duration are synthesized in Table 1. Drug solution is infused in peritoneal cavity by catheters appropriately positioned (fig.5). Infusion is performed under a constant temperature of 41-43°.

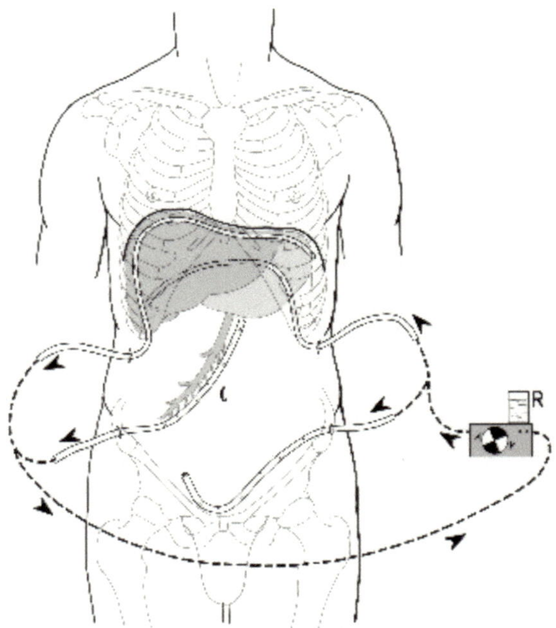

Figure 5. Intra-abdominal catheter position for HIPEC

Open and closed techniques are used for HIPEC but no proven advantage is related to a specific method.

Procedure duration varies from 60 to 90 minutes and CDDP is drug prevailingly administered.

No specific prospective studies have been conducted to verify differences in outcome by specific technique or to test the role of different chemotherapy regimens or drugs.

STUDY	HYPER-O [44]	DERACO [45]	BAKRIN [42]	DI GIORGIO [48]	DE BREE [43]
HIPEC DRUG					
CDDP	37.2%	-	41%	100%	nr
Oxaliplatin	-	-	21.3%	-	nr
MMC	38.7%	-	2.1%	-	nr
CarboTaxol	14.6%	-	-	-	nr
Doxorubicin	-	-	0.2%	-	nr
Combination (≥2)	9.5%	100%	35.4%	-	nr
HIPEC DURATION					
60 min	-	-	-	100%	nr
60-90 min	45.4%	100%	-	-	nr
90-120 min	54.6%	-	-	-	nr
HIPEC TECHNIQUES					
Open	12.1%	-	68.4%	-	nr
Closed	87.9%	100%	31.6%	100%	nr

Table 1. HIPEC drugs, duration and techniques. nr: not reported.

11. Inclusion and exclusion criteria

General criteria provide to include in the therapeutic program patients without extrabdominal disease with optimal ASA and Performance Status scores and with surgically cytoreducible peritoneal carcinomatosis. Isolated and easy resectable liver metastases are not contraindication to procedure performing when complete cytoreduction can be achieved. High level of PCI is not an absolute contraindication if surgery can obtain optimal cytoreduction although some authors identify levels beyond which the procedure is not advisable[14, 41-42].

Exclusion criteria include:

- great vessels involvement
- massive involvement of small bowel for over 50% of the length or of its mesenteric root
- infiltration of duodenum, pancreas or first jejunal loop
- infiltration of cardia or diaphragmatic pillars
- metastastic lymphadenopathy above the renal vessels
- extra-abdominal metastases

Age and comorbidity are relative exclusion criteria, being ASA and Performance Status scores the most reliable criteria to be considered even in patient in their eighties or suffering of other concomitant diseases.

12. Settings

Peritonectomy combined with HIPEC can be used as primary cytoreduction or as secondary. Primary cytoreduction can be performed as frontline or after neoadjuvant chemotherapy as interval debulking surgery. Secondary cytoreduction is performed in patients with recurrent or persistent disease after previous cytoreductive surgery combined or not with various forms of chemotherapy. Tertiary and quaternary cytoreduction combined or not with HIPEC can be performed in patient with repeated intraperitoneal relapses. PRT + HIPEC can be used as consolidation in primary setting during a second look in patients optimally treated with neoadjuvant chemotherapy or in secondary setting during a second look after any combination of surgery and locoregional or systemic chemotherapy.

13. Results

Over the last 15 years the use of peritonectomy combined with HIPEC has progressively widespread as treatment of peritoneal carcinomatosis from ovarian cancer. Phase III trials about the efficacy of such integrated procedure compared to traditional treatments based on CRS and systemic or normothermic intraperitoneal chemotherapy (IP CHT) are not available. Therefore the role and limits of application of PRT+HIPEC are inferable by results of phase I and mainly phase II studies. At present an overall analysis of the literature allows us to manage data from over 1900 treated cases (Table 2). Collective reviews, multicentric and monocentric case studies are the most available bases to verify the role of PRT combined with HIPEC in treating peritoneal carcinomatosis from ovarian cancer.

Among available collective reviews, the study of de Bree and Helm of 2012 is the more recent and complete. This study is based on 1102 cases collected from 22 monocentric studies and includes the three major previous reviews conducted by Bjelic, Chua and de Bree himself [43, 46-47]. The three multicenter study published between 2010 and 2013 are reported; their study designs were retrospective or prospective phase II. As for monocentric studies, results of a clinical phase II prospective study about the use of PRT and HIPEC in treating peritoneal ovarian carcinomatosis performed by the authors of this chapter is reported. This study is based on 130 cases treated between November 2000 and December 2013 in the same center and by the same staff [48]. This is the largest monocentric case study compared to all other reports included in the collective review of de Bree, the major of which consists of 81 cases.[49]

The multicenter study of Deraco includes exclusively cases undergoing primary CRS as front line, while that of Bakrin comprises prevailingly cases treated for recurrence (83,8%). In the other studies the rates of primary and secondary CRS were almost similar.

Author Year	De Bree 2012 [43]	Helm (HYPER-O) 2010 [44]	Deraco 2011 [45]	Bakrin 2013 [42]	Di Giorgio 2014 [48]
Type of study	Collective Reviews	Multicenter	Multicenter	Multicenter	Monocentric
Study Design	Collection of phase II studies	Retrospective	Prospective phase II	Retrospective	Prospective phase II
Frontline	18.4%	18.5%	100%	2.1%	17.7%
Interval debulking	5.6%	13.6%	-	4.2%	29.2%
Consolidation	8.9%	8,6%	-	9.9%	5.4%
Recurrence	67.1%	5.3%	-	83.8%	47.7%
No. Cases	1102	141	26	566	130

Table 2. PRT + HIPEC for peritoneal carcinomatosis from EOC: literature review.

PCI mean ranged from 10.6 to 16.3 and in all series the rate of patients classified as FIGO stage III and IV exceeded 90 %(Tab.3).

Author Year	De Bree 2012 [43]	Helm (HYPER-O) 2010 [44]	Deraco 2011 [45]	Bakrin 2013 [42]	Di Giorgio 2014 [48]
No. Cases	1102	141	26	566	130
PCI mean	nr	nr	15.5(5-26)	10.6(0-31)	16.3(0-39)
CC score 0 =1 >1	nr	58.3% 15.1% 26.6%	57.7% 42.3%	74.9% 17.9% 7.2%	66.7% 20% 13.3%
Platinum response *resistant* *sensitive* *undetermined*	nr	34% 53.9% 12.1%	nr	52.1% 47% 0.9%	36.8% 53.8% 9.4%
Adjuvant Chemotherapy yes no	nr	93.6% 6.4%	100%	28.3% 71.7%	71.5% 28.5%

Table 3. Patients characteristics. nr: not reported.

Peritonectomy was able to achieve optimal cytoreduction in most cases and the rates of complete cytoreduction ranged from 57,7 to 74,9, being the better scores related to lower level of PCI mean.

Platinum based drugs were the most used during HIPEC, alone or in combination with other chemotherapics. Adjuvant systemic chemotherapy was administered in post HIPEC phase in the vast majority of cases.

14. Survival

Results related to survival are synthesized in Tab 4 - 6.

Author - Year	**Helm (HYPER-O) 2010 [44]**								**Bakrin 2013 [42]**			
Survival	5 yr OS %		Median OS months		5 yr PFS %		Median PFS months		5 yr OS %		Median OS months	
Frontline	33.3		41.7		19.7		24.8		33.7		52.7	
Interval debulking	50.2	25.4	68.6	30.3	9.6	13	16.8	13.7	16	17	36.5	35.4
Consolidation	42.4		53.7		24.2		29.6		12.5		33.4	
Recurrence	18		23.5		9.6		13.7		37		45.7	
CC0 Primary	26.7		37		-		-		23.6		41.5	
CC0 Recurrence					-		-		40.2		51.5	
Author – year	Deraco 2011 [45]											
Survival	5 yr OS %		Median OS months		5 yr PFS %		Median PFS months					
Frontline	60.7		not reached		15.2		30					

Table 4. PRT + HIPEC for peritoneal carcinomatosis from EOC: survival in multicentre studies.

Author - Year	**De Bree 2012 [43]**							
Survival	5 yr OS %		Median OS Months		5 yr PFS %		Median PFS months	
Frontline	47		33		17,5		25	
Interval debulking	54	58.5	69	66.5	10	36.5	17	35
Consolidation	84		64		63		35	
Recurrence	33		42.5		11.5		20.5	
CC 0 Primary	-		66 (only frontline)		-		-	
CC 0 Recurrence	-		-		-		-	

Table 5. PRT + HIPEC for peritoneal carcinomatosis from EOC: survival in collective reviews

Author – year	**Di Giorgio 2014 [48]**							
Survival	5 yr OS %		Median OS Months		5 yr PFS %		Median PFS Months	
Frontline	57.6		63.1		38		38.5	
Interval debulking	41.2	50.7	37.4	61.1	39.7	43.1	21	38.5
Consolidation	-				-			
Recurrence	45		40		29.5		17.7	
CC0 (primary)	59.6		50.5		53.7		56.8	
CC0 (recurrence)	61.3		66		42.2		52	

Table 6. PRT + HIPEC for peritoneal carcinomatosis from EOC: survival in author's monocentric study.

In all studies except one, patients treated in primary setting tend to survive more than recurrent; only Bakrin reported better 5- year overall survival in secondary setting (Fig 6).

In an half of reports, 5- year overall survival rate was about 50 % after primary CRS and about 40% after secondary CRS. Overall PF survival ranged across the reported studies between 13 to 43.1% at 5 years.

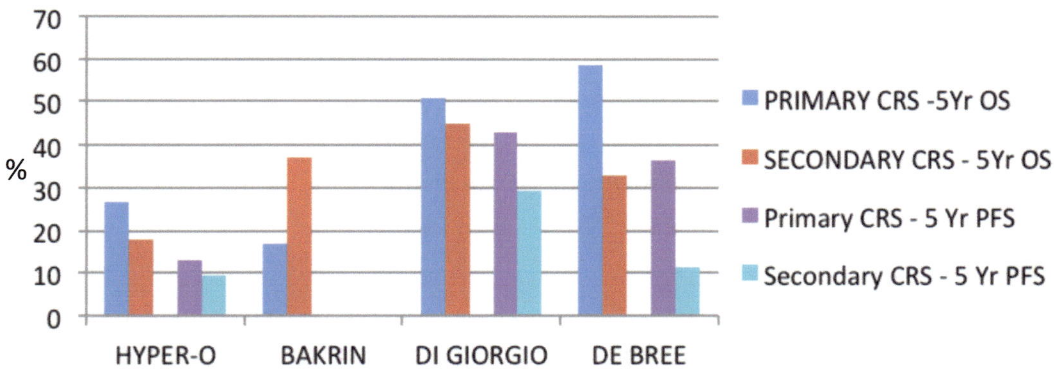

Figure 6. yr Overall and Progression Free survival after primary and secondary CRS +HIPEC

The values of median survival, both overall and progression free, reflected the general trend of 5-year survival: except for Bakrin's study, patients treated in primary setting survived more than patients treated for recurrence (Fig. 7).

Among patients treated in primary setting, patients undergoing PRT and HIPEC as front line tended to survive more than those neoadjuvated. Data from HYPER-O report are not available by admission of their Authors because of the small number of events

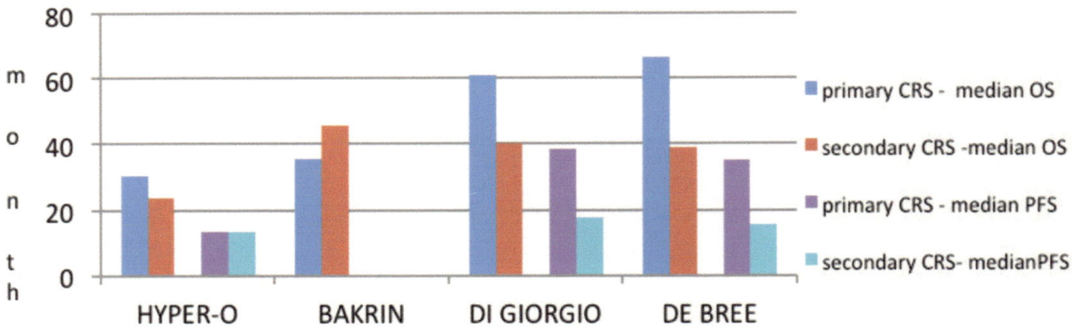

Figure 7. Median Overall and Progression Free survival after primary and secondary CRS+HIPEC

Results about long term prognosis in patients with PRT and HIPEC administered as consolidation during a second look are not useful for an advisable evaluation because of scarce number of treated cases in all analyzed studies.

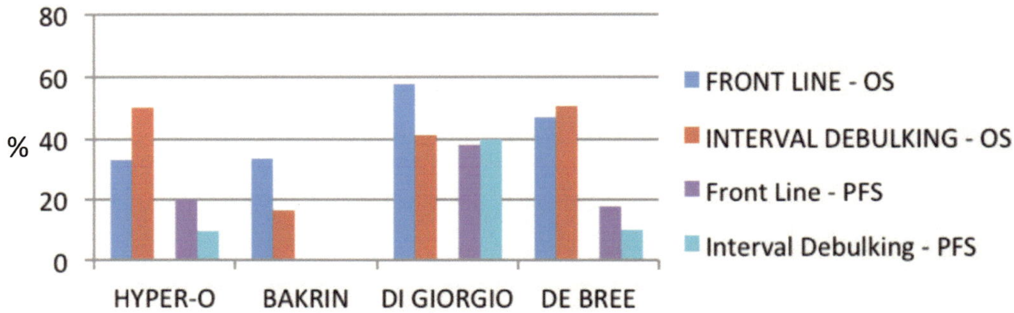

Figure 8. yr Overall and Progression Free survival in primary setting

14.1. Prognostic factors

A lot of potential prognostic factors have been analyzed by uni- and multivariate analyses and completeness of surgical cytoreduction (CC) resulted as the most significant prognostic factor in all series. Among the others, PCI was significantly related to survival in 3 of the 4 studies where has been analyzed.

Platinum response, blood loss, level of bowel wall infiltration by tumor implants, lymph node metastases, use of carboplatin and duration of perfusion, correlated significantly with survival at least once across the study by uni- or multivariate analyses.

14.2. The role of completeness of cytoreduction and PCI

Since 1970s results of treatment of locally advanced epithelial ovarian cancer emphasized the role of surgical debulking aimed not only at palliation of clinical status borned from intraper-

Author Year	De Bree and Helm 2012 [43]	Helm (HYPER-O) 2010 [44]	Deraco 2011 [45]	Bakrin 2013 [42]		Di Giorgio 2014 [48]	
Prognostic Factors				Primary	Recurrence	Primary	Recurrence
CC score	nr	0.025	nr	0.005	0.0001	0.003	0.009
PCI	nr	nr	nr	0.0012	0.0001	0.008	0.007
PS	nr	nr	nr	ns	0.0224	ns	0.006
Setting	nr	ns	nr	nr	nr	ns	ns
Platinum response	nr	0.048	nr	nr	ns	0.0005	ns
Blood loss	nr	0.005	nr	nr	nr	ns	0.0004
Ca125	nr	nr	nr	0.0241	0.2131	ns	ns
Lymph node metastases	nr	nr	nr	nr	nr	0.002	ns
Age	nr	nr	nr	0.0574	0.0314	ns	ns
Bowel wall infiltration	nr	nr	nr	nr	nr	0.0002	0.01
HIPEC drugs number	nr	nr	nr	0.9689	0.0176	ns	ns
HIPEC drug type	nr	0.011	nr	0.2653	0.7098	ns	Ns
Duration of perfusion	nr	0.047	nr	nr	nr	ns	ns

Table 7. PRT + HIPEC for peritoneal carcinomatosis from EOC: prognostic factors by uni or multivariate analyses. [nr: not reported; ns: not significant]

itoneal disease spread but also to improve long term survival. [50]. The concept of optimal cytoreduction correlated to the dimension of tumor residuals among gynecologic oncologist has progressively induced to reduce from 2 cm to 0.5 cm the maximum acceptable limit. Among surgical oncologist according to Sugarbaker classification such limit is up to 2.5 mm. The role of cytoreduction level in primary resection for locally advanced EOC is well highlighted by the most relevant retrospective and prospective studies reported in literature [51-53].

A meta-analysis of 6.855 cases confirmed these data [54]. The most significant gap was observed between patient without any residue and those with residues of any size. Even in patients undergoing cytoreductive surgery for recurrent disease a lot of retrospective studies [21-30] and a meta-analysis including 2.019 patients [55] confirmed the prognostic role of maximal cytoreduction. Maximal or optimal cytoreductive surgery are correlated to evident advantages improving patients quality of live, decreasing drug resistance clones entity and improving chemotherapy efficacy. Complete removal of peritoneal disease proves to be the most relevant prognostic factor in all setting even in all analyzed studies on HIPEC here reported (Tab 6).

Some authors argued about the role of PCI in selecting patients to be treated with peritonectomy and HIPEC, identifying level of diffusion of peritoneal disease by scores beyond which such combined procedures should be avoided. In particular Bakrin identified in a value of PCI equal to 10 that limit in relation to related poor prognosis, while other authors [14] identify specific laparoscopic scoring of diffusion of peritoneal carcinomatosis to predict the achievement of an optimal cytoreduction.

Results of our monocentric study show that in PC from ovarian cancer high degrees of PCI are not an absolute limit to the execution of the procedure, if it is possible to obtain an optimal cytoreduction. We believe that high degree of PCI does not constitute an absolute contraindication to cytoreduction, as some claim [41, 56] and that rather one should take greater account of technical feasibility, quality of carcinomatosis of the individual case and possibility of obtaining an optimal cytoreduction. In our series, which had a PCI mean of 16.3, patients with PCI> 16 have nevertheless demonstrated a 5-year overall survival of 24.3%, with no difference between primary and secondary CRS, and a 5 year survival of 50.2 % (median 61.1 months) when in these patients with high PCI a complete cytoreduction (CC0) was obtained.

14.3. The role of NACT

Diffuse Peritoneal Carcinomatosis in primary setting is ideal target for neoadjuvant chemotherapy with carboplatin and taxol, due to high rate or responsiveness when administered as first line treatment (> 80%).

Nevertheless advantages of such strategy are not clear and results are conflicting, both in patients treated with and without HIPEC.

In patients undergoing NACT and successively treated with standard cytoreductive surgery and systemic chemotherapy, preoperative chemotherapy failed to improve survival. In EORTC 55971 phase III trial, NACT increased the rate of optimal Cytoreduction and decreased post-operative morbidity compared to front line CRS, but did not influence Overall or PF survival [57-58].

Similar results have been observed also in the studies related to the role of NACT in patients treated with PRT + HIPEC[59-60].

A better comprehension of significance of this strategy may drawn from analysis of chemosensitivity during NACT. In our monocentric series more than 50% of patients treated in primary setting undergo carbo-taxol-based NACT. 26,3 % didn't respond to this regimen and demonstrated a significant worse prognosis (29,4% 5-yr OS) compared to cases treated front line or NACT responders (56,4% 5-yr OS).

Some studies envisage for NACT disadvantages related to increased risk of platinum resistance during post-CRS adjuvant chemotherapy [61] or post-NACT histological changes occurring in tumor tissue that correlate with a poor prognosis [62]. These data are reflected in our cases: neoadjuvated patients showed a higher percentage of chemoresistance during post-HIPEC treatment with platinum derivatives (41.7%) than those not neoadjuvated (31.8%) and survived less.

In the near future the results of ongoing trials will better highlight the optimal strategy in using NACT. Based on results of studies now available, NACT regimen should be personalized and administered to patients with bulky intraperitoneal disease at risk of incomplete CRS, or to patients with small metastatic pleural effusion or with small isolated liver metastasis easily resectable during CRS.

14.4. The role of platinum chemoresistance

The role of platinum chemoresistance has been analyzed in three studies and in two of them chemoresistance resulted as a negative prognostic factor [44, 48 - Tab 6]

In two studies platinum chemoresistance was analyzed in pre-HIPEC phase in patients treated for recurrence while in our monocentric study we have evaluated the chemoresistance by referring to the recurrence/progression within six months after the end of post-HIPEC adjuvant treatment with platinum-based drugs, both in primary and in recurrent forms.

In the two multicenter studies where chemoresistance was analyzed in pre- HIPEC phase, it didn't influence survival in Bakrin's report while resulted marginally significant in HYPER-O registry.

In our series,Platinum chemoresistance so assessed was related to a worse prognosis only after primary CRS plus HIPEC, with both univariate and multivariate analyses (Table 6). The negative correlation between platinum chemoresistance and prognosis in primary forms can be partly explained by the possibility that NACT determines chemoresistance against the platinum used in systemic form after CRS as described above [62].

In our series, post-HIPEC chemoresistance did not influence significantly survival of recurrent patients, whose rates of platinum chemoresistance and chemosensitivity were similar (47.2% vs 52.8%).

In patients treated for recurrence, PRT combined with HIPEC may induce, especially for cases CC0, a reset of previous oncologic situation and that the chemosensitivity assessment to platinum based drugs chemotherapy post-HIPEC more faithfully represents the new relationship between patient and such chemotherapics. Moreover, the possibility that the CRS associated with HIPEC may lead to a retrieval of chemoresistance to platinum is theorized by some authors [54].

14.5. The role of bowel wall infiltration

Among the analyzed studies carcinomatous infiltration of intestinal wall has been analyzed only in our monocentric study. Progressive infiltration of bowel wall influenced negatively long term survival. The impact of the degree of parietal layers infiltration like the T role in TNM staging of gastro-intestinal tumor but in an inverse sense has been analyzed in previous report by us and other authors in relation to only colorectal resection [63-65]

Recently the evaluation of bowel wall infiltration up to the mucosa has been included in new 2014 FIGO stage for ovarian cancer identifying mucosal infiltration as FIGO stage IVb [1,2].

14.6. The role of lymphadenectomy

The role of lymphadenectomy and significance of lymph node metastatic involved in locally advanced EOC is controversial. Lymphadenectomy is supported from some authors on the basis of its positive influence on survival [66-67], while other authors are skeptical [68]. The high rate of loco-regional lymph node metastases justify systematic lymphadenectomy in primary setting on principle and in secondary setting when not performed during primary cytoreduction.

The significance of lymph node metastasis was analyzed only in our monocentric study, where iliac-obturatory and lumbar lymphadenectomy was performed routinely in primary settings and when not done in previous CRS in patients treated for recurrence. Colorectal resections were routinely performed with radical technique as previously reported. Lymphadenectomy in other districts such as the hepatic pedicle, perigastric or mesenteric stations were performed when necessary.

In our study, overall 52,6% of patients had lymph node metastases without significant differences between primary or recurrent forms, similarly to what reported in the literature [45]. Although lymph node involvement worsened prognosis, related 5-year Overall survival reached 39,6% corroborating the role of lymphadenectomy.

15. The role of HIPEC — Comparison of HIPEC vs no HIPEC

Overall, the results so far obtained by using of PRT combined with HIPEC in treating peritoneal carcinomatosis from ovarian cancer even available mainly if not exclusively from non randomized prospective studies show progressive improvement of long term survival both in primary or recurrent forms in high volume activity centers [55].

Although general consensus about the role of maximum cytoreduction is at present undisputable, criticism about HIPEC role is diffuse because of its potential high morbidity risk and lack of prospective controlled studies.

At present both in primary and recurrent settings, a series of cases / controls studies has demonstrated the major efficacy of the association between CRS and HIPEC compared to traditional treatments [69-76]. Results of the first phase III prospective study recently published [77] about this topic confirmed a significant improvement in long term survival in patients treated with HIPEC compared with those undergoing traditional treatment with CRS and adjuvant systemic chemotherapy.

16. Morbidity and mortality

Peritonectomy and HIPEC are integrated in a complex and aggressive procedure whose specific related complications are difficult to distinguish, being the overall morbidity reasonably related to the whole procedure. Therefore if renal and haematological toxicity have to be related specifically to chemotherapy activity, even for most common surgical complications like anastomotic leak, intestinal fistulas or endoperitoneal haemorrhage, HIPEC influence can't be undervalued.

Overall the incidence of major complications (grade 3 and 4) ranged from 14% to 56% whose treatment provided surgical, radiological or endoscopic re-intervention in a percentage ranging from 13% to 19,2%.

Haematological and renal toxicity accounted for a maximum incidence of 11 and 8 % respectively.

Mortality rate was extremely variable ranging from 0 to 10%.

It is difficult to compare various experiences mainly because of different criteria by which complications are defined and of different classifications with which morbidity levels are synthetized. The number of possible complications after PRT + HIPEC is high and the likely to have a complete scenarios of all adverse events is difficult and depends on the accuracy with which databases are prepared and on the prospective or retrospective modalities with which data are updated.

A detailed example of database dedicated to morbidity is described in the book edited in 2013 by Sugarbaker about the treatment of peritoneal carcinomatosis [78] with an indication of 48 adverse events arranged within 9 categories. Each adverse event is graded with a score from I to IV, and 14 prognostic indicators have been used in uni and multivariate analyses with the aim to identify the most significant risk factors for postoperative morbidity and mortality.

It is an interesting try to organize the adverse events but results difficult to reproduce and not yet used in other studies. Its use can be considered particularly important for studies dedicated to this problem. An acceptable compromise to obtain comparable data can be gained by using of more simplified and diffused classifications of complications, such as that of Dindo's or CTCAE, and by performing multivariate analyses to infer the risk factors for various complications.

Among the analyzed studies, only Bakrin's multicentre study and the author's monocentric study reported the results of uni or multivariate analyses on risk factors and PCI and CC score resulted as the most significant parameters correlated to an increased occurrence of major complications. Cascales Campos on 91 patients treated with PRT + HIPEC for ovarian carcinomatosis in various settings [76] has confirmed with multivariate analysis the role of PCI as risk factor for major complications, associated to the performing of digestive anastomoses.

These results reliably correlate with operative mortality and re-intervention rates, as reported in Deraco and Di Giorgio's studies that include cases with highest mean of PCI, and with lowest morbidity rate in patients treated as consolidation which are free of disease at second look. An exception is represented by Pomel's prospective study dedicated to cases treated as consolidation with Oxaliplatin based-HIPEC (CHIPOVAC); the study was stopped for excessive morbidity. (70)

The duration of procedure resulted as risk factor in the monocentric study, as in other reports about using of PRT + HIPEC in both ovarian and extra-ovarian PC [72-74].

Among major complications, the anastomotic dehiscences are the most dangerous for concomitant risk of severe sepsis and postoperative mortality. Risk factors for these events are numerous and correlate with the extension of carcinomatosis, the number of intestinal resections required for cytoreduction, the duration of procedure, the blood loss, the extensive use of in situ destruction of parietal implants, the type of anastomosis, in particular, colorectal, the lack of adequate bowel cleaning in occluded and sub-occluded patients, the previous treatment with bevacizumab.

The containment of the risks lies in reducing the number of anastomoses with appropriate evaluation of the intestinal tracts to be resected and avoiding the simultaneous performing of multiple digestive anastomoses in conjunction with low colorectal anastomosis. In these cases it is strategically correct to perform a colorectal resection according to Hartmann and delay recanalization in a second intervention after the end of adjuvant treatment and after further 6 months follow up [65].

In summary, also in presence of remarkable variability of data from the analyzed studies, the incidences of complication and mortality appear limited and comparable to those related to major abdominal and pelvic surgery. Morbidity rate control is possible in highly active centers with consolidated experience and specialized medical, nursing and logistic organization. Results of trials in progress on the specific role of HIPEC shall furnish also significant data about HIPEC related morbidity, while the use of specific protocols and prospective databases, connected to multi-institutional experiences, can give useful data to limit morbidity in medium period.

17. Future

The use of PRT combined with HIPEC for treating peritoneal carcinomatosis from ovarian cancer is being widely diffused thanks to promising results in terms of survival but is not without its critics that are primarily focused on the role of HIPEC. To date, the major criticisms about HIPEC involve its potential influence on survival and morbidity and the lack of prospective randomized studies as support of results of this procedure. The differing opinions between oncological surgeons, who are more likely to use HIPEC, and oncologic gynecologists and medical oncologists, who are more likely to use standard treatment with CRS and systemic CHT or, more rarely, isothermic IP-CHT, plays a relevant role in such a scenario. Therefore, it is necessary to verify whether PRT plus HIPEC can guarantee better survival compared with standard treatments and whether the incidence of related morbidity is acceptable in comparison with other types of treatment. At present many clinical trials are ongoing about the efficacy of PRT and HIPEC, most of them are focused specifically on HIPEC role, both in primary and in recurrent patients (Tab 8).

Studies	Time	Drug	Type of study	Identification number*
Safety and Pharmacokinetics of Intraoperative Hyperthermic Intraperitoneal Chemoperfusion (HIPEC) With Cisplatin to Treat Platinum-sensitive Recurrent Ovarian Cancer	Recurrence	Cisplatin	Non-Randomized	NCT01387399
Hyperthermic Intra-peritoneal Chemotherapy (HIPEC) in Ovarian Cancer Recurrence (HORSE)	Recurrence	Cisplatin	Randomized	NCT01539785
Intraoperative Hyperthermic Intraperitoneal Chemotherapy With Ovarian Cancer	Primary Recurrence	Cisplatin	Randomized	NCT01091636
Phase 3 Trial Evaluating Hyperthermic Intraperitoneal Chemotherapy in Upfront Treatment of Stage IIIC Epithelial Ovarian Cancer (Chorine)	Primary	CDDP+ Paclitaxel	Randomized	NCT01628380
Secondary Debulking Surgery +/- Hyperthermic Intraperitoneal Chemotherapy in Stage III Ovarian Cancer	Recurrence	-	Randomized	NCT00426257
Hyperthermic Intra-Peritoneal Chemotherapy (HIPEC) in Relapse Ovarian Cancer Treatment (CHIPOR)	Recurrence	Cisplatin	Randomized	NCT01376752
Feasibility Study of HIPEC for Patients With Stage III or Only Pleural Stage IV Ovarian Carcinoma in First Line Therapy	Primary	Cisplatin	Safety/Efficacy	NCT01709487
WCC# 59 Hyperthermic Intraperitoneal Chemotherapy Utilizing Carboplatin in First Recurrence Ovarian Cancer	Recurrence	Carboplatin	Safety/Efficacy	NCT01144442
Outcomes After Secondary Cytoreductive Surgery With or Without Carboplatin Hyperthermic Intraperitoneal Chemotherapy (HIPEC) Followed by Systemic Combination Chemotherapy for Recurrent Platinum-Sensitive Ovarian, Fallopian Tube, or Primary Peritoneal Cancer	Recurrence	Carboplatin	Randomized	NCT01767675
A Phase II Combined Modality Protocol of Debulking Surgery With HIPEC Followed by Intraperitoneal Chemotherapy for the Treatment of Recurrent Ovarian, Primary Peritoneal & Fallopian Tube Cancers	Recurrence	Cisplatin	Safety/Efficacy	NCT01659554

Studies	Time	Drug	Type of study	Identification number*
Quality of Life and Survivorship Care in Patients Undergoing Hyperthermic Intraperitoneal Chemotherapy (HIPEC)	Primary Recurrence	-	Efficacy	NCT01126346
Surgery and Chemotherapy With or Without Chemotherapy After Surgery in Treating Patients With Ovarian, Fallopian Tube, Uterine, or Peritoneal Cancer	Primary Recurrence	Cisplatin	Safety	NCT01970722

Table 8. Ongoing clinical trials on HIPEC in EOC. [79-90]

Results of such trials may help to confirm the role of HIPEC in various subsets of patients treated in primary setting and contribute to specify also the prognostic role of NACT and chemoresistance.

An half of ongoing studies are referred to recurrent patients. In the most of such trials, only platinum sensitive recurrences are considered. All of these studies are aimed to evaluate the prognostic role of HIPEC in terms of OS, PFS and DFS, having a variety of secondary outcomes such as the role of different combinations of chemotherapy drugs, the use of IP CHT after HIPEC, the QoL, toxicity and morbidity.

18. Conclusions

At present, lacking results of prospective randomized phase III studies, the role of PRT and HIPEC in treating peritoneal carcinomatosis from EOC can be reliably evaluated by the studies reported in this research which include over 1900 treated cases. The overall size of these case studies is a solid base to reliably identify the trend of results regardless of the study limitations discussed above.

On the basis of analysed results, following conclusions can be drawn:

- PRT plus HIPEC guarantee significant percentage of long-term overall and progression free survival in primary and recurrent settings.
- In all settings, complete cytoreduction represents the most significant prognostic factor.
- High PCI levels do not constitute a limitation for this procedure if optimal CRS is technically feasible.
- The prognostic role of NACT and Platinum-based chemoresistance is uncertain; but NACT and platinum chemoresistance should be better assessed, the first for when to be applied and the other for its application even in post-HIPEC setting

- Major complications and mortality rates are similar to those related to major abdominal pelvic surgery and are not different after primary or secondary cytoreduction. PCI and CC scores represent the most significant risk factors for major complications.

Author details

Angelo Di Giorgio[1*], Daniele Biacchi[1], Antonio Ciardi[2], Alessio Impagnatiello[1], Maurizio Cardi[1], Simone Sibio[1], Bianca Sollazzo[1], Joseph Maher Fouad Atta[1], Giuseppe Naso[1], Fabio Accarpio[1] and Paolo Sammartino[1]

*Address all correspondence to: angelo.digiorgio@uniroma1.it

1 Department of Surgery "Pietro Valdoni", Sapienza University of Rome, Italy

2 Department of Radiology, Oncology and Human Pathology, Sapienza University of Rome, Italy

References

[1] Prat J (2014). Staging classification for cancer of the ovary, fallopian tube, and peritoneum. Int J Gynecol Obstet 124(1): 1-5

[2] Zeppernick F, Meinhold-Heerlein I (2014). The new FIGO staging system for ovarian, fallopian tube, and primary peritoneal cancer. Arch Gynecol Obstet. 2014 Nov;290(5): 839

[3] Morgan, R. J., Alvarez, R. D., Armstrong, D. K., Robert, A., Chen, L., Copeland, L.,... Hughes, M. (2013). Ovarian Cancer, Version 2. 2013 Featured Updates to the NCCN Guidelines.

[4] Hennessy BT, Coleman RL, Markman M. Ovarian cancer. Lancet. 2009 Oct 17;374(9698):1371-82

[5] Maringe C, Walters S, Butler J, Coleman MP, Hacker N, Hanne L, and the ICBP Module 1 Working Group. Stage at diagnosis and ovarian cancer survival: evidence from the International Cancer Benchmarking Partnership. Gynecologic Oncology in press. [DOI: 10.1016/ j.ygyno.2012.06.033]

[6] Muzii L, Angioli R, Zullo M, Panici PB. The unexpected ovarian malignancy found during operative laparoscopy: incidence, management, and implications for prognosis. Journal of Minimally Invasive Gynecology 2005;12(1):81–9.

[7] Lawrie TA, Medeiros LR, Rosa DD, da Rosa MI, Edelweiss MI, Stein AT, Zelmanowicz A, Ethur AB, Zanini RR. Laparoscopy versus laparotomy for FIGO stage I ovarian cancer. Cochrane Database Syst Rev. 2013 Feb 28;2:CD005344.

[8] Stephen A. Cannistra, M.D Cancer of the ovary. N Engl J Med 2004; 351:2519-2529December 9, 2004DOI: 10.1056/NEJMra041842

[9] Armstrong DK, Bundy B, Wenzel L, Huang HQ, Baergen R, Lele S, Copeland LJ, Walker JL, Burger RA; Gynecologic Oncology Group. Intraperitoneal cisplatin and paclitaxel in ovarian cancer. N Engl J Med. 2006 Jan 5;354(1):34-43.

[10] Jaaback K, Johnson N, Lawrie TA. Intraperitoneal chemotherapy for the initial management of primary epithelial ovarian cancer. Cochrane Database Syst Rev. 2011 Nov 9;(11):CD005340

[11] Parkin DM, Bray F, Ferlay J, Pisani P. Global cancer statistics, 2002.CA Cancer J Clin. 2005 Mar-Apr;55(2):74-108

[12] Dubeau L, Drapkin R. Coming into focus: the nonovarian origins of ovarian cancer. Ann Oncol. 2013 Nov;24 Suppl 8:28-35.

[13] Jacquet P, Sugarbaker PH. Clinical research methodologies in diagnosis and staging of patients with peritoneal carcinomatosis. Cancer Treat Res. 1996;82:359-74.

[14] Fagotti A, Ferrandina G, Fanfani F, Ercoli A, Lorusso D, Rossi M, Scambia G. A laparoscopy-based score to predict surgical outcome in patients with advanced ovarian carcinoma: a pilot study. Ann Surg Oncol. 2006 Aug;13(8):1156-61.

[15] Fagotti A, Vizzielli G, De Iaco P, Surico D, Buda A, Mandato VD, Petruzzelli F, Ghezzi F, Garzarelli S, Mereu L, Viganò R, Tateo S, Fanfani F, Scambia G. A multicentric trial (Olympia-MITO 13) on the accuracy of laparoscopy to assess peritoneal spread in ovarian cancer. Am J Obstet Gynecol. 2013 Nov;209(5):462.e1-462.e11.

[16] Varnoux C, Huchon C, Bats AS, Bensaid C, Achouri A, Nos C, Lécuru F. Diagnostic accuracy of hand-assisted laparoscopy in predicting resectability of peritoneal carcinomatosis from gynecological malignancies. Eur J Surg Oncol. 2013 Jul;39(7):774-9.

[17] Garofalo A, Valle M. Laparoscopy in the management of peritoneal carcinomatosis. Cancer J. 2009 May-Jun;15(3):190-5.

[18] Wang PH, Yuan CC, Lin G et al. Risk factors contributing to early occurrence of port site metastases of laparoscopic surgery for malignancy. Gynecol Oncol 1999; 72:38-84

[19] Van Dam PA, DeClodet J, Tjalma WA et al. Trocar implantation metastasis after laparoscopy in patients with advanced ovarian cancer: can the risk been reduced?. Am J Obste Gynecol 1999; 181:536-541

[20] Nagarsheth NP, Rahaman J, Cohen CJ et al. the incidence of port-site metastases in gynecologic cancers. JSLS 2004; 8:133-139

[21] Eisenkop SM, Friedman RL, Wang HJ. Secondary cytoreductive surgery for recurrent ovarian cancer. A prospective study. Cancer 1995; 76: 1606-14.

[22] Cormio G, di Vagno G, Cazzolla A, Bettocchi S, di Gesu G, Loverro G, et al. Surgical treatment of recurrent ovarian cancer: report of 21 cases and a review of the literature. Eur J Obstet Gynecol Reprod Biol 1999; 86: 185-8.

[23] Eisenkop SM, Friedman RL, Spirtos NM. The role of secondary cytoreductive surgery in the treatment of patients with re- current epithelial ovarian carcinoma. Cancer 2000; 88: 144-53.

[24] Gadducci A,Iacconi P, Cosio S, Fanucchi A, Cristofani R,Riccardo Genazzani A. Complete salvage surgical cytoreduction improves further survival of patients with late recurrent ovar- ian cancer. Gynecol Oncol 2000; 79: 344-9.

[25] Gronlund B, Lundvall L, Christensen IJ, Knudsen JB, Hogdall C. Surgical cytoreduction in recurrent ovarian carcinoma in pa- tients with complete response to paclitaxel-platinum. Eur J Surg Oncol 2005; 31: 67-73.

[26] Onda T, Yoshikawa H, Yasugi T, Yamada M, Matsumoto K, Taketani Y. Secondary cytoreductive surgery for recurrent epi- thelial ovarian carcinoma: proposal for patients selection. Br J Cancer 2005; 92: 1026-32.

[27] Benedetti Panici P, De Vivo A, Bellati F, Manci N, Perniola G, Basile S, et al. Secondary cytoreductive surgery in patients with platinum-sensitive recurrent ovarian cancer. Ann Surg Oncol 2007; 14: 1136-42

[28] Oksefjell H, Sandstad B, Trope C. The role of secondary cytoreduction in the management of the first relapse in epithelial ovarian cancer. Ann Oncol 2009; 20: 286-93.

[29] Tian WJ, Jiang R, Cheng X, Tang J, Xing Y, Zang RY. Surgery in recurrent epithelial ovarian cancer: benefits on Survival for patients with residual disease of 0.1-1 cm after secondary cytoreduction. J Surg Oncol 2010; 101: 244-50.

[30] Tay EH, Grant PT, Gebski V, Hacker NF. Secondary cytoreductive surgery for recurrent epithelial ovarian cancer. Obstet Gynecol 2002; 99: 1008-13.

[31] Sugarbaker PH.Complete Parietal and Visceral Peritonectomy of the Pelvis for advanced primary and recurrent ovarian cancer. Cancer Treat Res 1996. 81: 75-87

[32] Van der Speeten, Kurt MD *; Stuart, Oswald A. BS +; Sugarbaker, Paul H. MD Institution From the *Department of Surgical Oncology, Ziekenhuis Oost-Limburg, Genk, Belgium; and +Washington Cancer Institute, Washington Hospital Center, Washington, DC. Pharmacokinetics and Pharmacodynamics of Perioperative Cancer Chemotherapy in Peritoneal Surface Malignancy. Cancer Journal. 15(3):216-224, May/June 2009.

[33] Laird A. K. "Dynamics of tumor growth". Br J of Cancer 1964. 18 (3): 490–502. DOI: 10.1038/bjc.1964.55.

[34] Simpson-Herren L, Sanford L, Holmquist JP. Effects of surgery on the cell kinetics of residual tumor. Cancer Treat Rep 1976;60:1749-60.

[35] Gundaz N, Fisher B, Saffer EA. Effects of surgical removal on the growth and kinetics of residual tumor. Cancer Res 1979;39:3661-865.

[36] Goldie JH, Coldman JA. A mathematic model for relating the drug sensitivity of tumors to their spontaneous mutation rate. Cancer Treat Rep 1979;63:1727–33

[37] Di Giorgio, A., Cardi, M., Biacchi, D., Sibio, S., Accarpio, F., Ciardi, A.,... Sammartino, P. (2013). Depth of colorectal-wall invasion and lymph-node involvement as major outcome factors influencing surgical strategy in patients with advanced and recurrent ovarian cancer with diffuse peritoneal metastases. World Journal of Surgical Oncology, 11(1), 64.

[38] Burghardt E, Pickel H, Lahousen M, Stettner H (1986) Pelvic lymphade- nectomy in operative treatment of ovarian cancer. Am J Obstet Gynecol 155: 315–319

[39] Spirtos NM, Gross GM, Freddo JL, Ballon SC (1995) Cytoreductive surgery in advanced epithelial cancer of the ovary: the impact of aortic and pelvic lymphadenectomy. Gynecol Oncol 56: 345–352

[40] Kigawa J, Minagawa Y, Ishihara H, Kanamori Y, Itamochi H, Terakawa N. Evaluation of cytoreductive surgery with lymphadenectomy including para-aortic nodes for advanced ovarian cancer. Eur J Surg Oncol. 1993 Jun;19(3):273-8.

[41] Bakrin N, Cotte E, Golfier F, Gilly FN, Freyer G, Helm W, Glehen O, Bereder JM. Cytoreductive surgery and hyperthermic intraperitoneal chemotherapy (HIPEC) for persistent and recurrent advanced ovarian carcinoma: a multicenter, prospective study of 246 patients. Ann Surg Oncol. 2012 Dec;19(13):4052-8.

[42] Bakrin N, Bereder JM, Decullier E, Classe JM, Msika S, Lorimier G, Abboud K, Meeus P, Ferron G, Quenet F, Marchal F, Gouy S, Morice P, Pomel C, Pocard M, Guyon F, Porcheron J, Glehen O; FROGHI (FRench Oncologic and Gynecologic HIPEC) Group. Peritoneal carcinomatosis treated with cytoreductive surgery and Hyperthermic Intraperitoneal Chemotherapy (HIPEC) for advanced ovarian carcinoma: a French multicentre retrospective cohort study of 566 patients. EJSO 39 (2013) 1435e1443

[43] de Bree E, Helm CW. Hyperthermic intraperitoneal chemotherapy in ovarian cancer: rationale and clinical data. Expert Rev Anticancer Ther. 2012 Jul;12(7):895-911.

[44] Helm, C. W., Richard, S. D., Pan, J., Bartlett, D., Goodman, M. D., Hoefer, R.,... Rai, S. N. (2010). Hyperthermic intraperitoneal chemotherapy in ovarian cancer: first report of the HYPER-O registry. International Journal of Gynecological Cancer : Official Journal of the International Gynecological Cancer Society, 20(1), 61–69.

[45] Deraco M, Kusamura S, Virzì S, Puccio F, Macrì A, Famulari C, Solazzo M, Bonomi S, Iusco DR, Baratti D. Cytoreductive surgery and hyperthermic intraperitoneal chemo-

therapy as upfront therapy for advanced epithelial ovarian cancer: multi-institutional phase-II trial. Gynecol Oncol. 2011 Aug;122(2):215-20.

[46] Bijelic L, Yan TD, Sugarbaker PH. Treatment failure following complete cytoreductive surgery and perioperative intraperitoneal chemotherapy for peritoneal dissemination from colorectal or appendiceal mucinous neoplasms. J Surg Oncol. 2008 Sep 15;98(4):295-9.

[47] Chua TC, Robertson G, Liauw W, Farrell R, Yan TD, Morris DL. Intraoperative hyperthermic intraperitoneal chemotherapy after cytoreductive surgery in ovarian cancer peritoneal carcinomatosis: systematic review of current results. J Cancer Res Clin Oncol. 2009 Dec;135(12):1637-45.

[48] Di Giorgio A, Pinto E (2014). Treatment of Peritoneal Surface Malignancies -Updates in Surgery: 295-328. Springer-Verlag Italia 2015

[49] Cotte, E., Glehen, O., Mohamed, F., Lamy, F., Falandry, C., Golfier, F., & Gilly, F. N. (2007). Cytoreductive surgery and intraperitoneal chemo-hyperthermia for chemoresistant and recurrent advanced epithelial ovarian cancer: prospective study of 81 patients. World Journal of Surgery, 31(9), 1813–1820. doi:10.1007/s00268-007-9146-8

[50] Griffith CT. Surgical resections of tumor bulk in the primary treatment of ovarian carcinoma. NCI Monogr. 1975;42:101–104

[51] Oskins WJ, McGuire WP, Brady MF et al. The effect of diameter of largest residual disease on survival after primary cytoreductive surgery in patients with suboptimal residual epithelial ovarian carcinoma. Am J Obstet Gynecol 170:974-979

[52] Chi DS, Eisenhauer EL, Lang J et al. what is the optimal goal of primary cytoreductive surgery for bulky stage IIIC epithelial ovarian cancer (EOC)? Gynecologic Oncology 2006; 105:559-564

[53] Wimberger P, Wehling M, Lehmann N, Kimmig R, Schmalfeldt B, Burges A, Harter P, Pfisterer J, du Bois A. Influence of residual tumor on outcome in ovarian cancer patients with FIGO stage IV disease: an exploratory analysis of the AGO-OVAR (Arbeitsgemeinschaft Gynaekologische Onkologie Ovarian Cancer Study Group). Ann Surg Oncol. 2010 Jun;17(6):1642-8.

[54] Bristow RE, Tomacruz RS, Armstrong DK, Trimble EL, Montz FJ. Survival effect of maximal cytoreductive surgery for advanced ovarian carcinoma during the platinum era: a meta-analysis. J Clin Oncol. 2002 Mar 1;20(5):1248-59

[55] Bristow RE, Puri I, Chi DS. Cytoreductive surgery for recurrent ovarian cancer: a meta-analysis. Gynecol Oncol. 2009 Jan;112(1):265-74.

[56] Passot, G., Bakrin, N., Isaac, S., Decullier, E., Gilly, F. N., Glehen, O., & Cotte, E. Postoperative outcomes of laparoscopic vs open cytoreductive surgery plus hyperthermic intraperitoneal chemotherapy for treatment of peritoneal surface malignancies. European Journal of Surgical Oncology : The Journal of the European Society of Sur-

gical Oncology and the British Association of Surgical Oncology 2013, 1–6. doi: 10.1016/j.ejso.2013.10.002

[57] Barlin JN, Dao F, Bou Zgheib N, Ferguson SE, Sabbatini PJ, Hensley ML, Bell-McGuinn KM, Konner J, Tew WP, Aghajanian C, Chi DS. Progression-free and overall survival of a modified outpatient regimen of primary intravenous/intraperitoneal paclitaxel and intraperitoneal cisplatin in ovarian, fallopian tube, and primary peritoneal cancer. Gynecol Oncol. 2012 Jun;125(3):621-4.

[58] Vergote I, Tropé CG, Amant F et al. Neoadjuvant chemotherapy or primary surgery in stage IIIC or IV ovarian cancer. N. Engl. J. Med. 363(10), 943–953 (2010).

[59] Onda, T., & Yoshikawa, H. (2011). Neoadjuvant chemotherapy for advanced ovarian cancer: overview of outcomes and unanswered questions. Expert Review of Anticancer Therapy, 11(7), 1053–1067. doi:10.1586/era.11.24

[60] Goff BA. Advanced ovarian cancer: what should be the standard of care? J Gynecol Oncol. 2013 Jan;24(1):83-91.

[61] Rauh-Hain, J. A., Nitschmann, C. C., Worley, M. J., Bradford, L. S., Berkowitz, R. S., Schorge, J. O.,... Horowitz, N. S. (2013). Platinum resistance after neoadjuvant chemotherapy compared to primary surgery in patients with advanced epithelial ovarian carcinoma. Gynecologic Oncology, 129(1), 63–8.

[62] Samrao D, Wang D, Ough F, Lin YG, Liu S, Menesses T, Yessaian A, Turner N, Pejovic T, Mhawech-Fauceglia P. (2012). Tr a n s l a t i o n a l O n c o l o g y Histologic Parameters Predictive of Disease Outcome in Women with Advanced Stage Ovarian Carcinoma Treated with neoadjuvant chemotherapy. 5(6), 469–474.

[63] Di Giorgio, A., Cardi, M., Biacchi, D., Sibio, S., Accarpio, F., Ciardi, A.,... Sammartino, P. (2013). Depth of colorectal-wall invasion and lymph-node involvement as major outcome factors influencing surgical strategy in patients with advanced and recurrent ovarian cancer with diffuse peritoneal metastases. World Journal of Surgical Oncology, 11(1), 64.

[64] Park, J.-Y., Seo, S.-S., Kang, S., Lee, K. B., Lim, S. Y., Choi, H. S., & Park, S.-Y. (2006). The benefits of low anterior en bloc resection as part of cytoreductive surgery for advanced primary and recurrent epithelial ovarian cancer patients outweigh morbidity concerns. Gynecologic Oncology, 103(3), 977–984.

[65] Scarabelli C, Gallo A, Franceschi S, Campagnutta E, De G, Giorda G, Visentin MC, Carbone A. Primary cytoreductive surgery with rectosigmoid colon resection for patients with advanced epithelial ovarian carcinoma. Cancer. 2000 Jan 15;88(2):389-97.

[66] Chan JK, Urban R, Hu JM, Shin JY, Husain A, Teng NN, Berek JS, Osann K, Kapp DS. The potential therapeutic role of lymph node resection in epithelial ovarian cancer: a study of 13918 patients. Br J Cancer. 2007 Jun 18;96(12):1817-22.

http://dx.doi.org/10.5772/60844

[67] Pereira A, Pérez-Medina T, Magrina JF, Magtibay PM, Millan I, Iglesias E. The role of lymphadenectomy in node-positive epithelial ovarian cancer. Int J Gynecol Cancer. 2012 Jul;22(6):987-92.

[68] Sakai K, Kajiyama H, Umezu T, Shibata K, Mizuno M, Suzuki S, Kawai M, Nagasaka T, Kikkawa F. Is there any association between retroperitoneal lymphadenectomy and survival benefit in advanced stage epithelial ovarian carcinoma patients? J Obstet Gynaecol Res. 2012 Jul;38(7):1018-23.

[69] Bae JH, Lee JM, Ryu KS, Lee YS, Park YG, Hur SY, Ahn WS, Namkoong SE. Treatment of ovarian cancer with paclitaxel- or carboplatin-based intraperitoneal hyperthermic chemotherapy during secondary surgery. Gynecol Oncol. 2007 Jul;106(1): 193-200.

[70] Pomel C, Ferron G, Lorimier G, Rey A, Lhomme C, Classe JM, Bereder JM, Quenet F, Meeus P, Marchal F, Morice P, Elias D. Hyperthermic intra-peritoneal chemotherapy using oxaliplatin as consolidation therapy for advanced epithelial ovarian carcinoma. Results of a phase II prospective multicentre trial. CHIPOVAC study. Eur J Surg Oncol. 2010 Jun;36(6):589-93.

[71] Frenel JS, Leux C, Pouplin L, Ferron G, Berton Rigaud D, Bourbouloux E, Dravet F, Jaffre I, Classe JM. Oxaliplatin-based hyperthermic intraperitoneal chemotherapy in primary or recurrent epithelial ovarian cancer: A pilot study of 31 patients. J Surg Oncol. 2011 Jan 1;103(1):10-6.

[72] Di Giorgio A, Naticchioni E, Biacchi D, Sibio S, Accarpio F, Rocco M, Tarquini S, Di Seri M, Ciardi A, Montruccoli D, Sammartino P. Cytoreductive surgery (peritonectomy procedures) combined with hyperthermic intraperitoneal chemotherapy (HIPEC) in the treatment of diffuse peritoneal carcinomatosis from ovarian cancer. Cancer. 2008 Jul 15;113(2):315-25.

[73] Ryu KS, Kim JH, Ko HS, Kim JW, Ahn WS, Park YG, Kim SJ, Lee JM. Effects of intraperitoneal hyperthermic chemotherapy in ovarian cancer. Gynecol Oncol. 2004 Aug; 94(2):325-32.

[74] Rubin SC, Randall TC, Armstrong KA, Chi DS, Hoskins WJ. Ten-year follow-up of ovarian cancer patients after second-look laparotomy with negative findings. Obstet Gynecol. 1999 Jan;93(1):21-4.

[75] Harter P, Hahmann M, Lueck HJ, Poelcher M, Wimberger P, Ortmann O, Canzler U, Richter B, Wagner U, Hasenburg A, Burges A, Loibl S, Meier W, Huober J, Fink D, Schroeder W, Muenstedt K, Schmalfeldt B, Emons G, du Bois A. Surgery for recurrent ovarian cancer: role of peritoneal carcinomatosis: exploratory analysis of the DESKTOP I Trial about risk factors, surgical implications, and prognostic value of peritoneal carcinomatosis. Ann Surg Oncol. 2009 May;16(5):1324-30.

[76] Cascales Campos P, Gil J, Parrilla P. Morbidity and mortality outcomes of cytoreductive surgery and hyperthermic intraperitoneal chemotherapy in patients with pri-

mary and recurrent advanced ovarian cancer. Eur J Surg Oncol. 2013 Sep 12. pii: S0748-7983(13)00752-X.

[77] Glehen O, Osinsky D, Cotte E, Kwiatkowski F, Freyer G, Isaac S, Trillet-Lenoir V, Sayag-Beaujard AC, François Y, Vignal J, Gilly FN. Intraperitoneal chemohyperthermia using a closed abdominal procedure and cytoreductive surgery for the treatment of peritoneal carcinomatosis: morbidity and mortality analysis of 216 consecutive procedures. Ann Surg Oncol. 2003 Oct;10(8):863-9.

[78] Sugarbaker PH(Ed): Cytoreductive Surgery & Perioperative Chemotherapy for Peritoneal Surface Malignancy. Ciné-Med; 2013: 183-206.

[79] http://www.clinicaltrials.gov/ct2/show/ NCT01387399

[80] http://www.clinicaltrials.gov/ct2/show/NCT01539785

[81] http://www.clinicaltrials.gov/ct2/show/NCT01091636

[82] http://www.clinicaltrials.gov/ct2/show/NCT01628380

[83] http://www.clinicaltrials.gov/ct2/show/NCT00426257

[84] http://www.clinicaltrials.gov/ct2/show/NCT01376752

[85] http://www.clinicaltrials.gov/ct2/show/NCT01709487

[86] http://www.clinicaltrials.gov/ct2/show / NCT01144442

[87] http://www.clinicaltrials.gov/ct2/show/NCT01767675

[88] http://www.clinicaltrials.gov/ct2/show/NCT01659554

[89] http://www.clinicaltrials.gov/ct2/show/NCT01126346

[90] http://www.clinicaltrials.gov/ct2/show/NCT01970722

Chapter 5

Individualized Novel Therapies for Patients with Tumor Suppressor Genes *BRCA1* and *BRCA2* Mutated Epithelial Ovarian Cancer

Sandra García-Nieto, Carmen Guillén-Ponce, Carmen Alonso, María-Carmen Rodríguez-Soriano, María-Luz Pombo, Earl Julie and Samir A. Farghaly

Additional information is available at the end of the chapter

http://dx.doi.org/10.5772/61938

Abstract

Ovarian cancer is the leading cause of death in women with gynecological cancer, since a large proportion of patients are diagnosed at later stages of the disease. The incidence of ovarian cancer in the general population is 2%, but patients with germline mutations in the *BRCA* genes have a risk of developing ovarian cancer of up to 2050% with a cumulative risk of ovarian cancer at 70 years of age of 40% in *BRCA1* and 18% in *BRCA2* mutation carriers. Although it is a chemosensitive tumor, most of the patients after surgery and chemotherapy based on taxanes and platinum will relapse later in life. Due to the high risk of developing ovarian cancer in patients with *BRCA* germline mutations, new treatments rely increasingly on histological and molecular characteristics of the primary tumor, achieving greater selectivity and lower toxicity compared with standard cytotoxic agents. Poly (ADP-ribose) polymerase (PARPS) inhibitors are the first biologically active agents for patients with ovarian cancer with alterations in the DNA repair pathway, particularly in the high-grade serous subtype of ovarian cancer.

The results of clinical trials published so far mean that olaparib has been approved, pending the results of the Phase III trials. The European Medicines Agency (EMA) adopted olaparib (lynparza ®) on the December 18, 2014, as a maintenance therapy after response to platinum-based chemotherapy in relapsed platinum-sensitive ovarian cancer patients with a *BRCA* mutation. By contrast, the Food and Drug Administration (FDA) approved olaparib on December 19, 2014, in patients with high-grade ovarian epithelial serous tumors and a *BRCA* mutation who have progressed during three or more lines of chemotherapy. Olaparib is also used in primary fallopian tube and peritoneal cancers with *BRCA* mutations.

Keywords: PARP inhibitors, Olaparib, Mutant epithelial ovarian cancer, Tumor suppressor Genes *BRCA1* and *BRCA2*, Novel therapies for ovarian cancer

1. Introduction

The usual treatment of advanced disease of ovarian cancer is surgery [1] followed by taxane and platinum-based chemotherapy, although a large proportion of patients will relapse throughout their lives. Therefore, current clinical trials focus on the detection of molecular targets that can act more selectively and efficiently on ovarian cancer [2].

It is known that chemotherapy treatments damage the DNA and there are molecules that are responsible for repair and proper maintenance of the genome such as poly (adenosine diphosphate-ribose) polymerase (PARP), which plays a key role in the repair of DNA single-strand breaks; so, researchers have focused on the mechanism for the development of new therapies, including the PARP inhibitors.

Olaparib is the first PARP-inhibitor class recently approved for the treatment of ovarian cancer with mutations in *BRCA* (breast cancer), delivered orally and with good tolerance, with myelosuppression and gastrointestinal toxicity as the most frequent adverse effects. Throughout the chapter, we describe the features of hereditary ovarian cancer with *BRCA* mutation, and the steps to follow once the mutation is detected in patients at risk of ovarian cancer. The characteristics of PARP inhibitors are discussed, focusing on olaparib, and their use and dosage recommendations after reviewing the main Phase II trials for which it has been approved; also, we comment on Phase III olaparib trials that are currently underway.

2. *BRCA1* and *BRCA2* genes

Most breast cancers and hereditary ovarian cancers are associated with mutations in two genes, breast cancer type 1 and 2 susceptibility genes (*BRCA1* and *BRCA2*), whose prevalence varies among different geographical areas and ethnic groups, being known as the founder effect among Ashkenazi Jews, whose descendants have an increased risk with any of the three founder mutations (two *BRCA1* mutations, 187delAG and 5385insC, and one *BRCA2* mutation, 6174delT). Founder mutations come from a single carrier ancestor initially extending from a small town with some degree of inbreeding, highly recurrent alterations, or even characteristics of an ethnic group [3].

BRCA1 and *BRCA2* are tumor suppressor genes and are involved in the repair of double-strand breaks of DNA, maintaining genome integrity. Germline mutations in the *BRCA1* and *BRCA2* genes are caused by the loss of one of their wild type alleles, and therefore have a single functioning allele, promoting genomic instability and tumorigenesis [4].

Studies suggest that mutation in p53 favor loss of functionality of the *BRCA 1/2* genes inducing tumorigenesis [5,6]. The function of p53 is to detect DNA damage during the cell cycle, allowing repair; so if p53 is altered, DNA repair is incomplete or inadequate, causing cell death in normal cells [7]. The p53 mutation was detected in almost 90% of patients with high-grade serous carcinoma (HGSC) in patients with *BRCA 1/2* mutation.

The *BRCA1* is located on the long arm of chromosome 17 (17q21) gene. It has a sequence of 5,592 nucleotides, divided into 24 exons. The *BRCA1* protein is localized with *BRCA2*, PALPB2, and RAD51 (essential proteins in homologous recombination) in areas of repair of double-strand breaks of DNA. *BRCA1* is part of BASC (*BRCA1* Associated genome surveillance) complex multiprotein complex responsible for the detection, removal, and repair of DNA breaks. In conclusion, *BRCA1* interacts with other oncogenes, repressors, and activators of transcription, cell cycle regulators, etc., involved in genomic stability. It has also been linked to the development of other cancers, particularly pancreas, uterus, and prostate cancers [8].

The *BRCA2* gene is located on chromosome 13q (13q12), and has a sequence of 11,385 nucleotides in 27 exones. *BRCA2* plays a key role in the cell cycle, especially in cytokinesis and meiosis, as well as in homologous recombination DNA repair [9]. Mutations in this gene have been linked to other cancers such as cancer of the gallbladder, pancreas, stomach, and malignant melanoma.

Hereditary breast and ovarian cancer (HBOC) syndrome is characterized by an autosomal dominant inheritance with high penetrance, presenting increased susceptibility to breast and ovarian cancer, although it has been shown that *BRCA1* and *BRCA2* genes are expressed in most tissues and cells analyzed, suggesting that the pathological impact of a mutation is tissue-specific and that there must be alternative pathways that compensate for their loss of function in other tissue types [10].

Women with hereditary ovarian cancer may have higher rates of response to chemotherapy and improved survival rates in cases of sporadic cancer.

In 2012, the results of an analysis were published [11] in which data from 26 observational studies on the survival of women with ovarian cancer with germline mutations in *BRCA1* and *BRCA2* mutations.

Data from 1,213 cases with a germline mutation in *BRCA1* ($n = 909$) and *BRCA2* ($n = 303$) and 2,666 no mutation carriers were included. The observed overall survival (OS) for 5 years was 36% in non-carriers of mutation patients versus 44% for patients with a *BRCA1* mutation and 52% for patients with a mutation in *BRCA2*. There was an increased survival in *BRCA* mutation carriers versus non-carriers. *BRCA2* carriers had a better prognosis. There were several significant differences in the clinical characteristics of *BRCA1* and *BRCA2* compared with non-carriers. The *BRCA1* and *BRCA2* tumors were more likely to be serous histology and less likely to be mucinous histology. Patients with *BRCA1* and *BRCA2* mutation were more likely to have a tumor stage III/IV and present greater degree of differentiation compared to non-carriers. *BRCA1* carriers were also younger at diagnosis.

Detection of *BRCA1* and *BRCA2* genes is accomplished by DNA extraction from peripheral blood lymphocytes. Detection techniques must be able to identify everything from small changes to large duplications or deletions of exons.

There are over one thousand different mutations to *BRCA1* and *BRCA2*, most of them being small insertions or deletions causing a change in the reading frame (frameshift) and producing a stop codon. However, amino acid substitutions producing a stop codon (nonsense) or mutations located at sites of exon splicing that alter the splicing of the genes and producing full or partial loss of exons [12] can also be found to occur.

It is known that the mutation in the *BRCA1* gene presents a risk of ovarian cancer throughout life of up to 40%, while the *BRCA2* gene has a 20% risk. Although penetrance may vary in the same family carrying a mutation, suggesting that the risk can be influenced by allelic heterozygosity, modifier genes, and environmental and hormonal cofactors [13,14].

After the diagnosis of breast cancer in a patient with a *BRCA* mutation, there is a subsequent risk of developing ovarian cancer of up to 12.7% in women for *BRCA1* and 6.8% for *BRCA2* [15].

Diagnosis in elderly or the absence of family history does not exclude the presence of a germline mutation as approximately 35% of the *BRCA* mutation carriers have no family history. Genetic tests are expensive, so you should select the most appropriate individuals for genetic testing, varying recommendations between populations and countries.

The presence of *BRCA* somatic and germline mutations are predictors of response to different chemotherapy treatments because they exhibit greater sensitivity and response to platinum-type drugs or PARP inhibitors, which are involved in the repair of DNA single-strand breaks [16].

It is important that families carrying this mutation are informed about the risks of developing various types of cancer, including education about prenatal diagnosis and assisted reproduction. Another option is IVF with previously selected embryos. Although, the decision should finally be made on an individual basis and will depend on the preference of each patient.

3. Patients with ovarian cancer *BRCA* genes mutations syndrome

Ovarian cancer is the principal cause of death in women with gynecological cancer, due to the late onset of symptoms and the absence of a method for early detection. Nulliparity, early menarche, and late menopause are associated with an increased risk of occurrence; however, the strongest risk factor is the history of ovarian cancer in a first-degree relative [17].

Malignant primary ovarian tumors fall into three main groups: epithelial, sex cord / stromal, and germ cell tumors. Epithelial tumors being ovarian carcinomas (CBs), which are the most common group, represent up to 90% of ovarian cancers. Low-grade and high-grade serous carcinoma (LGSC and HGSC), mucinous carcinoma (MC), endometrioid carcinoma (EC), and clear cell carcinoma (CCC) are the five histological subtypes of OCs that are known. It is important to make a proper histological typing to determine the prognosis and response to different treatments, including cisplatin [18].

A large proportion of ovarian tumors are sporadic, and only a minority is due to an inherited cause. *BRCA1* and *BRCA2* mutations have been identified in approximately 15% of all epithelial ovarian cancers and up to 22.6% in HGSC. Somatic mutations in *BRCA1* and *BRCA2* have also been identified in as much as 7% of all ovarian cancers [19,20]. Although up to 50%

http://dx.doi.org/10.5772/61938

of patients with HGSC harbor homologous recombination defects including the homologous recombination pathway independent of *BRCA 1/2*, this is known as *BRCA*-like behavior.

BRCA-like behavior is similar to when there is a loss of function or mutation of the *BRCA* genes with the same clinical and molecular characteristics. Examples include promoter methylation *BRCA1* (observed up to 35% of patients with epithelial ovarian cancer) and p53 mutation,

c-myc amplification or other proteins are needed for proper homologous recombination [21–24]. The loss of function of suppressor gene *PTEN* has also been shown to produce *BRCA*-like behavior [25], more common in breast and prostate cancers [26,27].

The HGSC subtype has a greater sensitivity to PARP inhibitors without a *BRCA* mutation, probably due to changes in DNA repair that occur up to 50% of cases as we have mentioned previously [28,18,29].

Studies describe that *BRCA* mutation carriers diagnosed with ovarian cancer have higher survival rates compared with sporadic cases [30–32]. This could be due to increased sensitivity to cisplatin.

In HBOC syndrome, mutations in the *BRCA-1* and *BRCA-2* genes associated with the development of ovarian cancer [29] occur. Other inherited syndromes have also been associated with an increased occurrence of ovarian cancer such as Lynch syndrome (hereditary nonpolyposis colorectal cancer syndrome), characterized by mutations in the DNA repair genes *MLH1*, *MSH2*, *MSH6*, and *PMS2* genes [33].

3.1. Prevention of ovarian cancer in women who have mutations in *BRCA1* and *BRCA2* genes

Primary prevention strategies consist of primarily risk-reducing surgeries, the procedure of choice being prophylactic salpingo-oophorectomy bilateral from 35 to 40 years, or after childbearing. Some experts also recommend prophylactic hysterectomy to dry the small portion of remaining fallopian knotweed, although 92% of fallopian tube neoplasms originate in the middle or distal portion of the tube [34]. Although the final decision will be made by the patient.

Patients with *BRCA1* mutation are at increased risk of developing ovarian cancer from the age of 40; the recommendations as explained above are made from that age. This is not so with patients carrying the *BRCA2* mutation; the increased risk of ovarian cancer starts after age 50, so surgery can be postponed for a few years and secondary effects of surgery reduced [35].

After prophylactic surgery, one of the most important side effects which can deteriorate the quality of life of patients is premature menopause, with increased risk of osteoporosis and cardiovascular diseases such as hypertension, diabetes, and hypercholesterolemia. So that closer monitoring is recommended for cardiovascular risk [36].

Secondary prevention is early detection strategies in women carrying mutations in the *BRCA1* and *BRCA2* genes. Current recommendations include performing transvaginal ultrasound twice a year (preferably day 1–10 of the menstrual cycle), together with detection of serum CA-125 levels (after day 5 of the menstrual cycle for), from age 30 or five to ten years earlier than the earliest age of first diagnosis of ovarian cancer in the family. But these methods have limited sensitivity and specificity, with no observed benefit in women carrying mutation since no mortality was reduced. All women who refuse to perform prophylactic surgeries should undergo screening every six months [37].

Despite the greatly reduced risk of developing ovarian cancer after prophylactic surgery, patients should know that a minority (from 3.9% to 4.3%) of them will develop primary peritoneal carcinoma 20 years after the last oophorectomy in patients with *BRCA*-1 mutations. So before you perform these procedures, patients should be informed of the risks and morbidities associated with these interventions [38,39].

4. Inhibitors of poly (ADP -ribose) polymerase

The preservation of the genetic code by DNA repair is essential for proper cell function. Currently, there is a better understanding of the DNA repair pathways, so it has been studied more carefully for potential drug targets [40].

There are at least five ways engaged in DNA repair, two of them involved in the repair of double-strand breaks (error-prone, non–homologous, end–joining, predominantly active in G1 cells, and error-free HRR, which predominates in dividing cells) [41].

The major DNA repair pathways are direct repair, mismatch repair (MMR), the base excision repair (BER), nucleotide excision repair (NER), and double-strand break repair recombination, which includes both non-homologous, end-joining and homologous recombination repair (HRR) [41,42].

There are certain external agents such as ionizing radiation producing damaging DNA strand breaks. Normal cells have the ability to repair this damage by a protection mechanism maintaining its normal function, but the tumor cells' ability to repair DNA is a radio-resistance mechanism. In recent years, studies have identified a number of agents in these pathways such as PARP inhibitors [43].

Poly (ADP-ribose) polymerase (PARP) inhibitors are a new class of targeted agents against ovarian cancer [44–46]. PARP is a nuclear enzyme whose function is to repair single-stranded DNA.

There are three generations of PARP inhibitor. The first generation of inhibitors included nicotinamide analogs. 3-Aminobenzamide was the first PARP inhibitor but was not considered powerful enough compared to the second generation [47]. Currently, clinical trials are aimed at third-generation inhibitors with greater potency and specificity, decreasing side effects, this includes olaparib.

DNA repair is essential for proper cell function. Each cell sustains many thousands of episodes of DNA damage every day, which will be repaired by a wide variety of repair mechanisms [48,49].

The *BRCA 1/2* genes are responsible for DNA repair known as homologous recombination (HR) repair. HR is a form of double-strand break repair that occurs in the G2 phase of the cell cycle where the second double-stranded copy of the DNA is used as a template to form an error-free repair [49].

Other DNA repair pathway, such as the non-homologous, end-joining (NHEJ) pathway, also plays a role in the anti-cancer mechanism of action of PARP inhibitors [50].

PARP inhibitors act by trapping PARP-1 and PARP-2 on the double-strand break and blocks DNA replication, which is more toxic to cells than the accumulation of DNA breaks [51]. Overall, in tumors in where there is an apparent defect in homologous DNA repair (and thus a defect in the repair of double-stranded breaks), they seem to be susceptible to PARP-inhibitor therapy. These include tumors associated with germline or somatic mutations in *BRCA 1/2* [52].

There are at least 17 PARP counterparts, with only three PARP-1, PARP-2, and PARP-3s that play a critical role in DNA repair [53,54]. The best known are PARP-1 and PARP-2 [55, 56], and the most studied PARP-1.

PARP-1 was the first to be reported in 1963 [57]. Durkacz [58] stated that modulating PARP1 could enhance the effect of chemotherapy.

PARP-1 contains three functional domains: the N-terminal DNA-binding domain (DBD), the center self-modification domain (DMA), and the C-terminal catalytic domain (CD). The DBD is involved in recognition of DNA-strand breakage and in the binding of PARP-1 to DNA. AMD can interact with many DNA damage response proteins and the CD includes a PARP signature motif and catalyzes the formation of PAR [59]. PARP-1 is essential for base excision repair (BER).

PARP-1 also contributes to other cellular processes such as gene transcription, and the regulation of the chromatin structure, to restart stalled replication forks due to nucleotide depletion or collisions with bulky lesions [52].

PARP-1 has been used in in vitro studies in combination with chemotherapy, to demonstrate its ability to inhibit the classical mechanisms of DNA repair, showing also increased distribution of cytotoxicity to the tumor, increasing their exposure by improving vascular perfusion. This resulted in further studies with PARP-1.

The DNA repair biology has allowed us to identify patients most likely to respond to treatment with PARP inhibitors [60].

PARP inhibitors act by synthetic lethality, which occurs when two independent conditions alone do not cause cell death but in combination are lethal. It occurs when a patient has an alteration in the homologous recombination (HR) such as in carriers of a mutation in *BRCA1* and *BRCA2* genes and the application of PARP inhibitors, causing cell death [61,62]. Up to 5% of cutaneous melanomas and gastric cancers, 1% of prostate cancers, and even 19% of familial pancreatic cancers will carry a germline mutation in *BRCA 1/2*, thus they have an altered HR and therefore they may also respond to PARP inhibitors [63].

PARP-2 cooperates with PARP-1 to synthesize poly (ADP-ribose) [pADPr] after damage in the DNA chain [41]. PARP-3 suppresses error-prone NHEJ [52, 64,65] while associated with

PARP-1 for DNA repair. The clinical development of PARP-inhibitors has lead to its use as monotherapy or in combination with chemotherapy agents. Olaparib has been recently approved for the treatment of hereditary breast ovarian cancer syndrome, and other PARP-inhibitors such as veliparib, rucaparib, or niraparib are being studied [66].

4.1. Combination therapy of PARP inhibitors and radiotherapy

The efficacy of radiotherapy in the treatment of cancer have been known for several years either concomitantly with chemotherapy or as adjuvant use in therapy.

New clinical trials not only focus on researching new systemic treatments alone or in combination with other chemotherapy agents but also study their association with radiotherapy. These new therapies are the PARP inhibitors that have shown activity in conjunction with radiation therapy in several cancer cell lines. Data suggest that PARP inhibitors may enhance the effects of radiation in various types of tumors, such as lung cancer, colorectal, and cervical among others [67]. However, the mechanism of action is still unknown, one hypothesis is that it is due to mutual damage (of PARP-inhibitors and radiotherapy) of DNA or whether tumor re-oxygenation contributes to this radio sensitization via the vasoactive effects of the PARP inhibitors remains to be fully determined [43].

A recently published Phase I clinical trial [68] combined low-dose abdominal level fractionated radiotherapy with increasing doses of the PARP-inhibitor veliparib in patients with peritoneal carcinomatosis secondary to advanced malignant solid tumors. Patients were treated with veliparib (80–320 mg daily) for a total of 3 cycles.

The dose of radiotherapy consisted of 21.6 Gy in 36 fractions, 0.6 Gy twice daily on days 1 and 5 for weeks 1–3 of each cycle. Twenty-two patients were included. Disease stabilization (≥24 weeks) was observed in 7 patients (33%). Median progression-free survival (MPFS) was 4.47 months and median overall survival (MOS) was 13.04 months. In the trial, there were 8 patients with ovarian and fallopian cancers with an observed MPFS of 6.77 months and an MOS of 17.54 months, combined with a higher quality of life. The toxicity grade 3 and 4 lymphopenia were more frequent (68%), anemia (9%), and thrombocytopenia (14%). With these results, the authors concluded that the combination of radiotherapy and veliparib resulted in a stabilization of the response in patients with solid tumors and peritoneal carcinomatosis, especially in the subgroup of patients with ovarian cancer, besides being a well-tolerated regimen.

5. OLAPARIB

Because many cytotoxic agents work by damaging the DNA, there has been a great deal of interest in the use of inhibitors of DNA repair such as new treatments against cancer, especially in patients with mutations in the *BRCA* genes with altered function, and will be more likely to develop different types of neoplasms due to increased tumorigenesis [69].

Olaparib is a member of the class of N-acylpiperazines formally obtained by condensation of the carboxyl group of 2-fluoro-5 - [(4-oxo-3,4-dihydrophthalazin-1-yl) methyl] benzoic acid with the free amino group of N- (cyclpropylcarbonyl) piperazine.

5.1. Initial clinical trials with OLAPARIB

In 2008, Rottenberg et al. [70] postulated the hypothesis of the use of olaparib (then called AZD2281, KU-0059436) in cancer triple negative breast, because these tumors harbor defects in DNA repair and mutations in *BRCA1*. To do this, they used PARP inhibitors (AZD2281) in genetically engineered mouse models of breast cancer *BRCA1*, resulting in an inhibition of tumor growth and increased overall survival with no signs of toxicity. Drug resistance developed after long-term treatment due to upregulation of efflux pumps; however, this was overcome by co-administration of the P-glycoprotein inhibitor tariquidar. They observed that the combination of AZD2281 with cisplatin or carboplatin increased progression-free survival, suggesting the effectiveness of AZD2281 as DNA-damaging agents.

Evers et al. [71] studied sensitivity to conventional cytotoxic drugs AZD2281 in cell lines with *BRCA2* mutations. AZD2281 was observed to be the drug that caused greater tumor reduction in the presence of *BRCA2* mutations, alone or in combination with cisplatin.

Fong et al. [60] conducted a Phase I clinical trial with escalating doses of mg to 600mg olaparib, in a population of 60 patients, including 22 mutation carriers in the *BRCA1* and *BRCA2* gene. Dose-limiting toxicity was observed in one of eight patients receiving 400 mg twice daily (grade 3 fatigue and mood alteration) and two of five patients who received 600 mg twice daily (grade 4 thrombocytopenia and drowsiness grade 3). In 63% of patients with cancer and carriers of *BRCA* mutations, a clinical benefit for a period of 4 months or more was observed and 8 patients had ovarian cancer.

In this study, patients resistance to platinum response was observed.

A year later, the same team of Fong et al. confirmed previous results by expanding a cohort of patients with mutations in *BRCA1* and *BRCA2*, including primary peritoneal cancer with ovary, and fallopian tube cancers (13 platinum-sensitive, 24 platinum-resistant, and 13 platinum-refractory) observing a clinical benefit response of up to 46%. The overall clinical benefit rate decreased due to insensitivity to platinum (platinum-sensitive patients: 69%, platinum-resistant: 46% refractory to platinum: 23%). The median response duration was 28 weeks, concluding that patients who were platinum-sensitive present a greater response to olaparib, in addition to showing a benefit in resistant and refractory patients [72].

Seventy five percent of *BRCA1*-mutated breast cancers are classified as triple-negative breast and *BRCA1* or *BRCA2* mutation carriers and have the tendency to develop ovarian cancer. In a Phase II clinical trial [63], the investigators administered 400 mg of olaparib twice daily in patients with ovarian cancer HGSC and triple-negative breast cancer. Patients were stratified according to whether they were carriers of *BRCA1*, *BRCA2*, and *BRCA* wild-type gene. The primary endpoint was objective response rate by Response Evaluation Criteria In Solid Tumors (RECIST). It was observed that 41% of patients with *BRCA* mutation carrier ovarian cancer and 24% of patients with wild-type *BRCA* showed no response to olaparib RECIST criteria. No confirmed objective responses were reported in patients with breast cancer and they concluded that olaparib is an efficient drug for treatment of *BRCA* mutant ovarian cancer.

Kaye et al. published the results of a Phase II trial in 2012. The study included 97 patients with ovarian cancer and *BRCA1* or *BRCA2* germline mutations that had recurred within 12 months of prior platinum therapy. They randomized in a 1:1:1 ratio to receive olaparib 200 mg or 400 mg bd or pegylated liposomal doxorubicin (PLD) 50 mg / m2 intravenously. The median PFS was 6.5 months, 8.8 months, and 7.1 months for the olaparib 200 mg, 400 mg olaparib, and PLD groups, respectively. Objective response rates were 25, 31, and 18% for olaparib 200 mg, 400 mg olaparib, and PLD, respectively. Proving that olaparib 400 mg twice daily is an appropriate dose. A surprising finding was the effectiveness of PLD [74]. These results affirm the data published by Adams et al. [75] which show increased PLD activity in patients carrying a *BRCA* mutation.

Lederman et al. [76] reported on a Phase II trial; they administered olaparib as a maintenance therapy in patients with recurrent ovarian cancer or fallopian tube or primary peritoneal cancer of high-grade, which was platinum-sensitive. Patients were randomized to receive olaparib 400 mg twice daily or placebo within 8 weeks after the last dose of platinum-based chemotherapy. The primary endpoint was progression-free survival (PFS). A first analysis performed after progression in 57.7% of patients showed that PFS was significantly longer in the olaparib group than in the placebo group. Median PFS was 8.4 months in the olaparib group versus 4.8 months in the placebo group ($P < 0.001$). Subgroup analysis of progression-free survival showed that, in the olaparib group, patients had a lower risk of progression than those in the placebo group. Having had a complete response to the treatment of platinum-based chemotherapy before entering the study was a significant prognostic factor for longer progression-free survival (hazard ratio, 0.46; $P<0.001$). Time to progression according to the RECIST guidelines or CA-125 level was significantly longer in the olaparib group than in the placebo group (median, 8.3 months vs. 3.7 months ($P < 0.001$). The response rate was 12% (7 of 57 with measurable disease patients at study entry) in the olaparib group, as compared with 4% ($P = 0.12$).

In the interim analysis of overall survival (OS), 101 patients (38%) had died: 52 in the olaparib group and 49 in the placebo group. No significant difference in overall survival was observed ($P = 0.75$). The median overall survival was similar in the two study groups (29.7 months in the olaparib group and 29.9 months in the placebo group). Although *BRCA* mutation status was known for 37% of all patients who entered the study, a subgroup analysis suggested that olaparib could increase PFS in patients with a *BRCA* mutation.

The incidence of adverse events grade 3 or 4 was higher in the olaparib group (35.3%) compared to the placebo group (20.3%). The most common adverse events leading to discontinuation or dose reduction of olaparib were vomiting, nausea, and fatigue. There were no statistically significant differences in quality of life test performed patients.

In another study, Lederman et al. [77] presented test data 19, a second retrospective analysis of OS, and *BRCA* mutation status of the Phase II trial published by them in 2012. The primary endpoint was PFS, analyzed for the overall population and by *BRCA* status. *BRCA* mutation status was known in 96% of patients in the group of olaparib compared to 95% in the placebo group, of whom 56% versus 50% had a deleterious or suspected tumor or deleterious *BRCA* germline mutation. The median PFS was significantly longer in the olaparib group compared to the placebo group, 11.2 months vs. 4.3 months; in the wild-type *BRCA* patients the findings were similar, 7.4 months vs. 5.5 months. In a second interim analysis (58% maturity), the OS was similar in patients with mutated *BRCA* and wild-type *BRCA*, this may be secondary to the fact that 23% of patients receiving placebo could subsequently receive an inhibitor of PARP. In the results, they observed that some patients responded to olaparib in the absence of a *BRCA* mutation, this could be due to epigenetic silencing of *BRCA* or homologous recombination genes such as RAD51D.

There were more treatment interruptions and dose reductions in the olaparib group compared to placebo. Adverse effects grade 3 or 4 in the olaparib group were fatigue in 7% vs. 3% in the placebo group, and anemia 5% vs. <1%, respectively. Serious adverse effects were reported in 18% of patients receiving olaparib compared to 9% on placebo. Tolerability was similar regardless of the mutational status.

Although the number of patients treated with somatic *BRCA* mutations was lower, responses were also seen during maintenance therapy.

The test of olaparib superiority over the placebo in platinum-sensitive patients demonstrated that patients relapsed after treatment. In addition, it was shown that *BRCA* mutations, whether somatic or germ line, are the main determinants of response to olaparib.

After the results of test data19 were published, olaparib was approved by EMA as a maintenance therapy after response to platinum-based chemotherapy in relapsed platinum-sensitive ovarian cancer, fallopian tube, and primary peritoneal cancers patients with a *BRCA* mutation. In contrast, the FDA-approved olaparib in patients with high-grade serous ovarian epithelial tumors, primary fallopian tube and peritoneal cancers with a *BRCA* mutation who had progressed during three or more lines of chemotherapy.

Before starting treatment with olaparib, they confirmed the presence of a *BRCA* germline or somatic mutation, using a valid method of analysis in a specialized laboratory.

It also assessed the efficacy and tolerability of olaparib in combination with chemotherapy followed by maintenance olaparib versus chemotherapy alone in patients with high-grade serous ovarian cancer, including primary peritoneal and fallopian tubes, platinum-sensitive who had received three or more lines of platinum-based chemotherapy. AM Oza et al. [78] published data based on chemotherapy combination of carboplatin (area under the curve [AUC] 4 mg / mL per min) plus paclitaxel (175 mg / m2) every 21 days with olaparib 200 mg twice daily (during days 1--10 of each cycle of 21 days), 6 total cycles followed olaparib maintenance monotherapy (400 mg twice daily) until disease progression or unacceptable toxicity, compared to chemotherapy alone (carboplatin AUC 6 mg / mL paclitaxel 175 mg / m2) without maintenance. The primary endpoint was PFS, the secondary efficacy endpoints were overall survival; percentage change in tumor size; the proportion of patients with an objective response according to RECIST; cancer antigen 125 (CA-125) response.

The results concluded that the PFS was higher in the olaparib plus chemotherapy group (median 12.2 months) compared with chemotherapy alone (median of 9.6 months). *BRCA* mutation status was known in 107 patients. *BRCA* mutations were observed in 41 (38%) of 107 patients (20 in the chemotherapy group and 21 in more olaparib chemotherapy alone); of the 41 patients with *BRCA* mutation, the PFS at 12 months was 70% for patients in the combination arm vs. 12.5% in the chemotherapy alone arm. There were no statistically significant differences in OS or percentage change in tumor size. The proportion of patients with an objective response by the central review was similar between treatment groups. The two treatment groups had a similar proportion of patients with a CA-125 response and ovarian cancer response. The most frequent grade 3 or 4 adverse effects in the combination arm were neutropenia (43%) vs. (35%) in patients with chemotherapy alone and anemia ([9%] vs. [5%]). The most frequent adverse effects of mild or moderate intensity were alopecia, nausea, diarrhea, headache, and peripheral neuropathy among others, they were all more common in the combination group.

Not only olaparib has been studied in combination with chemotherapy, but their association was also analyzed with cediranib, an anti-angiogenic agent with activity against the VEGF receptor (VEGFR) 1, VEGFR2, and VEGFR3. In Phase I clinical trials, combination responses and manageable toxicities were observed, so that a Phase II clinical trial was developed aimed at demonstrating whether their combination would result in increased PFS versus olaparib monotherapy in women with recurrent platinum-sensitive ovarian cancer. The trial was conducted by Liu [79].

They recruited women with ovarian (HGSC and EC), fallopian tube or primary peritoneal cancer, or patients with a *BRCA* germ line mutation. Patients were randomized to receive olaoparib in 400 mg capsules twice daily or the combination of cediranib 30 mg daily and olaparib 200 mg capsules twice daily. The primary endpoint was PFS. 46 women received 44 olaparib monotherapy and combination therapy women. Median PFS was 17.7 months for the women treated with cediranib plus olaparib compared with 9 months in patients receiving olaparib monotherapy. Grade 3 and 4 adverse events were more common with the combination therapy, including fatigue, diarrhea, and hypertension. Thus, the authors concluded that PFS increases considerably with the combination therapy, so Phase III clinical trials are necessary to confirm these results, including assessments of quality of life.

Because of the mechanism of action of olaparib, the use of PARP inhibitor in other tumors with mutations in the *BRCA 1/2* gene could be effective, a Phase II clinical trial with different tumors was performed, all patients had *BRCA 1/2* mutations and recurrent cancer. The study was conducted by Kaufman et al. [52]. It was a prospective, multi-center, randomized trial, and patients were recruited in several centers in Israel, Australia, Germany, Spain, Sweden, and the United States between February 21, 2010, and July 31, 2012. It included patients with ovarian cancer resistant to prior platinum; with three breast cancer chemotherapy regimens for metastatic disease; pancreatic cancer progression during treatment with gemcitabine; with prostate cancer progression or on hormonal and one systemic therapy. Olaparib was administered 400 mg twice per day. The primary efficacy end point was tumor response rate according to RECIST. Secondary end points included: objective response rate (in those with measurable disease at baseline), PFS, duration of response, safety, and tolerability.

And 298 patients were evaluated, of whom 193 had ovarian cancer, 62 had breast cancer, 23 had advanced pancreatic cancer, and 8 patients with advanced prostate cancer. The remaining 12 patients had a range of cancers, including cancers of the biliary tract, bladder, colorectum, lung, esophagus, and uterus.

The tumor response rate was 26.2% (78 of 298; 95% CI, 21.3 to 31.6) overall and 31.1% (60 of 193; 95% CI, 24.6 to 38.1) in patients with ovarian cancer, 12.9% (eight of 62; 95% CI, 5.7 to 23.9) in breast, 21.7% (five of 23; 95% CI, 7.5 to 43.7) in pancreatic, and 50.0% (four of eight; 95% CI, 15.7 to 84.3) in prostate cancers. In 42% of all patients, stable disease was observed after 8 weeks of treatment, up to 46.8% having achieved stabilization in cases of breast cancer. Overall median duration of the response was 208 days (ovarian cancer, 225 days; breast cancer, 204 days; pancreatic cancer, 134 days; prostate cancer, 327 days). Median time to onset of response was 56.0 days (ovarian cancer, 56.5 days; breast cancer, 54.5 days; pancreatic cancer, 113.0 days; prostate cancer, 54.5 days). The objective response rate (restricted to those with measurable disease at baseline) was 29.3% (95% CI, 23.9 to 35.2).

A similar response rate for patients with a *BRCA1* mutation (26.3 % ; 95 % CI, 20.3 to 33.0) and those with a *BRCA2* mutation was also noted.

The most common side effects were fatigue, nausea, and vomiting. About 54% of patients experienced grade 3 toxicity, most frequently fatigue and anemia, 40.3 % of patients had to modify (interruption and / or reduction) olparib dose due to adverse effects. Nine patients died as a result of severe adverse effects.

After these results, they concluded that the response to olaparib is independent of the anatomical organ of origin, provided that there is a mutation in *BRCA 1/2*.

Despite the demonstrated efficacy of PARP inhibitors in patients with *BRCA 1/2* mutation, there has been less activity in patients with breast cancer, perhaps due to the biologic heterogeneity and low *BRCA 1/2* mutation rate in somatic triple negative breast cancer [80–83].

5.2. Phase III clinical trials

Currently, there are two Phase III trials underway with olaparib, both sponsored by Astra Zeneca: SOLO 1 (NCT01844986) and SOLO2 (NCT01874353). Both are multi-center, double-blind, in which randomly assigned patients (2: 1) receive 300 mg of olaparib daily maintenance in patients diagnosed with high-grade serous or endometrioid ovarian cancer, primary peritoneal including and / or fallopian tube cancer with a *BRCA* mutation, and having partial or complete response after completion of platinum-based chemotherapy. To be included in SOLO1 trial, patients must have been newly diagnosed, with advanced (FIGO stage III-IV) disease, and responding to first-line treatment with platinum. To be included in SOLO2, patients must have completed ≥2 lines of platinum therapy. The main objective for both clinical trials is progression-free survival [84].

Not only they are testing olaparib, but there are also other Phase III trials with PARP inhibitors, such as veliparib, rucaparib, and niraparib, trying to improve the identification of patients who might best respond to PARP inhibitors [80] and reducing associated toxicities.

5.3. Combination therapy of OLAPARIB with other therapeutic agents

Olaparib has been tested in several clinical trials in combination with other chemotherapy because it was thought that it could increase sensitivity to chemotherapy by inhibiting DNA repair which could be responsible for drug resistance. This has been associated with topotecan [85], dacarbazine [86], paclitaxel [87], and cisplatin and gemcitabine [88]. In several Phase I clinical trials, myelosuppression increased in the combination therapy versus monotherapy, especially with topotecan and cisplatin.

Olaparib has also been studied in combination with bevacizumab. Dean et al. [89] designed a Phase I clinical trial, as they hypothesized that bevacizumab antiangiogenic activity and hypoxia inducing DNA damage may enhance olaparib therapeutic activities. They showed that a dose of olaparib 400 mg twice daily in combination with Avastin 10mg / kg every two weeks was tolerated well. They are considering the combination for future clinical trials.

5.4. Dosage

The recommended lynparza® (olaparib) dose is 400 mg (eight capsules) twice a day, i.e., a total daily dosage of 800 mg. Treatment should begin before eight weeks of completion of the last cycle of chemotherapy with a regimen containing platinum. Continual treatment is recommended until disease progression. The recommended dose is reduced to 200 mg orally twice daily (total daily dose 400 mg). Elderly patients require a dose reduction initially, and it can be administered in patients with mild renal impairment (creatinine clearance> 50 mL / min).

5.5. Adverse reactions

Among the most frequent toxicities in clinical trials are hematologic toxicity with mild to moderate anemia, lymphopenia, neutropenia, and thrombocytopenia at manageable levels. Other frequently observed side effects are headache, fatigue, decreased appetite, abdominal discomfort, nausea, vomiting, diarrhea, and dyspepsia.

Another event that was observed was the development of myelodysplastic / AML syndrome, in only a small number of patients receiving olaparib alone or in combination with other antineoplastic during clinical trials. All had previously received platinum-based chemotherapy regimens, radiation, and other DNA-damaging agents.

There have been cases of pneumonitis, some of them being fatal. If patients are treated with Lynparza, respiratory symptoms such as cough, dyspnea, and fever should be closely monitored. If there is any alteration in the chest radiography, treatment must be stopped and the patient is treated appropriately. Paralyzer can cause birth defects if given to pregnant women. A reliable contraception should be recommended during treatment and one month after the last dose [90,63].

6. Mechanisms of resistance to PARP inhibitors

Targeted therapy based on the patient's mutation status is the future of the treatment of ovarian cancer. *BRCA* deficiency may be reversed by mutational changes in the reading frame, resulting in wild-type *BRCA* protein production. A second mutation (compensatory mutations or crossovers) can cause changes in the reading frame *BRCA* mutation, HR rebuilding, and restoring its functionality, explaining why not all tumors with *BRCA* mutation respond to PARP inhibitors [91]. Some *BRCA1* mutant alleles encode functional proteins but are degraded,

http://dx.doi.org/10.5772/61938

stabilizing the activity of the mutated protein and can reset the HR [92]. Another mechanism could be the upregulation of the pump glycoprotein efflux reducing concentrations of the intracellular PARP inhibitor [93,94] or loss of 53BP1, a key protein in the NHEJ pathway.

7. Conclusions

The context of the *BRCA 1/2*-mutant genotype has a significant impact on disease behavior and outcome. An encouraging data on responses to PARP inhibitors in *BRCA 1/2*-mutant carriers with prostate, pancreatic, and breast cancer have been reported and are likely to be associated with platinum sensitivity. It is apparent that establishing the germ-line and/or tumor *BRCA 1/2* mutation status in patients with cancers known to be associated with *BRCA 1/2* mutations is of notable importance due to the potential therapeutic options. Chemotherapy recommendation for patients with *BRCA 1/2* mutant epithelial ovarian cancer ought to be based on rechallenging these patients with platinum-based treatment, and prolonging the platinum-free interval in the event of early relapse following platinum-based treatment. The timing and sequence of therapy, and the indications for rechallenging patients with platinum-based chemotherapy, including routes and schedules of administration (IV vs. IP, weekly vs. thrice weekly), olaparib plus paclitaxel and carboplatin followed by laparib maintenance monotherapy, significantly improved progression-free survival versus paclitaxel plus carboplatin alone, in patients with *BRCA*-mutated recurrent platinum-sensitive ovarian cancer, with acceptable tolerability profile. It differs as more data emerges from analyses of the mutation status of *BRCA 1/2* genes and other HR-related genes in tumor samples from previously completed studies. In addition, stratification based on HR-deficiency phenotype/genotype may become the standard in future clinical trials involving patients with *BRCA 1/2* mutant epithelial ovarian cancer. It has been established that olaparib plus paclitaxel and carboplatin followed by olaparib maintenance monotherapy significantly improved progression-free survival versus paclitaxel plus carboplatin alone, in patients with *BRCA*-mutated recurrent platinum-sensitive ovarian cancer, with acceptable tolerability profile.

8. Future directions

Tumors with alterations in DNA repair lead to a defective HR, based on synthetic lethality and being very sensitive to PARP inhibitors. This happens with HGSC *BRCA* mutation carriers demonstrating its response to olaparib. We still need to better identify patients who will respond to PARP inhibitors because a proportion of patients developed resistance to these treatments, so research is needed to understand the mechanisms of action of PARP inhibitors and mechanisms of resistance. The only biomarkers that have been shown to be predictive of response while using PARP inhibitors are the *BRCA 1/2* mutations both somatic and germ line, in the absence of other biomarkers, we are limited to using the PARP inhibitors only in patients with *BRCA* mutation 1/2, although it may be effective in other tumors despite the absence of *BRCA* mutation.

We have studied the operation of Rad5 using antibody detection of Rad5 as new response PARP-inhibitors biomarkers, although initial results suggest that is not sufficient, specific and sensitive for use in clinical application, so we need to keep looking for new biomarkers or methods that help us to identify the appropriate patients for treatment with PARP inhibitors [52]. As not all genes responsible for DNA repair are known, another option that has not yet been implemented is to apply functional tests of DNA-repair capability, this would help us identify the abnormalities and tumors suitable for treatment with PARP inhibitors [95], the molecules involved in *BRCA*-like tumors whose information is essential to broaden the scope of action of PARP-inhibitors, without limiting its use for patients with *BRCA* 1/2 mutations. A current research topic is whether these new drugs work better alone or in combination with standard cytotoxic agents, avoiding toxicities and resistance mechanisms [96]. They have been shown to be well tolerated with manageable toxicity, but the long-term action is unknown. Some experts question whether inhibiting DNA repair can lead to deleterious effects such as an increased risk of developing other types of cancer in the future. Another topic of interest is its effect in combination with radiotherapy or as maintenance therapy. As of now, we do not know what effect PARP inhibitors may have in patients with low tumor burden, and what would be the benefit when these agents are used as maintenance therapy or chemoprevention.

Author details

Sandra García-Nieto[1], Carmen Guillén-Ponce[3*], Carmen Alonso[1], María-Carmen Rodríguez-Soriano[2], María-Luz Pombo[1], Earl Julie[3] and Samir A. Farghaly[4]

*Address all correspondence to: carmenguillenponce@gmail.com

1 Oncology Department. Hospital General Universitario de Albacete. Albacete, Spain

2 Oncology Department. Hospital Virgen de la Luz. Cuenca, Spain

3 Oncology Departmen. Hospital Universitario Ramón y Cajal. Madrid, Spain

4 Joan and Sanford I. Weill Medical College/ The Graduate School of Medical Sciences, and The New York Presbyterian Hospital-Weill Cornell Medical Center, Cornell University, New York, NY, USA

References

[1] Chi DS, Eisenhauer EL, Zivanovic O, etal. Improved progression-free and overall survival in advanced ovarian cancer as a result of a change in surgical paradigm. Gynecol Oncol 2009;114:26–31.

[2] Jemal A, Bray F, Center MM, et al. Global cancer statistics.CA Cancer J Clin 2001;61:69–90.

[3] Diez O, Osorio A, Duran M, et al. Analysis of *BRCA1* and *BRCA2* genes in Spanish breast/ovarian cancer patients: a high proportion of mutations unique to Spain and evidence of founder effects. Hum Mutat 2003;22:301–12.

[4] Vicus D, Finch A, Cass I, et al. Prevalence of *BRCA1* and *BRCA2* germline mutations among women with carcinoma of the fallopian tube. Gynecol Oncol 2010.

[5] Jonkers J, Meuwissen R, van der Gulden H, et al. Synergistic tumor suppressor activity of *BRCA2* and p53 in a conditional mouse model for breast cancer. Nat Genet 2001;29:418–25.

[6] Liu X, Holstege H, van der Gulden H, et al. Somatic loss of *BRCA1* and p53 in mice induces mammary tumors with features of human *BRCA1*-mutated basal-like breast cancer. Proc Natl Acad Sci USA 2007;104:12111–6.

[7] Meek DW. Tumour suppression by p53: a role for the DNA damage response? Nat Rev Cancer 2009;9:714–23.

[8] Miki Y, Swensen J, Shattuck-Eidens D, et al. A strong candidate for the breast and ovarian cancer susceptibility gene *BRCA1*. Science 1994;266:66–71.

[9] Wooster R, Bignell G, Lancaster J, et al. Identification of the breast cancer susceptibility gene *BRCA2*. Nature 1995;378:789–92.

[10] Elledge SJ, Amon A. The *BRCA1* suppressor hipothesis: an explanation for the tissue-specific tumor development in *BRCA1* patients. Cancer Cell 2002;1:129–32.

[11] Kelly L. Bolton; Georgia Chenevix- Trench; Cindy Goh, BA, et al. Association Between *BRCA1* and *BRCA2* Mutatiions and Survival in Women with invasive Epithelial Ovarian Cancer. J Am Med Assoc January 25, 2012;307:4.

[12] Hoeijmakers JH. Genome maintenance mechanisms for preventing cancer. Nature 2001;411:366–74.

[13] Narod SA, Foulkes WD. *BRCA1* and *BRCA*-2:1994 and beyond. Nat Rev Cancer 2004;665–76.

[14] King MC, Marks JH, Mandello JB. Breast and ovarian cancer risks to due to inherited mutationes in *BRCA1* and *BRCA2*. Science 2003;302:643–46.

[15] Metkalfe KA, Lynch HT, Ghadirian P, et al. The risk of ovarian cancer after breast cancer in *BRCA1* and *BRCA2* carriers. Gynecol Oncol 2005;96:222–6.

[16] Burk RD. *BRCA1* mutations and survival in women with ovarian cancer 6. N Engl J Med 1997;336:1255–7.

[17] Jemal A, Bray F, Center MM, Ferlay J, Ward E, Forman D. Global cancer statistics. CA Cancer J Clin 2011;6:69–90.

[18] Pennington KP, Walsh T, Harrell MI, Lee MK, Pennil CC, Rendi MH, et al. Germline and somatic mutations in homologous recombination genes predict platinum response and survival in ovarian, fallopian tube, and peritoneal carcinomas. Clin Cancer Res 2014;20:764–75.

[19] Alsop K, Fereday S, Meldrum C, DeFazio A, Emmanuel C, George J, et al. *BRCA* mutation frequency and patterns of treatment response in *BRCA* mutation-positive women with ovarian cancer: a report from the Australian Ovarian Cancer Study Group. J Clin Oncol 2012;30:2654–63.

[20] Hennessy BT, Timms KM, Carey MS, Gutin A, Meyer LA, Flake DD, et al. Somatic mutations in *BRCA1* and *BRCA2* could expand the number of patients that benefit from poly (ADP ribose).

[21] Press JZ, De Luca A, Boyd N, et al. Ovarian carcinomas with genetic and epigenetic *BRCA1* loss have distinct molecular abnormalities. BMC Cancer 2008;8:17.

[22] Turner N, Tutt A, Ashworth A. Hallmarks of '*BRCA*ness' in sporadic cancers. Nat Rev Cancer 2004;4:814–9.

[23] Long KC, Kauff ND. Hereditary ovarian cancer: recent molecular insights and their impact on screening strategies. Curr Opin Oncol 2011;23:526–30.

[24] Walsh T, Casadei S, Lee MK et al. Mutations in 12 genes for inherited ovarian, fallopian tube, and peritoneal carcinoma identified by massively parallel sequencing. Proc Natl Acad Sci USA 2011;108:18032–7.

[25] Malkin D, Li FP, Strong LC et al. Germline p53 mutations in a familial syndrome of breast cancer, sarcomas, and other neoplasms. Science 1990;250:1233–8.

[26] Saal LH, Gruvberger-Saal SK, Persson C, et al. Recurrent gross mutations of the *PTEN* tumor suppressor gene in breast cancers with deficient DSB repair. Nat Genet 2008;40:102–7.

[27] Fraser M, Zhao H, Luoto KR, et al. *PTEN* deletion in prostate cancer cells does not associate with loss of RAD51 function: implications for radiotherapy and chemotherapy. Clin Cancer Res 2012;18:1015–27.

[28] Gelmon KA, Tischkowitz M, Mackay H, Swenerton K, Robidoux A, Tonkin K, et al. Olaparib in patients with high grade serous or poorly differentiated ovarian carcinoma or triple negative breast cancer: a phase 2, multicenter, open-label, nonrandomized study. Lancet Oncol 2011;12:852–61.

[29] Pennington KP, Swisher EM. Hereditary ovarian cancer: beyond the usual suspects. Gynecol Oncol 2012;124:347–53.

[30] Ben DY, Chetrit A, Hirsh-yechezkel G, et al. Effect of *BRCA* mutations on the length of survival in epithelial ovarian tumors. J Clin Oncol 2002;20:463–6.

[31] Majadak EJ, Debniak J, Milczek T, et al. Pronostic impact of *BRCA1* pathogenic and *BRCA1/BRCA2* unclassified variant mutations in patients with ovarian carcinoma. Cancer 2005;104:1004–12.

[32] Pharoah PD, Easton DF, Stockton DL, Gaytner S, Ponder BA. Survival in familial, *BRCA*-ASSOCIATED, and *BRCA2*-associated epithelial ovarian cancer. Unite Kingdom Coordinating Committee for Cancer Research (UKCCCR) Familial Ovarian Cancer Study Group. Cancer Res 1999;59:868–71.

[33] Lynch HT, Smyrk T, Lynch J. An update of HNPCC (Lynch syndrome). Cancer Genet Cytogenet 1997;93:84–99.

[34] Varado-Cabrero I, Young RH, Vamvakas EC, Scully RE. Carcinoma of the fallopian tube: a clinicopathological study of 105 cases with observations on staging and prognostic factors. Gynecol Oncol 1999;72:367–79.

[35] Rebbeck TR, Levin AM, Eisen A, et al. Breast cancer risk after bilateral prophylactic oophorectomy in *BRCA1* mutation carriers. J Natl Cancer Inst 1999:91:1475–9.

[36] Madalinska JB, Hollenstein J, Bleiker E, et al. Quality-of-life effects of propuhylactic salpingo-oophorectomy versus gynecologic screening among women at an increased risk of hereditary ovarian cancer. J Clin Oncol 2005;23:6890–8.

[37] Casey MJ, Synder C, Bewtra C, Narod SA, Watson P, Lynch HT. Intra-abdominal carcinmatosis after prophylactic oophorectomy in women of hereditary breast ovarian cancer syndrome kindreds associated with *BRCA1* and *BRCA2* mutations. Gynecol Oncol 2005;97:457–67.

[38] Finch A, Shaw P, Rosen B, Murphy J, Narod SA, Colgan TJ. Clinical and pathologic findings of prophylactic salpingo-oophorectomies in 159 *BRCA1* and *BRCA2* carriers. Gynecol Oncol 2006;100:58–64.

[39] Powell CB, Kenley E, Chen LM, et al. Risk-reducing Salpingo-oophorectomiy in *BRCA*mMutation carriers: role of serial sectioning in the detection of occult malignancy. J Clin Oncol 2005;23:127–32.

[40] Hansen K, Kelly M. Review of mammalian DNA repair and translational implications. J Pharmacol Exp Ther 2000;295:1e9.

[41] Plummer R. Poly (ADP- ribose) polymerase (PARP) inhibitors: from bench to bedside. Clin Oncol 2014;26:250–6.

[42] Christmann M, Tomicic MT, Roos WP, Kaina B. Mechanisms of human DNA repair: an update. Toxicology 2003;19:3e34.

[43] Pernin V, Mégnin-Chanet F, Pennaneach V, et al. Inhibiteurs de PARP et radiothérapie: rationnel et perspectives pour une utilisation en clinique. Cancer/Radiothérapie 2014 Dec;18:790–8.

[44] Do K, Chen AP. Molecular pathways: targeting PARP in cancer treatment. Clin Cancer Res 2012;19:977–84.

[45] Lord CJ, Ashworth A. The DNA damage response and cancer therapy. Nature 2012;481:287–94.

[46] Liu JF, Konstantinopoulos PA, Matulonis UA. PARP inhibitors in ovarian cancer: Current status and future promise. Gynecol Oncol 2014;133:362–9.

[47] Bauer PI, Buki KG, Hakam A, Kun E. Macromolecular association of ADP-ribose osyltransferase and its correlation with enzymic activity [J]. Biochem J 1990;270:17–26.

[48] Hoeijmakers JH. Genome maintenance mechanisms for preventing cancer. Nature 2001;411:366–74.

[49] Calvert H, Azzariti A. The clinical development of inhibitors of poly(ADPribose) polymerase. Ann Oncol 2011;22(1):53–9.

[50] LoRusso P, Ji J, Li J, et al. Phase I study of the safety, pharmacokinetics and pharmacodynamics of the poly(ADP-ribose)polymerase (PARP) inhibitor veliparib (ABT-888) in combination with irinotecan (CPT- 111) in patients with advanced solid tumors. J Clin Oncol 2011;29 [Suppl.: abstract 3000].

[51] Tan AR, Toppmeyer D, Stein MN, Moss RA, Gounder M, Lindquist DC, et al. Phase I. trial of veliparib (ABT-888), a poly(ADP-ribose)polymerase (PARP) inhibitor in combination with doxorubicin and cyclophosphamide in breast cancer and other solid tumors. J Clin Oncol 2011;29 [Suppl.: abstract 3041].

[52] Kaufman B, Shapira-Frommer R, Schmutzler RK, et al. Olaparib monotherapy in patients with advanced cancer and a germline *BRCA1*/2 mutation. J Clin Oncol: Official J Am Soc Clin Oncol 2015;33:244–50.

[53] Sousa FG, Matuo R, Soares DG, et al. PARPs and the DNA damage response. Carcinogenesis 2012;33:1433–40.

[54] De Vos M, Schreiber V, Dantzer F. The diverse roles and clinical relevance of PARPs in DNA damage repair: Current state of the art. Biochem Pharmacol 2012;84:137–46.

[55] Lord CJ, Ashworth A. The DNA damage response and cancer therapy. Nature 2012;481:287–94.

[56] Rouleau M, Patel A, Hendzel MJ, Kaufmann SH, Poirier GG. PARP inhibition: PARP1 and beyond. Nat Rev Cancer 2010;10:293–301.

[57] Chambon P, Weill JD, Mandel P. Nicotinamide mononucleotide activation of new DNA-dependent polyadenylic acid synthesizing nuclear enzyme [J]. Biochem Biophys Res Commun 1963;11:39–43.

[58] Durkacz BW, Omidiji O, Gray DA, et al. (ADP- ribose)n participates in DNA excision repair [J]. Nature 1980;283(5747):593–6.

[59] Hassa PO, Haenni SS, Elser M, Hottiger MO. Nuclear ADP-ribosylation reactions in mammalian cells: where are we today and where are we going? Microbiol Mol Biol Rev 2006;70:789–829.

[60] Fong PC, Boss DS, Yap TA, Tutt A, Wu P, Mergui-Roelvink M, et al. Inhibition of poly(ADP-ribose) polymerase in tumors from *BRCA* mutation carriers. N Engl J Med 2009;361:123–34.

[61] Bryant HE, Schultz N, Thomas HD, et al. Specific killing of*BRCA2*-deficient tumors with inhibitors of poly (ADP-ribose) polymerase [J]. Nature 2005;434:913–7.

[62] Bryant HE, Petermann E, Schultz N, et al. PARP is activated at stalled forks to mediate Mre11-dependent replication restart and recombination [J]. EMBO J 2009;28:2601–15.

[63] Gelmon KA, Tischkowitz M, Mackay H, Swenerton K, Robidoux A, Tonkin K, et al. Olaparib in patients with recurrent highgrade serous or poorly differentiated ovarian carcinoma or triplenegative breast cancer: a phase 2, multicentre, open-label, non-randomised study. Lancet Oncol 2011;12:852–61.

[64] Rulten SL, Fisher AE, Robert I, et al. PARP-3 and APLF function together to accelerate nonhomologous end-joining. Mol Cell 2011;41:33–45.

[65] Boehler C, Gauthier LR, Mortusewicz O, et al. Poly(ADP-ribose) polymerase 3 (PARP3), a new comer in cellular response to DNA damage and mitotic progression. Proc Natl Acad Sci USA 2011;108:2783–8.

[66] Lee J-M, Ledermann JA, Kohn EC. PARP-inhibitors for *BRCA* 1 / 2 mutation-associated and *BRCA*-like malignancies. Ann Oncol 2014;25:32–40.

[67] Powell C, Mikropoulos C, Kaye SB, et al. Pre-clinical and clinical evaluation of PARP inhibitors as tumour-specific radiosensitisers. Cancer Treat Rev 2010;36:566–75.

[68] Kim A. Reiss, Joseph M. Herman, Marianna Zahurak et al. A phase I study of veliparib (ABT-888) in combination with low-dose fractionated whole abdominal radiation therapy in patients with advanced solid malignancies and peritoneal carcinomatosis. Clin Cancer Res 2015;January 1(21):68.

[69] Simon R, Zhang X. On the dynamics of breast tumor development in women carrying germline *BRCA1* and *BRCA2* mutations. Int J Cancer 2008;122:1916–7. Ali M, Telfer BA, McCrudden C, et al. Vasoactivity of AG014699, a clinically active small molecule inhibitor of poly(ADP-ribose) polymerase: a contributory factor to chemopotentiation in vivo? Clin Cancer Res 2009;15:6106–12.

[70] Rottenberg S, Jaspers JE, Kersbergen A, et al. High sensitivity of *BRCA1*-deficient mammary tumors to the PARP inhibitor AZD2281 alone and in combination with platinum drugs. Proc Natl Acad Sci USA 2008;105:17079–84.

[71] Evers B, Drost R, Schut E, et al. Selective inhibition of *BRCA2*-deficient mammary tumor cell growth by AZD2281 and cisplatin. Clin Cancer Res 2008;14:3916–25.

[72] Fong PC, Yap TA, Boss DS, et al. Poly (ADP)-ribose polymerase inhibition: frequent durable responses in *BRCA* carrier ovarian cancer correlating with platinum-free interval. J Clin Oncol 2010;28:2512–9.

[73] Audeh MW, Carmichael J, Penson RT, et al. Oral poly(ADP-ribose) polymerase inhibitor olaparib in patients with *BRCA1* or *BRCA2* mutations and recurrent ovarian cancer: a proof-of-concept trial. Lancet 2010;376:245–251.

[74] Kaye SB, Lubinski J, Matulonis U, et al. Phase II, openlabel, randomized, multicenter study comparing the efficacy and safety of olaparib, a poly (ADP-ribose) polymerase inhibitor, and pegylated liposomal doxorubicin in patients with *BRCA1* or *BRCA2* mutations and recurrent ovarian cancer. J Clin Oncol 2012;30(4):372–9.

[75] Adams SF, Marsh EB, Elmasri W, et al. A high response rate to liposomal doxorubicin is seen among women with *BRCA* mutations treated for recurrent epithelial ovarian cancer. Gynecol Oncol 2011;123(3):486–91.

[76] Ledermann JA, Harter P, Gourley C, Friedlander M, Vergote I, Rustin G, et al. Olaparib maintenance therapy in platinum-sensitive relapsed ovarian cancer. N Engl J Med 2012;366:1382–92.

[77] Ledermann J, Harter P, Gourley C. Olaparib maintenance therapy in patients with platinumsensitive relapsed serous ovarian cancer: a preplanned retrospective analysis of outcomes by *BRCA* status in a randomised phase 2 trial. Lancet Oncol 2014;15:852–61.

[78] Oza AM, Cibula D, Benzaquen AO, et al. Olaparib combined with chemotherapy for recurrent platinum-sensitive ovarian cancer: a randomised phase 2 trial. Th lancet Oncology 2015;16:87–97.

[79] Joyce F Liu, William T Barry, Michael Birrer, et al. Combination cedirani and olaparib versus olaparib alone for women with recurrent platinum- sensitive ovarian cancer: a randomised phase 2 study. Lancet Oncol 2014;15:1207–14.

[80] Scott CL, Elizabeth M, Scott HK. Poly (ADP-ribose) Polymerase inhibitors: recent advances and future development. J Clin Oncol 33.

[81] Lehmann BD, Bauer JA, Chen X, et al. Identification of human triple-negative breast cancer subtypes and preclinical models for selection of targeted therapies. J Clin Invest 2011;121:2750–67.

[82] Balko JM, Giltnane JM, Wang K, et al. Molecular profiling of the residual disease of triple-negative breast cancers after neoadjuvant chemotherapy identifies actionable therapeutic targets. Cancer Discov 2014;4:232–45.

[83] Gonzalez-Angulo AM, Timms KM, Liu S, et al. Incidence and outcome of *BRCA* mutations in unselected patients with triple receptor-negative breast cancer. Clin Cancer Res 2011;17:1082–9.

[84] Kathleen NM, DiSilvestro P, Elizabeth S, Sally G, Pujade-Lauraine E. SOLO1 and SOLO2: Randomized phase III trials of olaparib in patients (pts) with ovarian cancer and a *BRCA1/2* mutation (*BRCA*m). J Clin Oncol 2014;32:5s(suppl; abstr TPS5616).

[85] Samol J, Ranson M, Scott E, et al. Safety and tolerability of the poly(ADP-ribose) polymerase (PARP) inhibitor, Olaparib (AZD2281) in combination with topotecan for the treatment of patients with advanced solid tumours: a phase I study. Invest New Drugs 2011;30(4):1493–500.

[86] Khan OA, Gore M, Lorigan P, et al. A phase I study of the safety and tolerability of olaparib (AZD2281, KU0059436) and dacarbazine in patients with advanced solid tumours. Br J Cancer 2011;104:750–5.

[87] Dent RA, Lindeman GJ, Clemons M, et al. Safety and efficacy of the oral PARP inhibitor Olaparib (AZD2281) in combination with paclitaxel for the first or second-line treatment of patients with metastatic triple-negative breast cancer: results from the safety cohort of a phase I/II multicenter trial. J Clin Oncol 2011;28(15S):1018 (abstract).

[88] Rajan A, Carter CA, Kelly RJ, et al. A phase I combination study of olaparib with cisplatin and gemcitabine in adults with solid tumours. Clin Cancer Res 2012;18(8): 2344–51.

[89] Dean E, Middleton MR, Pwint T, et al. Phase I study to assess the safety and tolerability of Olaparib in combination with Bevacizumab in patients with advanced solid tumours. Br J Cancer 2012;106(3):468–74.

[90] Chen Y, Zhang L, Hao Q. Olaparib: a promising PARP inhibitor in ovarian cancer therapy. Arch Gynecol Obstet 2013;288:367–74.

[91] Norquist B, Wurz KA, Pennil CC, Garcia R, Gross J, Sakai W, et al. Secondary somatic mutations restoring *BRCA1*/2 predict chemotherapy resistance in hereditary ovarian carcinomas. J Clin Oncol 2011;29:3008–15.

[92] Johnson N, Johnson SF, Yao W, et al. Stabilization of mutant *BRCA1* protein confers PARP inhibitor and platinum resistance. Proc Natl Acad Sci U S A 2013;110:17041–6.

[93] Sakai W, Swisher EM, Karlan BY, et al. Secondary mutations as a mechanism of cisplatin resistance in *BRCA2*-mutated cancers [J]. Nature 2008;451:1116–20.

[94] Rottenberg S, Jaspers JE, Kersbergen A, et al. High sensitivity of *BRCA1*-deficient mammary tumors to the PARP inhibitor AZD2281 alone and in combination with platinum durgs. PROC Natl Acad Sci USA 2008;105:17079–84.

[95] Pennington KP, Walsh T, Harrell MI, et al. Germline and somatic mutations in homologous recombination genes predict platinum response and survival in ovarian, fallopian tube, and peritoneal carcinomas. Clin Cancer Res 2014;20:764–75.

[96] Liu JF, Konstantinopoulos PA, Matulonis UA. PARP inhibitors in ovarian cancer: Current status and future promise. Gynecol Oncol 2014;133:362–9.

Chapter 6

Ovarian Cancer Research in the Post Genomic Era — Challenges and Opportunities

Alicia A. Goyeneche and Carlos M. Telleria

Additional information is available at the end of the chapter

http://dx.doi.org/10.5772/60600

Abstract

The field of ovarian cancer research is undergoing major re-examination. Pathologists are defining the disease in new terms, and—having observed discrepancies in its actual cell(s) and tissue(s) of origin—are asking whether or not ovarian cancer truly represents one disease or a complex group of diseases. Further complexity was unveiled after sequencing a large number of high-grade serous ovarian cancer tumor samples (the most frequent ovarian cancer histotype). The experiments uncovered the existence of at least four different molecular subtypes, which standard pathological assessment cannot determine. These discoveries propelled a need for designing novel model systems to study the disease and to develop therapies tailored to the molecular genetics of the tumor. Though there has been no major breakthrough as regards overall patient survival of ovarian cancer in the last 50 years, this chapter summarizes the many challenges and fascinating opportunities scientists face in altering the fatal course of this disease.

Keywords: Epithelial ovarian cancer (EOC), the cancer genome atlas (TCGA), patient-derived xenografts (PDXs), peritoneal ovarian carcinomatosis, tumor burden, ; tumor dormancy, minimal residual disease (MRD), high-grade serous ovarian cancer (HGSOC), Genetically engineered mouse models (GEMM), single nucleotide polymorphisms (SNPs), Calculator of Ovarian Carcinoma Subtype Prediction (COSP)

1. Introduction

1.1. Ovarian cancer represents various diseases

Epithelial ovarian cancer (EOC) is the deadliest gynecological disease. Over 70% of patients are diagnosed at late stages when the disease has disseminated within the abdominopelvic cavity. This is due to a lack of specific symptoms and valid biomarkers to look out for in early screenings, a consequence of the poor understanding of the disease's pathobiology. Upon late diagnosis, the standardized treatment is surgery (to remove all macroscopic disease within the abdominal cavity), followed by 6 cycles of a platinating, DNA-damaging agent combined with a taxane that disrupts microtubule function. Ninety percent of patients with late diagnosis, despite showing a promising initial response to standard of care treatment, ultimately relapse and die of the disease. The 5-year survival rate for EOC has remained below 35% over the past 20 years (rev.in [1-6]).

EOC genetically and biologically represents various diseases with different sites of origin that share common anatomical locations in the abdominal cavity when symptomatic [6]. EOCs are histologically classified as low-grade serous carcinoma, endometrioid carcinoma, clear-cell carcinoma, mucinous carcinoma, and high-grade serous ovarian carcinoma (HGSOC) [4]. Mucinous ovarian tumors are frequently the result of metastatic gastrointestinal cancers. Clear ovarian cancers and endometrioid ovarian cancers likely originate from endometrioid lesions, whereas serous ovarian cancers have 3 likely sites of origin: (1) the secretory cells of the distal fallopian tubes, (2) the ovarian surface epithelium, and (3) a niche of cells found in the hilum region of the ovary in a transitional area among the ovarian surface epithelium, the mesothelium, and the tubal epithelium [7, 8]. Among serous ovarian cancers, the low-grade serous tumors often carry wild-type p53 gene, are chromosomally stable and frequently unresponsive to platinum therapy, and carry Ras mutations. In contrast, HGSOC are p53 mutant and usually highly responsive to platinum therapy, and carry widespread DNA copy changes and wild-type Ras [9].

HGSOC is the most aggressive subtype of EOC, represents the majority of cases of EOC, and causes almost 70% of all deaths from this disease [9]. The Cancer Genome Atlas (TCGA) network reported the genetic sequencing of 489 tumors histopathologically classified as HGSOC [10]. The study confirmed, in a larger cohort of patients, that the genetic signature of HGSOC involves mutation of tumor suppressor p53 in 96-97% of cases, as previously described in a smaller cohort [11], with almost 50% of the tumors having dysregulation of the homologous recombination DNA repair pathway. The study led to revisiting HGSOC in terms of its biology, response to chemotherapy, clinical outcome, and genetic subtypes [6, 9, 12].

2. There are insufficient model systems to study ovarian cancer in vivo

The stagnation in successfully treating patients with EOC is compounded with an insufficiency of model systems to study the disease when harbored within the abdominopelvic cavity. Four main approaches have been used to study EOC in vivo in mice: (1) genetically engineered mouse models (GEMM) that develop EOC from the epithelium of the ovaries [13-15] or the oviducts (fallopian tubes) [16, 17]; (2) syngeneic models in which mouse EOC cells are orthotopically xenografted into the ovarian bursa [18] or the peritoneal cavity [19] of immunocompetent mice; (3) patient-derived xenografts (PDX) models in which the tumors of the patients are transplanted into the peritoneal cavity of severe immunodeficient mice (deficient in T-cells, B-cells and NK cells) [20-22]); and (4) xenografts of human EOC cells into the flanks or the abdominal cavity of nude, T-cell deficient mice [23]. Current GEMM of EOC facilitate studying the disease from its inception. Yet, due to a lack of highly specific promoters to target the presumed cells of origin, the GEMM do not develop the same genetic lesions carried by patients, and, hence, do not recapitulate the human phenotype in its entirety (rev.in [24, 25]). The use of mouse EOC cells xenografted in immunocompetent mice is highly relevant since the disease can be assessed in the presence of an intact immune system; however, the number of available models is limited [18, 19]. PDX closely recapitulate the histology of the patient's sample when placed within the peritoneal cavity as a finely minced tumor with some variability depending on the host mice. For instance, when human ovarian cancer tissues are xenografted in SCID (C.B-17/IcrHsd-*Prkdc*^{scid} *Lyst*^{bg}) mice, the human stroma accompanying the cancer cells is rapidly replaced with mouse stroma [22]. In contrast, in severe immunodeficient NOD-SCID IL2Rγ^{null} (NSG) mice lacking acquired and innate immunities [26], the tumor associated human stromal cells (e.g. fibroblasts and lymphocytes) remain functional for an extended period of time [20]. Nevertheless, the xenograft of EOC into the peritoneal cavity of immunosuppressed mice recapitulates only a late phase of disease as the cells are directly deposited into the peritoneal cavity of a host. Clearly, each model system for recapitulating EOC in mouse models has shortcomings.

3. The progression of epithelial ovarian cancer within the abdominopelvic cavity is not easy to assess

Studies involving the implantation of EOC cells in the peritoneal cavity (intraperitoneally; i.p.) of host mice are limited when compared to the number of studies done using EOC cells xenografted subcutaneously (s.c.) (rev.in [25, 27]). One main reason for this discrepancy is that the growth of s.c. tumors can be monitored easily using precision calipers; yet, this site fails to represent the environment of the abdominal cavity in which EOC thrive. The struggle to analyze disease progression in the peritoneal cavity is that it requires sophisticated, non-invasive, imaging approaches to follow the development of internal tumor nodules in a context of a lack of well-defined parameters of tumor burden [28]. In most studies done with i.p. xenografts, tumor burden has been assessed by recording overall survival [23], noting volume of ascites accumulated [29], or calculating the total mass of what is considered tumoral tissue after collection from the abdominal cavity at necropsy [30]. More recently, non-invasive imaging methods to evaluate tumor progression in longitudinal studies have been developed, yet their application in evaluating EOC within the peritoneal cavity has been limited [25]. Overall, information as to how EOC develops within the abdominal cavity is scarce. Preferred sites of anatomical distribution of the tumors remain unknown as do their histopathology and molecular genetics.

4. Peritoneal ovarian cancer needs to be studied in different regions of the abdominopelvic cavity

It is feasible that solid nodules that develop, for instance, in the omentum, have a different genetic profile when compared with sibling nodules found in other sites, such as the diaphragm, the surface of the liver, the bowel, or the lower pelvic cavity. This might be due to tissues (to which each tumor foci must adapt) having different histological and physiological micro-environments, likely impinging on the behavior of the cancer cells. Depending on the nearby tissue microenvironment, cancer cells may hijack otherwise non-malignant cells in a different manner depending on the anatomical location of the foci. As a consequence, this differential tumor adaptation to the environment may explain the apparent heterogeneity observed in tumors found within the peritoneal cavity of patients at the moment of debulking surgery, sometimes leading to difficulties in making the correct histopathological diagnosis of the overall disease. Thus, there is an urgent need to (1) standardize, across a genetically-defined group of available EOC cell lines, a common set of histopathological and genetic biomarkers of disease growing in the abdominal cavity; and (2) determine if such biomarkers, despite being expressed from the same cell types of origin, show heterogeneity according to the site within the abdominal cavity where the tumor develops. For instance, evidence suggests that omental vs. ovarian sites of HGSOC patients show variability in the host stromal responses among the sites [31]. Another study using biopsies from different sites within the peritoneal cavity of patients with HGSOC show heterogeneity or clonal diversity among the tumor sites manifested by single nucleotide polymorphisms (SNPs) associated with differentially expressed genes [32].

One tool currently available for characterizing the histopathological subtype of ovarian carcinomas is the Calculator of Ovarian Carcinoma Subtype Prediction (COSP), which is an algorithm that encompasses 9 predictive biomarkers and is used to differentiate histotypes of EOCs. The algorithm is freely accessible [33] and permits the scoring by immunohistochemistry, using standardized antibodies and incubation procedures, the abundances of WT1 (Wilms Tumor 1), p16 (cyclin dependent kinase inhibitor 2A; CDKN2A), DKK1 (dickkopf homolog 1), VIM (vimentin), p53 (TP53), PRG (progesterone receptor), TFF3 (trefoil factor 3 [intestinal]), HNF1B (hepatocyte nuclear factor 1β) and MDM2 (mouse double minute 2). The scores for these markers are 0 or 1, except for p53 that has scores of 0 (no expression denoting null p53), 1 (low abundance for wild type p53), or 2 (high abundance for mutant p53). For instance, for the Kuramochi ovarian cancer cell line (see later Table 1), the algorithm predicts a HGSOC histotype with 97% probability, whereas for the popular A2780 ovarian cancer cell line (see later Fig.1), the algorithm predicts an endometrioid histotype with 94% probability [34]. A limitation to the algorithm is its difficulty in clearly differentiating between low-grade and high-grade serous histotypes. However, low-grade serous ovarian carcinomas only account for ~3% of all [35]. Furthermore, a combination of histological assessment and molecular genetic profiles should be able to distinguish between these two serous ovarian cancer subtypes.

5. Most popular epithelial ovarian cancer cell lines used to study peritoneal carcinomatosis in mouse models give rise to disparate intra-abdominal disease phenotypes

Common EOC cell lines, utilized for years in preclinical studies, were evaluated for their ability to cause i.p. tumors [23]. ES-2, A2780, and HEY cells (all originally diagnosed as undifferentiated carcinomas), OV2008 (likely originated from an endometrial carcinoma), and SKOV-3 (which depicts a clear-cell adenocarcinoma histotype in xenografts) all develop intra-abdominal tumors in less than 3 months. The tumors are described as "dense solid," often accompanied by accumulation of cellular ascites. Our experience with widely used EOC cell lines reveals different times for the establishment of the xenografts and highly diverse anatomical depiction of the solid growths within the abdominal cavity among the different cell lines. IGROV-1 cells generate large solid masses termed omental cakes that expand toward the lower pelvic cavity (Fig.1A). SKOV-3 cells develop small yet multiple nodules in the mesentery and the omentum (Fig.1B), while A2780 cells develop large solid masses, taking the ovaries and the lower pelvic cavity (Fig.1C). The diversity in anatomical growths is likely due to the varied histotypes and genetic profiles represented by these cell lines (see later) [36].

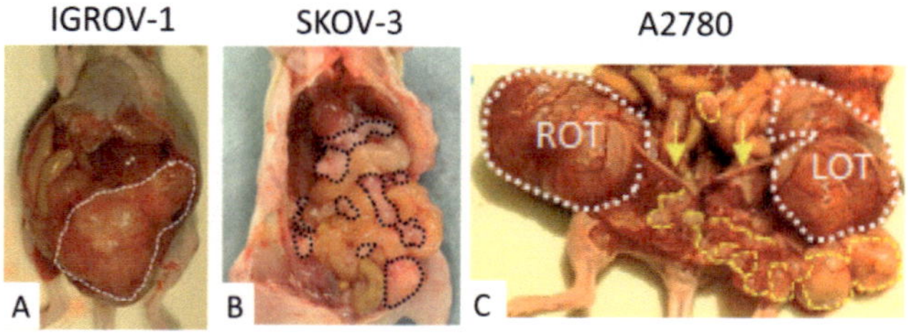

Figure 1. Peritoneal disease caused by IGROV-1 (A), SKOV-3 (B), and A2780 (C) EOC cells. The images were taken after 4 weeks of injection for IGROV-1, 10 weeks for SKOV-3, and 6 weeks for A2780 tumors. In A, the growth within the peritoneal cavity is mostly confined to an "omental cake" (white area). In B, dotted black areas show solid tumors adhering to fat in the pelvic region, intestines, and mesentery. In C, right (ROT) and left (LOT) ovarian tumors clearly are connected to the uterine horns (yellow arrows). Ovaries carrying tumors have more blood supply and are larger than the rest of the peritoneal, pale nodules (yellow pattern).

6. The majority of epithelial ovarian cancer cell lines used for preclinical studies do not embody the most frequent histotype of the disease

Based on the genetic signatures published from over 50 human ovarian cancer cell lines widely available, out of the approximately 100 that have been described in the literature [36-38], it is apparent that the vast majority of the cell lines overwhelmingly used for over 30 years to study the disease have a genotype which does not resemble the most predominant histotype of EOC, HGSOCs. This may be a major contributing factor in the failure to bring new and effective treatments of HGSOC to clinical practice.

The cell lines currently characterized as likely representing HGSOC [36-38] were developed in the 1970s and 1980s and have been poorly described. Oftentimes they lack information on the original histopathological diagnosis, are poorly linked to patient data, and were developed from ascites or solid nodules following an array of protocols not always clearly stated. It is imperative that biomedical researchers worldwide join efforts to develop new, highly standardized and annotated ovarian cancer cell lines. These cells lines should be developed under similar isolation and culture protocols as to prevent inter-laboratory variations in their behavior, thus accelerating the creation of new knowledge in the field of preclinical ovarian cancer modelling and therapy. By taking advantage of the progress made in the area of molecular genetics and ovarian cancer biology, it is time to generate new cell lines that genetically and histopathologically can be characterized as pertaining, for instance, to the HGSOC histotype, and, within it, to each one of the molecular subtypes described by Tothill et al. [39] and later on confirmed in a larger cohort of patients [10]. Additionally, there is a timely opportunity to utilize these biological resources with the objective of standardizing mouse models of intra-abdominal disease caused by genetically-identified HGSOC cells.

7. The need for an expanded definition of tumor burden when referring to peritoneal ovarian cancer carcinomatosis

Limiting preclinical analysis of tumor burden to overall survival, tumor mass, or volume of ascites accumulated is not sufficient if we are to find early metrics of response to new therapies as well as early signs and symptoms of the disease. Re-defining tumor burden in peritoneal ovarian cancer in a comprehensive manner should provide investigators worldwide with multifaceted metrics—anatomical, physiological, and behavioral—to be followed to understand the biology of the progression of EOC and, most importantly, that of the most frequent HGSOC type. The metrics should also allow inter-laboratory and inter-cell line comparisons of HGSOC as a unique disease, provide standardized benchmarks for testing new preclinical therapies, reveal markers of disease state with clinical implications for earlier diagnosis, and provide a baseline reference for the validation of new HGSOC cell lines established from patients with well-documented medical history and annotated histopathological diagnosis of HGSOC.

Based on recently published genotypes [36-38], it is feasible to begin redefining peritoneal ovarian tumor burden by utilizing the currently available cell lines that have the highest probability of genetically representing HGSOC (some examples are displayed in Table 1). Despite that each cell line was established using different culture conditions, we should standardize all cell lines to grow under the same culture conditions to avoid bias and proceed to authenticate them using DNA microsatellite short tandem repeats (STR) as recently recommended [37]. Only cell lines which match their STR public genetic database 90-100% should be used worldwide [40]. Validated cell lines may be injected i.p. in the lower pelvic region of widely available immunosuppressed female mice lacking T-cell function (Hsd: Athymic Nude-*Foxn1*^{nu}) or in severe immunodeficient NOD/SCID/IL2Rγ^{null} mice lacking acquired and innate immunities [26]. Disease progression can then be followed and the signs and symptoms contrasted against non-cancerous, age-matched controls studied in parallel.

The animals can be monitored to record body weight, abdominal circumference, body temperature, and food/water intake to build a clinical history of each animal as the disease progresses, using biomarkers of tumor progression [41]. The experimental animals and age-matched, non-cancer controls also can be subjected to a battery of behavioral tests to assess visceral pain, motor function, and depression-like behavior (helplessness and social withdrawal). In animal models of EOC, depressive-like behaviors may be facilitated by the production of inflammatory cytokines from the cancer cells acting at the level of brain regions like the hippocampus [42, 43] and thus, may be a sensitive marker of disease state. Finally, these parameters can be completed with longitudinal, intra-abdominal anatomy of the tumor-carrying mice using non-invasive imaging approaches (e.g. micro-ultrasound) [44, 45]. The recorded images can then be analyzed longitudinally to identify the formation and progression of intra-abdominal solid masses and accumulation of ascites fluid. On selected masses, it is also possible to study vascularity using 3D power Doppler ultrasound [46, 47].

Cell Line	Original Histological Classification
KURAMOCHI*	undifferentiated
OVSAHO*	serous
SNU119*	serous
COV362*	endometrioid
OVCAR4*	undifferentiated
COV318*†	serous
JHOS4*†	serous
PEO1**†	serous
PEO4**†	serous
PEO6**	serous
PEO14**†	serous
TO14**	serous
PEO23**†	serous
PEA1**†	serous
PEA2**†	serous

* [36]; ** [38]; † [37].

Table 1. Epithelial ovarian cancer cell lines with likely HGSOC genomic classification.

The accumulation of bloody ascites in the abdominopelvic cavity suggests that changes in vascular integrity, with possible effects on blood pressure and oxygen delivered, are taking place. Indeed, declines in oxygenation and blood pressure have been suggested as biomarkers of peritoneal tumor progression [28]. Thus, as part of a comprehensive approach for assessing tumor burden, we suggest determining the level of peripheral blood oxygen saturation [48] and blood pressure [49]. Finally, we propose completing the assessment of tumor burden by taking a blood sample from the animals in order to (1) measure cancer antigen CA-125 used as a biomarker of EOC disease progression [50]; (2) study hematological parameters that can be altered due to tumor burden—e.g. red and white blood cell counts, platelets, hemoglobin concentration, and hematocrit; (3) perform chemical analysis of GOT (glutamic oxaloacetic transaminase) and GPT (glutamic pyruvic transaminase) as surrogate markers of hepatic function; (4) measure serum levels of creatinine and urea as surrogate markers of renal function; and (5) measure serum levels of estradiol and progesterone, since they impact the outcome of the behavioral tests suggested above.

8. Understanding all cellular components of advanced disease

In ovarian cancer, metastasis through the vasculature is rare and a very late manifestation of the disease. Instead, ovarian cancer cells are prone to spread by direct extension from the ovaries to adjacent tissues, or to detach from the primary ovarian tumor directly into the peritoneal cavity where they seed the mesothelium of the omentum, diaphragm, bowel serosa, and the entire peritoneum [51-53]. Widespread visceral and intestinal wall metastases with formation of adhesions between the loops of the bowel cause intestinal obstruction, prevent normal nutrition, and become a primary cause of death [1].

The high incidence (65%) of peritoneal malignant effusions in ovarian cancer patients at advanced presentation [54, 55], and the development of symptoms due to ascites accumulation at diagnosis as well as recurrence [56], suggest that the "liquid" component is an active pathogenic manifestation of the disease. Ovarian cancer cells isolated from peritoneal ascites of major ovarian cancer histological types were described as organized structures of different sizes and heterogeneous morphology [57]. Furthermore, multicellular structures isolated directly from ascites were shown capable of adhering ex vivo to components of the extracellular matrix and to monolayers of mesothelial cells, suggesting their participation in the dissemination of ovarian cancer [58]. Cancer cells isolated from ascites and metastatic secondary sites exhibit a higher percentage of stemness markers when compared to their primary tumors [59-61]. Additionally, cancer-associated proteins and mRNAs are differentially expressed in peritoneal effusions when compared to primary carcinomas or solid metastases. Lastly, there is a differential gene expression among peritoneal effusions when comparing samples at diagnosis (pre-chemotherapy) vs. samples at recurrence (post-chemotherapy) [62]. Altogether, these data suggest that cancer cells within effusions—the "liquid" component of ovarian cancer—represent a biomarker of tumor evolution toward a more aggressive/ advanced disease phenotype of poor prognosis.

Most of our understanding of the biology of ovarian cancer multicellular structures is based on the premise that mono-dispersed ovarian cancer cells, when gathering together either by enforced gravity or prevention of adhesion, mimic the program of assembly followed by ovarian cancer multicellular structures found within malignant effusions [63, 64]. Therefore, it is of importance to define if ovarian cancer multicellular structures found in ascites represent aggregation following shedding from solid tumors or, instead, are active products of disease selection and critical drivers of disease advancement and prognosis (Fig.2).

While the presence of multicellular structures in ascites was reported over 25 years ago [57], their biology has been studied using in vitro platforms and multicellular structures that were forced to form from ovarian cancer cell lines by using either gravity or non-adherent conditions. We should investigate the pathogenic capacity of unforced, spontaneously arranged ovarian cancer multicellular structures in vivo. If a key mechanism for ovarian cancer progression takes place within the "liquid" component of the disease, then multicellular structures may represent a druggable target. Developing therapeutic interventions to interrupt formation of multicellular structures free-floating in the peritoneal fluid may be an efficient way of interrupting disease advancement.

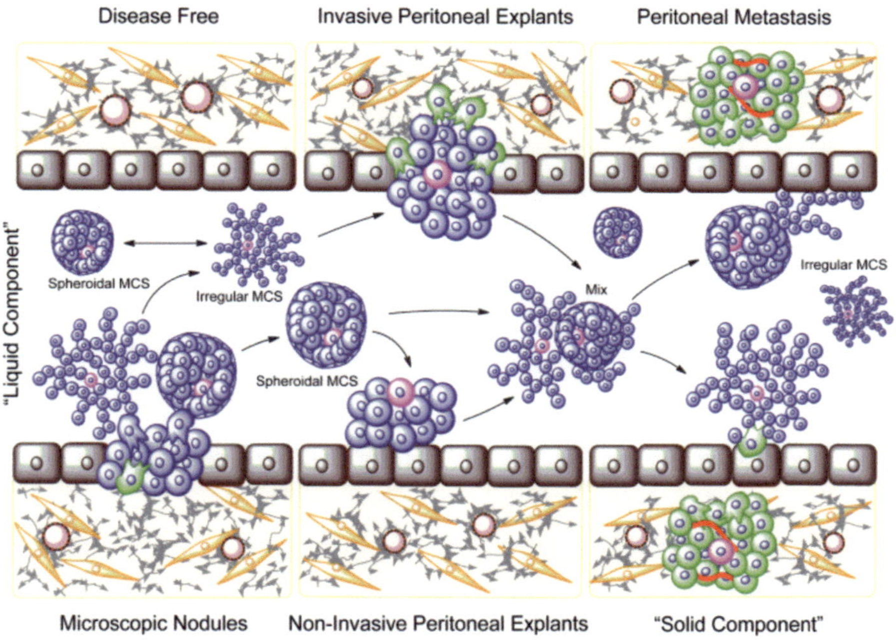

Figure 2. Proposed model for the role of ovarian cancer multicellular structures (MCS) in peritoneal carcinomatosis. Selected cells from microscopic nodules with distinctive capacity to form MCS, adapt, survive, and grow in the peritoneal fluid developing irregular and organized spheroidal MCS that might evade chemotherapy and/or preserve ovarian cancer initiating cells (CIC), leading to a feed-forward, chemo-resistant, and self-renewal recurrent seeding. MCS committed to develop the solid component of the disease will adhere, disaggregate, migrate, and invade the mesothelial cell layer covering the surface of the peritoneum (maroon), and form foci that neo-vascularize and grow (green). Other MCS might develop non-invasive nodules that amplify the cellularity within the "liquid" compartment causing ascites. Blue: highly differentiated ovarian cancer cells. Pink: less differentiated ovarian cancer cells with self-renewal capacity. Red: new blood vessels. Gray: extracellular matrix. Yellow: fibroblasts.

9. Understanding dormancy after "successful" standard of care (surgery and chemotherapy)

Although most patients diagnosed with ovarian cancer undergo remission after optimal surgical cytoreduction and platinum-taxane chemotherapy, microscopic foci of cells manage to survive within the peritoneal cavity and recreate the illness. Recurrence develops a more aggressive phenotype for which current therapies almost always fail (rev.in [1-6]). Thus, understanding the biology of minimal residual disease is crucial in developing effective therapies for ovarian cancer.

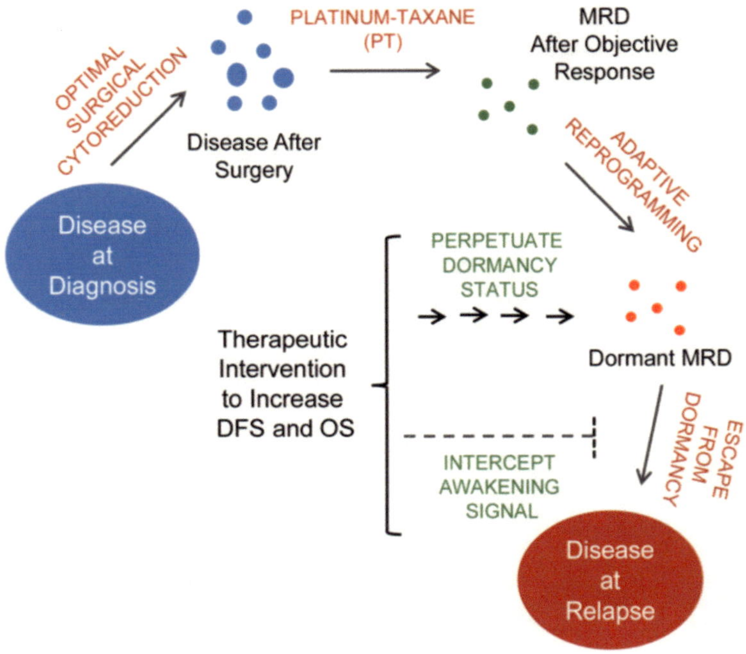

Figure 3. Hypothetical model of ovarian cancer dormancy after debulking surgery and platinum–taxane (PT) therapy, relapse after chemotherapy-associated dormancy, and potential stages of the disease where therapeutic intervention is envisioned. DFS, disease free survival; OS, overall survival. MRD, minimal residual disease.

Within the minimal residual disease, ovarian cancer cells are in a unique, subclinical, biological stage termed dormancy. Long recognized in the clinic, *dormancy* describes a period of time that can last many years between primary therapy and recurrence of metastatic disease (rev.in [65]). In ovarian cancer, dormancy was reported to be represented by small, poorly vascularized fibrotic nodules located on the surface of the peritoneum in patients undergoing second-look surgery after front-line debulking operation and chemotherapy [66]. Dormant cancer cells are usually defined as survivors of primary therapy likely containing drug-resistant, tumor-initiating cells. They are kept either in a status of cell cycle arrest (quiescence) or equilibrium among proliferating and dying cells to preserve constant micro-tumor mass (rev.in [65]). Attempts to eliminate dormant ovarian cancer cells with maintenance therapies have not been efficient: they extend progression-free survival but not overall survival [67, 68].

It is important to investigate the magnitude and location of the disease still present following an objective response to front-line therapy, and characterize the adaptive molecular reprogramming after chemotherapy leading to the dormant status of the cells comprising the minimal residual disease (Fig.3). Chemotherapy-associated tumor dormancy and awakening from dormancy likely have defined molecular signatures that can be unveiled by combined use of currently available transcriptomic, proteomic, and epigenomic platforms that can be integrated utilizing multipronged bioinformatic tools. Knowing the mechanism(s) ovarian cancer cells utilize to achieve dormancy in the peritoneum and awake from it will provide two potential avenues for intervention as follows: (1) perpetuation of the dormant status of the cancer; and/or (2) interception of the awakening signal that causes disease relapse (Fig.3).

Whereas total elimination of ovarian cancer cells is the ideal goal, the alternative approach of keeping ovarian cancer in a chronic dormant state is highly relevant as this would categorize ovarian cancer patients with an objective response to front-line standard of care as having a chronic manageable disease or "cancer without disease."

10. Conclusions

Progresses made in the field of molecular oncology within the last decade have been remarkable. The use of RNA sequencing, micro RNA expression profiles, mutation analysis, shotgun proteomics, reverse-phase protein arrays, and epigenomic platforms, together with novel imaging tools, should be applied in uncovering the hidden secrets of ovarian cancer initiation and progression, and in developing early diagnostic tools. Understanding the location and molecular behavior of the abdominopelvic minimal residual disease after otherwise efficient front-line chemotherapy should lead to the discovery of new molecular targets for disease interception that can be exploited to prevent recurrence. We are at a point in time in which we have a unique opportunity to utilize the vast state-of-the-art technological armamentarium developed in the past decade to revisit the basic biology of peritoneal ovarian cancer and renew hopes for bettering the prognosis of this deadly disease.

Acknowledgements

This research was supported by award CA164622 from the National Cancer Institute, the National Institutes of Health (NIH), funds from the Division of Basic Biomedical Sciences of the Sanford School of Medicine of the University of South Dakota, and a donation from the SuFuDu Drumline. We thank Nahuel Telleria for proofreading the manuscript.

Author details

Alicia A. Goyeneche and Carlos M. Telleria*

*Address all correspondence to: carlos.telleria@usd.edu

Division of Basic Biomedical Sciences, Sanford School of Medicine, The University of South Dakota, Vermillion, South Dakota, USA

References

[1] Bast RC, Jr., Hennessy B, Mills GB. The biology of ovarian cancer: new opportunities for translation. Nature Reviews Cancer. 2009;9:415-28.

[2] Bast RC, Jr. Molecular approaches to personalizing management of ovarian cancer. Annals of Oncology : Official Journal of the European Society for Medical Oncology / ESMO. 2011;22 Suppl 8:viii5-viii15.

[3] Coleman RL, Monk BJ, Sood AK, Herzog TJ. Latest research and treatment of advanced-stage epithelial ovarian cancer. Nature Reviews Clinical Oncology. 2013;10:211-24.

[4] Kurman RJ, Shih Ie M. Molecular pathogenesis and extraovarian origin of epithelial ovarian cancer--shifting the paradigm. Human Pathology. 2011;42:918-31.

[5] Romero I, Bast RC, Jr. Minireview: human ovarian cancer: biology, current management, and paths to personalizing therapy. Endocrinology. 2012;153:1593-602.

[6] Vaughan S, Coward JI, Bast RC, Jr., Berchuck A, Berek JS, Brenton JD, et al. Rethinking ovarian cancer: recommendations for improving outcomes. Nature Reviews Cancer. 2011;11:719-25.

[7] Auersperg N. The origin of ovarian carcinomas: a unifying hypothesis. International Journal of Gynecological Pathology : Official Journal of the International Society of Gynecological Pathologists. 2011;30:12-21.

[8] Flesken-Nikitin A, Hwang CI, Cheng CY, Michurina TV, Enikolopov G, Nikitin AY. Ovarian surface epithelium at the junction area contains a cancer-prone stem cell niche. Nature. 2013;495:241-5.

[9] Bowtell DD. The genesis and evolution of high-grade serous ovarian cancer. Nature Reviews Cancer. 2010;10:803-8.

[10] Cancer Genome Atlas Research N. Integrated genomic analyses of ovarian carcinoma. Nature. 2011;474:609-15.

[11] Ahmed AA, Etemadmoghadam D, Temple J, Lynch AG, Riad M, Sharma R, et al. Driver mutations in TP53 are ubiquitous in high grade serous carcinoma of the ovary. The Journal of Pathology. 2010;221:49-56.

[12] Berns EM, Bowtell DD. The changing view of high-grade serous ovarian cancer. Cancer Research. 2012;72:2701-4.

[13] Connolly DC, Bao R, Nikitin AY, Stephens KC, Poole TW, Hua X, et al. Female mice chimeric for expression of the simian virus 40 TAg under control of the MISIIR promoter develop epithelial ovarian cancer. Cancer Research. 2003;63:1389-97.

[14] Laviolette LA, Garson K, Macdonald EA, Senterman MK, Courville K, Crane CA, et al. 17beta-estradiol accelerates tumor onset and decreases survival in a transgenic mouse model of ovarian cancer. Endocrinology. 2010;151:929-38.

[15] Orsulic S, Li Y, Soslow RA, Vitale-Cross LA, Gutkind JS, Varmus HE. Induction of ovarian cancer by defined multiple genetic changes in a mouse model system. Cancer Cell. 2002;1:53-62.

[16] Karst AM, Levanon K, Drapkin R. Modeling high-grade serous ovarian carcinogenesis from the fallopian tube. Proceedings of the National Academy of Sciences of the United States of America. 2011;108:7547-52.

[17] Kim J, Coffey DM, Creighton CJ, Yu Z, Hawkins SM, Matzuk MM. High-grade serous ovarian cancer arises from fallopian tube in a mouse model. Proceedings of the National Academy of Sciences of the United States of America. 2012;109:3921-6.

[18] Roby KF, Taylor CC, Sweetwood JP, Cheng Y, Pace JL, Tawfik O, et al. Development of a syngeneic mouse model for events related to ovarian cancer. Carcinogenesis. 2000;21:585-91.

[19] McCloskey CW, Goldberg RL, Carter LE, Gamwell LF, Al-Hujaily EM, Collins O, et al. A new spontaneously transformed syngeneic model of high-grade serous ovarian cancer with a tumor-initiating cell population. Frontiers in Oncology. 2014;4:53.

[20] Bankert RB, Balu-Iyer SV, Odunsi K, Shultz LD, Kelleher RJ, Jr., Barnas JL, et al. Humanized mouse model of ovarian cancer recapitulates patient solid tumor progression, ascites formation, and metastasis. PloS One. 2011;6:e24420.

[21] Elkas JC, Baldwin RL, Pegram M, Tseng Y, Slamon D, Karlan BY. A human ovarian carcinoma murine xenograft model useful for preclinical trials. Gynecologic Oncology. 2002;87:200-6.

[22] Weroha SJ, Becker MA, Enderica-Gonzalez S, Harrington SC, Oberg AL, Maurer MJ, et al. Tumorgrafts as in vivo surrogates for women with ovarian cancer. Clinical Cancer Research : An Official Journal of the American Association for Cancer Research. 2014;20:1288-97.

[23] Shaw TJ, Senterman MK, Dawson K, Crane CA, Vanderhyden BC. Characterization of intraperitoneal, orthotopic, and metastatic xenograft models of human ovarian

cancer. Molecular Therapy : The Journal of the American Society of Gene Therapy. 2004;10:1032-42.

[24] Garson K, Gamwell LF, Pitre EM, Vanderhyden BC. Technical challenges and limitations of current mouse models of ovarian cancer. Journal of Ovarian Research. 2012;5:39.

[25] Lengyel E, Burdette JE, Kenny HA, Matei D, Pilrose J, Haluska P, et al. Epithelial ovarian cancer experimental models. Oncogene. 2014;33:3619-33.

[26] Ito M, Hiramatsu H, Kobayashi K, Suzue K, Kawahata M, Hioki K, et al. NOD/SCID/gamma(c)(null) mouse: an excellent recipient mouse model for engraftment of human cells. Blood. 2002;100:3175-82.

[27] Konstantinopoulos PA, Matulonis UA. Current status and evolution of preclinical drug development models of epithelial ovarian cancer. Frontiers in Oncology. 2013;3:296.

[28] Workman P, Aboagye EO, Balkwill F, Balmain A, Bruder G, Chaplin DJ, et al. Guidelines for the welfare and use of animals in cancer research. British Journal of Cancer. 2010;102:1555-77.

[29] Hu L, Hofmann J, Lu Y, Mills GB, Jaffe RB. Inhibition of phosphatidylinositol 3'-kinase increases efficacy of paclitaxel in in vitro and in vivo ovarian cancer models. Cancer Research. 2002;62:1087-92.

[30] Hu L, Hofmann J, Zaloudek C, Ferrara N, Hamilton T, Jaffe RB. Vascular endothelial growth factor immunoneutralization plus Paclitaxel markedly reduces tumor burden and ascites in athymic mouse model of ovarian cancer. The American Journal of Pathology. 2002;161:1917-24.

[31] Kobel M, Turbin D, Kalloger SE, Gao D, Huntsman DG, Gilks CB. Biomarker expression in pelvic high-grade serous carcinoma: comparison of ovarian and omental sites. International Journal of Gynecological Pathology : Official Journal of the International Society of Gynecological Pathologists. 2011;30:366-71.

[32] Cowin PA, George J, Fereday S, Loehrer E, Van Loo P, Cullinane C, et al. LRP1B deletion in high-grade serous ovarian cancers is associated with acquired chemotherapy resistance to liposomal doxorubicin. Cancer Research. 2012;72:4060-73.

[33] Kalloger SE, Kobel M, Leung S, Mehl E, Gao D, Marcon KM, et al. Calculator for ovarian carcinoma subtype prediction. Modern Pathology : An Official Journal of the United States and Canadian Academy of Pathology, Inc. 2011;24:512-21.

[34] Anglesio MS, Wiegand KC, Melnyk N, Chow C, Salamanca C, Prentice LM, et al. Type-specific cell line models for type-specific ovarian cancer research. PloS One. 2013;8:e72162.

[35] Kobel M, Kalloger SE, Huntsman DG, Santos JL, Swenerton KD, Seidman JD, et al. Differences in tumor type in low-stage versus high-stage ovarian carcinomas. Inter-

national Journal of Gynecological Pathology : Official Journal of the International Society of Gynecological Pathologists. 2010;29:203-11.

[36] Domcke S, Sinha R, Levine DA, Sander C, Schultz N. Evaluating cell lines as tumour models by comparison of genomic profiles. Nature Communications. 2013;4:2126.

[37] Beaufort CM, Helmijr JC, Piskorz AM, Hoogstraat M, Ruigrok-Ritstier K, Besselink N, et al. Ovarian cancer cell line panel (OCCP): clinical importance of in vitro morphological subtypes. PloS One. 2014;9:e103988.

[38] Cooke SL, Ng CK, Melnyk N, Garcia MJ, Hardcastle T, Temple J, et al. Genomic analysis of genetic heterogeneity and evolution in high-grade serous ovarian carcinoma. Oncogene. 2010;29:4905-13.

[39] Tothill RW, Tinker AV, George J, Brown R, Fox SB, Lade S, et al. Novel molecular subtypes of serous and endometrioid ovarian cancer linked to clinical outcome. Clinical Cancer Research : An Official Journal of the American Association for Cancer Research. 2008;14:5198-208.

[40] Marx V. Cell line authentication demystified. Nature Methods. 2014;11:483-8.

[41] Hunter JE, Butterworth J, Perkins ND, Bateson M, Richardson CA. Using body temperature, food and water consumption as biomarkers of disease progression in mice with Emu-myc lymphoma. British Journal of Cancer. 2014;110:928-34.

[42] Lamkin DM, Lutgendorf SK, Lubaroff D, Sood AK, Beltz TG, Johnson AK. Cancer induces inflammation and depressive-like behavior in the mouse: modulation by social housing. Brain, Behavior, and Immunity. 2011;25:555-64.

[43] Yang M, Kim J, Kim JS, Kim SH, Kim JC, Kang MJ, et al. Hippocampal dysfunctions in tumor-bearing mice. Brain, Behavior, and Immunity. 2014;36:147-55.

[44] Graham KC, Wirtzfeld LA, MacKenzie LT, Postenka CO, Groom AC, MacDonald IC, et al. Three-dimensional high-frequency ultrasound imaging for longitudinal evaluation of liver metastases in preclinical models. Cancer Research. 2005;65:5231-7.

[45] Wirtzfeld LA, Wu G, Bygrave M, Yamasaki Y, Sakai H, Moussa M, et al. A new three-dimensional ultrasound microimaging technology for preclinical studies using a transgenic prostate cancer mouse model. Cancer Research. 2005;65:6337-45.

[46] Jugold M, Palmowski M, Huppert J, Woenne EC, Mueller MM, Semmler W, et al. Volumetric high-frequency Doppler ultrasound enables the assessment of early antiangiogenic therapy effects on tumor xenografts in nude mice. European Radiology. 2008;18:753-8.

[47] Xuan JW, Bygrave M, Jiang H, Valiyeva F, Dunmore-Buyze J, Holdsworth DW, et al. Functional neoangiogenesis imaging of genetically engineered mouse prostate cancer using three-dimensional power Doppler ultrasound. Cancer Research. 2007;67:2830-9.

[48] Verhoeven D, Teijaro JR, Farber DL. Pulse-oximetry accurately predicts lung pathology and the immune response during influenza infection. Virology. 2009;390:151-6.

[49] Feng M, Whitesall S, Zhang Y, Beibel M, D'Alecy L, DiPetrillo K. Validation of volume-pressure recording tail-cuff blood pressure measurements. American Journal of Hypertension. 2008;21:1288-91.

[50] Rustin GJ, Bast RC, Jr., Kelloff GJ, Barrett JC, Carter SK, Nisen PD, et al. Use of CA-125 in clinical trial evaluation of new therapeutic drugs for ovarian cancer. Clinical Cancer Rresearch : An Official Journal of the American Association for Cancer Research. 2004;10:3919-26.

[51] Lengyel E. Ovarian cancer development and metastasis. The American Journal of Pathology. 2010;177:1053-64.

[52] Naora H, Montell DJ. Ovarian cancer metastasis: integrating insights from disparate model organisms. Nature Reviews Cancer. 2005;5:355-66.

[53] Tan DS, Agarwal R, Kaye SB. Mechanisms of transcoelomic metastasis in ovarian cancer. The Lancet Oncology. 2006;7:925-34.

[54] Davidson B, Risberg B, Reich R, Berner A. Effusion cytology in ovarian cancer: new molecular methods as aids to diagnosis and prognosis. Clinics in Laboratory Medicine. 2003;23:729-54, viii.

[55] Puls LE, Duniho T, Hunter JE, Kryscio R, Blackhurst D, Gallion H. The prognostic implication of ascites in advanced-stage ovarian cancer. Gynecologic Oncology. 1996;61:109-12.

[56] Kipps E, Tan DS, Kaye SB. Meeting the challenge of ascites in ovarian cancer: new avenues for therapy and research. Nature Reviews Cancer. 2013;13:273-82.

[57] Allen HJ, Porter C, Gamarra M, Piver MS, Johnson EA. Isolation and morphologic characterization of human ovarian carcinoma cell clusters present in effusions. Experimental Cell Biology. 1987;55:194-208.

[58] Burleson KM, Casey RC, Skubitz KM, Pambuccian SE, Oegema TR, Jr., Skubitz AP. Ovarian carcinoma ascites spheroids adhere to extracellular matrix components and mesothelial cell monolayers. Gynecologic Oncology. 2004;93:170-81.

[59] Alvero AB, Chen R, Fu HH, Montagna M, Schwartz PE, Rutherford T, et al. Molecular phenotyping of human ovarian cancer stem cells unravels the mechanisms for repair and chemoresistance. Cell Cycle. 2009;8:158-66.

[60] Bapat SA, Mali AM, Koppikar CB, Kurrey NK. Stem and progenitor-like cells contribute to the aggressive behavior of human epithelial ovarian cancer. Cancer Research. 2005;65:3025-9.

[61] Zhang S, Balch C, Chan MW, Lai HC, Matei D, Schilder JM, et al. Identification and characterization of ovarian cancer-initiating cells from primary human tumors. Cancer Research. 2008;68:4311-20.

[62] Davidson B, Reich R, Trope CG, Wang TL, Shih Ie M. New determinates of disease progression and outcome in metastatic ovarian carcinoma. Histology and Histopathology. 2010;25:1591-609.

[63] Burleson KM, Hansen LK, Skubitz AP. Ovarian carcinoma spheroids disaggregate on type I collagen and invade live human mesothelial cell monolayers. Clinical and Experimental Metastasis. 2004;21:685-97.

[64] Shield K, Ackland ML, Ahmed N, Rice GE. Multicellular spheroids in ovarian cancer metastases: Biology and pathology. Gynecologic Oncology. 2009;113:143-8.

[65] Goss PE, Chambers AF. Does tumour dormancy offer a therapeutic target? Nature Reviews Cancer. 2010;10:871-7.

[66] Gadducci A, Tana R, Landoni F, Ferrari F, Peiretti M, Perrone F, et al. Analysis of failures and clinical outcome of advanced epithelial ovarian cancer in patients with microscopic residual disease at second-look reassessment following primary cytoreductive surgery and first-line platinum-based chemotherapy. European Journal of Gynaecological Oncology. 2013;34:213-7.

[67] Markman M, Liu PY, Moon J, Monk BJ, Copeland L, Wilczynski S, et al. Impact on survival of 12 versus 3 monthly cycles of paclitaxel (175 mg/m2) administered to patients with advanced ovarian cancer who attained a complete response to primary platinum-paclitaxel: follow-up of a Southwest Oncology Group and Gynecologic Oncology Group phase 3 trial. Gynecologic Oncology. 2009;114:195-8.

[68] Perren TJ, Swart AM, Pfisterer J, Ledermann JA, Pujade-Lauraine E, Kristensen G, et al. A phase 3 trial of bevacizumab in ovarian cancer. The New England Journal of Medicine. 2011;365:2484-96.

Chapter 7

Analysing Molecular Mechanism Related to Therapy-Resistance in *In-vitro* Models of Ovarian Cancer

Jens C. Hahne, Arnd Honig, Jörg B. Engel,
Andrea Lampis and Nicola Valeri

Additional information is available at the end of the chapter

http://dx.doi.org/10.5772/60727

Abstract

Ovarian cancer is among the most common cause of cancer death and ranks first in the number of deaths each year in the field of gynaecological malignancies. This is due to its late diagnosis and the development of chemoresistance. Platinum derivates, including cisplatinum and carboplatin in combination with paclitaxel, are the first-line chemotherapeutic agents. Platinum derivates irreversibly intercalates into the DNA and creates inter- and intra-strand DNA cross-links. During cell division, platinum-DNA-adducts block the replication machinery, inducing DNA damage and apoptosis. Nearly all patients respond to first-line chemotherapy before it comes later to recurrence of the disease. At time of recurrence, tumours are usually more aggressive, form metastasis in secondary tissues and acquire resistance to conventional chemotherapeutics. Drug resistance is a common problem in tumour therapy not only restricted to ovarian cancer. It is characterized by gene mutations, increased DNA repair, reduced drug efficacy and enhanced drug clearance and detoxification. Up to now the complex molecular mechanism of chemoresistance is not well understood. Increasing evidence points towards AKT over-expression and alteration of the PI3K/AKT/mTOR cascade as a central mechanistic reason for this resistance.

Keywords: Ovarian cancer, cisplatinum resistance, AKT, PI3K

1. Introduction

There were 14,1 million new cancer cases, 8,2 million cancer deaths and 32,6 million people living with cancer (within 5 years of diagnosis) in 2012 world-wide [1].

Gynaecological tumours are among the most common cause of cancer death and currently causing more than 100,000 deaths per year [2]. Ovarian cancer is an important public health problem because it has the highest tumour-associated mortality of gynaecological malignancies and 239,000 women have been diagnosed with ovarian cancer in 2012 [2]. Furthermore there has been no appreciable improvement in survival for woman with advanced ovarian cancer over the past 40 years. The survival of ovarian cancer is poor and more than 70% of cases are diagnosed at late stage.

In ovarian cancer treatment platinum-based chemotherapy plays a pivotal role as first-line chemotherapy option alone or in combination with taxane [3]. Therefore platinum-resistance is the most crucial problem for treating ovarian cancer. Increasing evidence points towards AKT over-expression and alteration of the PI3K/AKT/mTOR cascade as a mechanistic reason for this resistance.

This chapter provides a short overview of the PI3K/AKT/mTOR-signalling network by summarizing *in-vitro* cell culture based studies that confirm the role of AKT as an important mediator of platinum resistance. The rationale for targeting this pathway in cancer will be discussed with a special focus on tumour immunological aspects also based on *in-vitro* studies. Moreover the PI3K/AKT/mTOR-signalling cascade other general mechanisms of resistance will be shortly addressed. Platinum-resistance can be also caused by differential expression of microRNAs as well as by detoxification of bioactive platinum-complexes by sulphur-containing peptides or proteins, cellular compartmentation, increased DNA repair and alteration in apoptotic signalling pathways [4]. Furthermore diminished drug accumulation caused by reduced uptake or increased efflux of platinum compounds via heavy metal transporter can result in platinum therapy failure [4].

A better understanding of the molecular mechanisms causing cancer therapy-resistance might result in new therapeutic options for patients suffering from tumours.

2. Phosphatidylinositol-3-Kinase (PI3K)/AKT/mTOR-signal transduction pathway

One of the most frequently altered signalling pathways involved in cancer as well as in development of resistance especially in ovarian cancer is the PI3K/AKT/mTOR pathway.

PI3K is a member of the lipid-kinase-family that can phosphorylate the 3′-OH-group of inositolphospholipids as phosphatidylinositol-4,5-bisphosphate (PIP_2) which is converted into the second messenger phosphatidylinositol-3,4,5-trisphosphate (PIP_3) [5]. According to different protein structure of the catalytic subunit, PI3Ks are subdivided into three classes.

Class I PI3Ks are the most studied class of PI3K and the most interesting with regard to signalling in tumours. Class I PI3Ks are activated by extracellular signal transduction via receptors with tyrosine-kinase activity or via G-protein coupled receptors (GPCR). In tumour cells growth-factors that bind to the specific receptors activate class 1 PI3Ks and this results in inhibition of autophagy [6].

PI3K activity is associated with cytoskeletal organization, cell division, inhibition of apoptosis and glucose uptake [7-9]. The second messenger PIP_3 in turn activates in the PI3K/AKT-pathway different proteins like AKT (protein kinase B), a serine-threonine kinase [5, 10]. PIP_3 itself is reconverted in PIP_2 via different phosphatases especially PTEN and SHIP [5]. AKT is the key protein in the PI3K/AKT signalling pathway; it binds PIP_3 over the plekstrin-homology-domain (PH-domain) and by this AKT translocates to cell membrane where it interacts with various phospholipids [10]. Cell membrane bound AKT is phosphorylated by phosphoinositide-dependent kinase-1 (PDK1) at threonine 308 and by PDK2 at serine 473 [5, 10, 11]. AKT can also be activated by mTOR2 [5, 12]. Phosphorylated AKT is the active form that modulates and regulates a huge range of proteins involved in diverse cellular processes such as cell cycle regulation, cell proliferation and cell viability [13]. Phosphorylation of AKT can be blocked by the carboxy-terminal modulator-protein (CTMP) and by this preventing the AKT activation as well as further signal transduction [5]. Phosphorylated AKT activates another serine-threonine-kinase, the mammalian target of rapamycin (mTOR) an important regulator for translation, cell growth and cell cycle [14, 15]. Furthermore mTOR has an important role in regulation of autophagy [6, 16, 17].

In general the PI3K/AKT-signal transduction pathway is of pivotal importance for mediating and controlling several cellular processes including cell growth, cell proliferation, survival, motility, adhesion, migration, differentiation, metabolic processes and cell cycle progression in cells [18, 19]. Amplifications, mutations, translocations and deregulation result in aberrant activation of this pathway [5, 20-23]. Furthermore the loss-of-function caused by mutation or deletion of phosphatase and tensin homolog (PTEN) protein results in an increased activity of the PI3K/AKT pathway [6]. The PTEN protein acts as a phosphatase and dephosphorylate PIP_3, resulting in the biphosphate product PIP_2. The dephosphorylation is essential as it triggers the inhibition of the AKT signalling pathway [24, 25].

3. Alteration of the PI3K/AKT/mTOR-signal transduction pathway in tumours

Recent studies indicate that numerous components of the PI3K/AKT/mTOR-pathway are deregulated by amplification, mutation and translocation more frequently than any other pathway in cancer patients with resultant activation of this pathway [20].

Both genetic and biochemical data suggest that activation of the PI3K/AKT/mTOR survival pathway contributes to ovarian cancer development and tumourigenesis [15]. Such activation is caused by different mechanisms and one mechanism is somatic alterations in PI3KCA gene that have been found in a substantial fraction of ovarian cancers [26]. PIK3CA amplifications are present in 40% of ovarian cancers [19]. Furthermore, activation of PI3K/AKT/mTOR signal transduction pathway is caused by mutations in the gene coding for PIK3CA. Another alteration that results in increased activity of the PI3K/AKT/mTOR pathway is PTEN loss-of-function. PTEN loss is observed in about 7% of all ovarian cancer cases and it seems to be more common in type I ovarian tumours [27-32].

For AKT a point-mutation in the PH-domain has been detected in ovarian cancer [33]. This point-mutation results in conformational change of the PH-domain so that AKT can be activated without the presence of PI3K [33].

Deregulation, mutation or over-expression of cell surface receptors can also result in an increased activity of the PI3K/AKT/mTOR signalling pathway in ovarian cancer [34]. Furthermore Ras mutations are found in 20% of low-grade ovarian cancers [35]. Since Ras has been shown to activate both the Ras/Raf/MEK/ERK and the PI3K/AKT/mTOR pathways, mutations of Ras should theoretically activate both pathways simultaneously. Nevertheless so far it has not been evaluated in detail if Ras mutations can result in an increased activity of the PI3K/AKT/mTOR-signalling pathway. Although one study demonstrates that some Ras mutations result in deregulated PI3K and downstream AKT activation [36]. Beside Ras mutations also the over-expression of several other proteins e.g. Rab25 [37], Twist2 [38] or MyD88 [39] seems to enhance activation of AKT. The fact that AKT can be activated by a number of different proteins underlines the key role of AKT signalling under physiological and pathophysiological conditions. As evidence, in human specimens of ovarian cancer AKT was found to be activated in 68% of cases [40].

4. Effects of altered PI3K/AKT/mTOR-signal transduction pathway in tumours

As mentioned before, AKT is an important regulator of various cellular pathways that promote cell survival, cell proliferation, angiogenesis and invasion. Furthermore, the epithelial-mesenchymal-transformation, an important step for tumour metastasis, has been shown to be related to AKT activation [41]. Deregulation of components of the PI3K/AKT-cascade not only contributes to ovarian cancer development and tumourigenesis but also to chemotherapeutic drug and radiation resistance as it was recently shown [4, 5, 18, 42-56]. The sensitivity of cells to radiation and chemotherapeutic drug-induced apoptosis is determined by the balance between cellular survival and apoptosis [5, 12]. Due to the well-known anti-apoptotic role of AKT, an AKT over-expression in cancer cells might be related to increased resistance to radiation and chemotherapy.

Beside the PI3K/AKT/mTOR signalling cascade other general mechanisms of resistance exist. However in this chapter other possibilities of platinum-resistance will be mentioned only shortly.

In general diminished drug accumulation caused by reduced uptake or increased efflux of platinum compounds via heavy metal transporter can result in platinum therapy failure [4].

Furthermore in some resistant cell lines with increased cisplatinum efflux an increased intracellular pH was detected [57]. Intra-cellularly, cisplatinum's chlorides are replaced by neutral hydroxyl or highly reactive positively charged aqua groups, with the pKa for the interconversion between chloro-hydroxy and chloro-aqua species being 6.56 [58]. Hence, if intracellular pH is high, a higher proportion of drug may be represented in the uncharged chloro-hydroxy form, with increased passive efflux of this form.

Another general resistance mechanism is detoxification of bioactive platinum-complexes by sulphur-containing peptides or proteins. Increased glutathione (GSH) level has been shown to cause resistance by binding and inactivating cisplatinum, enhancing DNA repair and reducing cisplatinum-induced oxidative stress [59-62].

Increased DNA repair and reduced apoptotic response are further possible reasons for platinum resistance [4, 63]. Cisplatinum may induce apoptosis through the Fas/Fas ligand signalling complex (with activation of caspase-8, then caspase-3), or by mitochondrial cytochrome-c release [64]. In the presence of ATP and cytochrome-c, apoptotic-protease-activating-factor-1 (Apaf-1) activates caspase-9, with subsequent caspase-3 activation [64]. Cisplatinum may also kill via a caspase-3 independent apoptotic pathway, by a defective apoptotic pathway or by necrosis [64]. Caspase-3, -8 and -9 are important in cisplatinum-induced apoptosis [62]. A cisplatinum-resistant cell showed global down-regulation of caspase and Bax expression, but increased Bcl-2 [65].

Recent reports describe that platinum-resistance can be also caused by differential expression of microRNAs (miRNAs) [66-69]. miRNAs belong to the family of small non-coding RNAs; they are generally 21-25 nucleotides long and play key role in post-transcriptional modulation of gene expression thus representing fine regulators in tumour development and progression as well as response and resistance to anti-tumour agents [70]. miRNA-152 was identified as an autophagy-regulating miRNA down-regulated in cisplatinum-resistant cell lines and also *in-vivo* in ovarian cancer tissues reduced expression has been associated with cisplatinum-resistance. miRNA-152 regulates autophagy by targeting ATG14 the key player in orchestrating autophagy. Thus over-expression of miRNA-152 sensitized cisplatinum-resistant ovarian cancer cells by reducing cisplatinum-induced autophagy, enhancing cisplatinum-induced apoptosis and by inhibition of cell proliferation [69]. Microarray analyses have been used to identify miRNAs involved in cisplatinum-resistance and it was demonstrated that miRNA-21-3p over-expression, the passenger strand of the known oncomiR 5p, increased resistance to cisplatinum in a range of ovarian cell lines [66]. Furthermore a high level of miRNA-490-3p expression was identified as involved in the development of drug resistance against paclitaxel [68]. Another miRNA, miRNA-449a, was found to be down-regulated in cisplatinum-resistant ovarian cancer cells and NOTCH1 was identified as direct target of its modulation [67]. Therefore it is evident that down-regulation as well as over-expression of miRNAs can result in resistance to anti-tumour agents. Recently it was demonstrated that miRNAs involved in platinum-resistance are directly involved in regulation of PTEN, AKT or other downstream molecules of the PI3K/AKT pathway [71-79].

The evidence that members of the PI3K/AKT/mTOR pathway are regulated by miRNAs involved in platinum-resistance increases the importance of the PI3K/AKT/mTOR signalling cascade as therapeutic target. Therefore inhibition of PI3K/AKT/mTOR signalling in ovarian carcinomas appears a promising target to enhance the efficacy of anticancer agents such as cisplatinum and to overcome the resistance of tumour cells against therapy. This hypothesis was tested in different preclinical *in-vitro* studies. Cancer cell lines are frequently used as *in-vitro* tumour models especially for analyzing and studying the effects related to a single gene modification. Nowadays approximately 100 ovarian cancer cell lines are publicly available [80]. Some of these cell lines are known to be platinum resistant e.g. SKOV-3/DDP and Caov-3. Among different ovarian cancer cell lines established there are also the parental A2780 cells and the cisplatinum-resistant A2780cis cells [81]. Both cell lines are p53 and K-Ras wild-type and they share the same genetic background. The cisplatinum-resistant A2780cis cell line has been developed by chronic exposure of the parental cisplatinum-sensitive A2780 cell line to increasing concentrations of the chemotherapeutic agent [81]. These cell lines are excellent models for analyzing the molecular basis for cisplatinum resistance in ovarian cancer [47-49, 82-85]. According to these studies AKT over-expression in ovarian cancer is strongly related to platinum resistance in this specific tumour [37, 47, 86]. It was shown that high AKT protein expression is strongly associated to cisplatinum-resistant A2780cis cell line compared to the parental A2780 cell lines [47, 48]. The platinum resistance in A2780cis cell line could be overcome by AKT down-regulation via siRNA [47]. This was demonstrated in several functional *in-vitro* assays, e.g. clonogenicity assays and irradiation assays (Figure 1), as by determination of the apoptosis rate. Furthermore the cytotoxicity of cisplatinum was addressed in proliferation assays. Stable increase of AKT amount in the cell lines results in an increased IC_{50} value for cisplatinum whereas a stable decrease of AKT results in an increased accessibility for cisplatinum treatment [47].

However in the same isogenic model it was shown that AKT-over-expression was able to transform platinum-sensitive A2780 cells into platinum-resistant. On the contrary, platinum-resistance of A2780cis cells could be reversed by down-regulation of AKT [47]. FACS analysis demonstrated also that cisplatinum induces cell cycle arrest predominantly in the S and the G2/M phase but also in the G1 phase regardless of the AKT-expression status (Figure 2). However, required doses of cisplatinum to induce cell cycle arrest were progressively higher in cell lines with AKT over-expressed [47, 87].

As already mentioned above the sensitivity of cells to radiation and drug-induced apoptosis is determined by the balanced expression between pro-apoptotic and anti-apoptotic proteins [5, 12]. Therefore the effect of the PI3K/AKT cascade on pro-apoptotic protein like BAD, a known substrate of AKT, has been studied in both cisplatinum-resistant Caov-3 and sensitive A2780 human ovarian cancer cells [88]. Treatment of Caov-3 and A2780 cells with cisplatinum was able to stimulate the activation of AKT, whereas the PI3K inhibitor wortmannin blocked the cisplatinum-induced AKT activation. Cisplatinum treatment was capable to activate phosphorylation of BAD at Ser-112 and Ser-136 sites in Caov-3 and A2780 cells. While phosphorylation of BAD at Ser-136 was blocked by treatment with wortmannin, its phosphorylation at Ser-112 was blocked by a MAP/ERK kinase inhibitor PD98059 [89]. Transient exogenous expression of a dominant-negative AKT in both Caov-3 and A2780 cells decreased cell viability after treatment with cisplatinum. In contrast, no sensitization to cisplatinum was

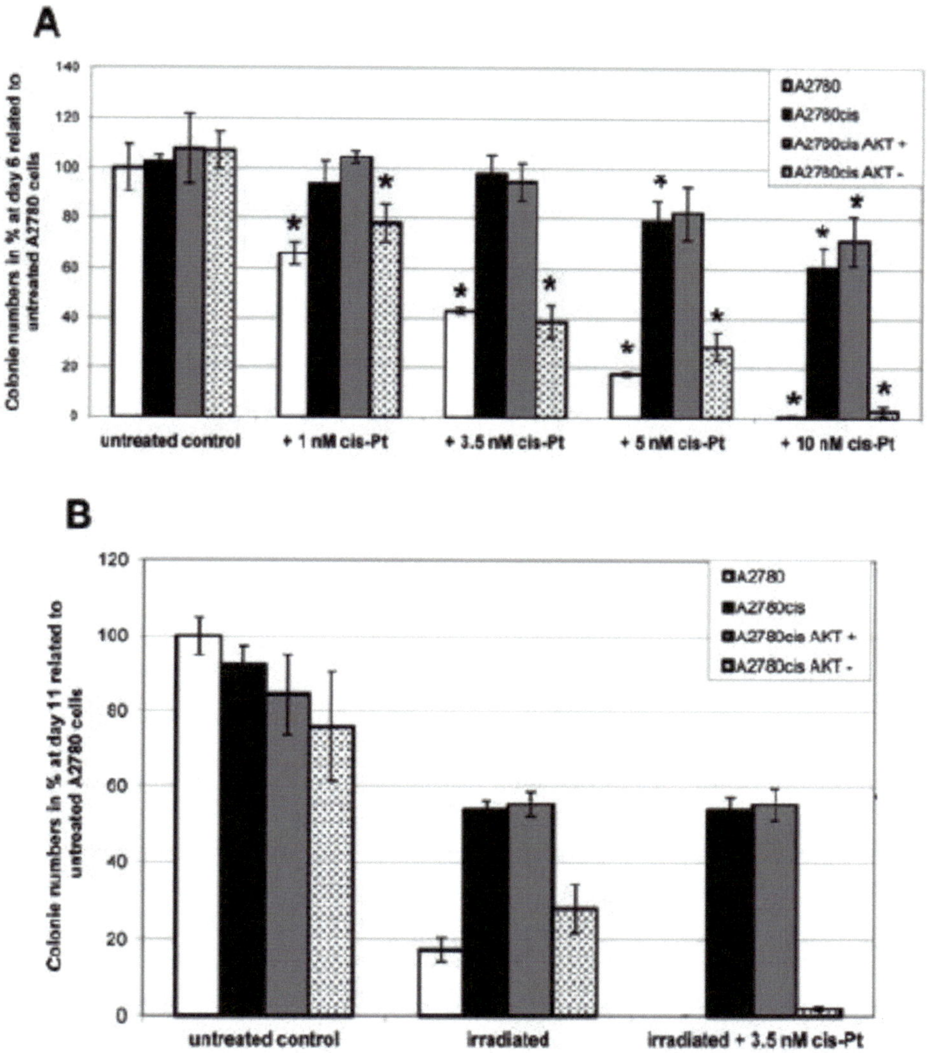

Figure 1. Clonogenicity-Assays. (A) Cells were treated with different concentrations of cisplatin (cis-Pt) for 6 days and (B) cells were first irradiated with 2.5 Gray and then treated with 3.5 nM cisplatin (cis-Pt) for 11 days. Cells were stained and fixed with crystal violet. The formed cell colonies were counted. The figure shows the colony numbers in relation to the colonies formed by untreated A2780 (set to 100%). Three independent experiments were performed, and each experiment was carried out in triplicate. Statistically significant difference ($p<0.05$) between a sample and the relevant control is indicated by *. All data were previously published in "Oncology Reports" [47] and is reprinted by permission of Spandidos Publications ©2012.

observed in cells expressing wild-type AKT. These findings suggested that cisplatinum-induced DNA damage causes phosphorylation of BAD via an extracellular signal-regulated protein kinase (ERK) cascade and via a PI3K/AKT/mTOR cascade. Inhibition of both cascades enhance the sensitivity of ovarian cancer cells to cisplatinum thus providing further evidence that AKT-pathway is involved in cisplatinum resistance in ovarian cancers [88]. Additional

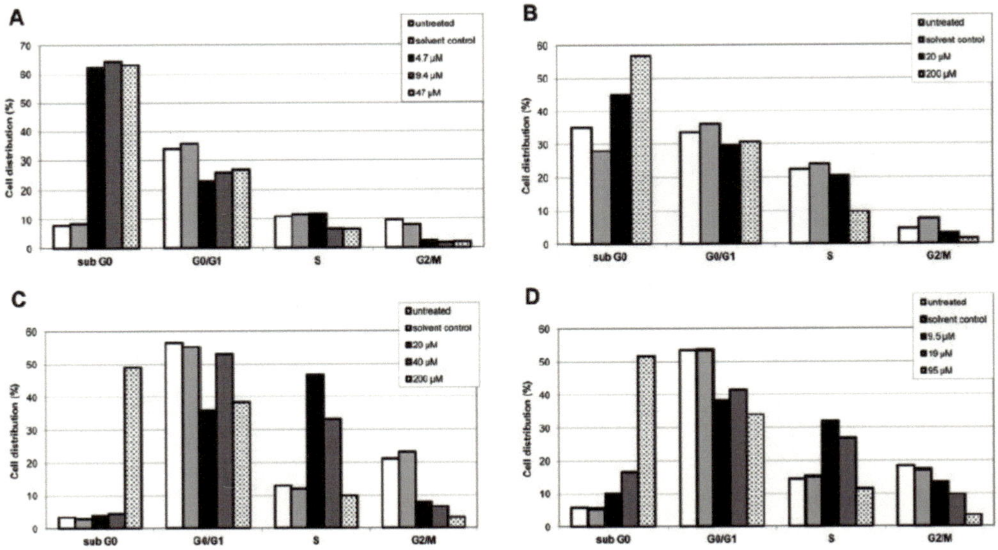

Figure 2. Effect of cisplatin (cis-Pt) on the cell cycle distribution. A2780 (A), A2780cis (B), A2780cis AKT+ (C) and A2780cis AKT- (D) cells were treated with different concentrations of cisplatin (cis-Pt) for 24 h, fixed, permeabilzed, stained with propidium iodide and analysed by flow cytometry. The figure shows the distribution of the cells to the different phases of cell cycle (%). All data were previously published in "Oncology Reports" [47] and is reprinted by permission of Spandidos Publications ©2012.

results suggest that AKT confers platinum-resistance in part by modulating the direction of p53 on the caspase-dependent mitochondrial death pathway [90]. Thus in ovarian cancers while p53 is a determinant for platinum sensitivity AKT contributes to chemoresistance in part by attenuating p53-mediated PUMA upregulation and phosphorylation of p53 [91]. Recent results suggest that in platinum sensitive ovarian cancer cells cisplatinum-induced apoptosis can also proceed to a lesser extent via a caspase-independent mechanism involving apoptosis inducing factor (AIF) and that AKT activation additionally confers resistance to cisplatinum-induced apoptosis by blocking this pathway [90].

A recent work evaluated the anti-tumour efficacy of the AKT inhibitor perifosine in platinum-sensitive and –resistant human ovarian cancer cells [45, 92]. In different ovarian cancer cell lines and *in-vivo* experiments it has been possible to show that cells with higher levels of phospho-AKT are more sensitive to treatment with AKT-inhibitor perifosine. Furthermore, coincubation with perifosine sensitized A2780cis cells to treatment with cisplatinum. AKT-inhibitor perifosine has already been tested in phase II studies in patients with breast, prostate, pancreatic, head and neck, colorectal cancer, malignant melanoma, multiple myeloma, and soft tissue sarcoma [93-99]. A recent phase I study with perifosine combined with radiotherapy performed in patients with advanced solid tumours has shown preliminary evidence of anti-cancer activity, including complete responses [100]. Thus, perifosine seems to be an attractive compound for further clinical studies in particular phenotypes tumour like platinum-resistant ovarian cancers.

New attractive therapeutic targets are presented by the PI3K/AKT/mTOR-pathway activating cell surface receptors like vascular endothelial growth factor (VEGF) receptors [101]. VEGF is a key activator of angiogenesis, a physiological multi-step process that includes endothelial cell growth and movement [102]. It plays important roles in wound healing and endothelial-cell-mediated degradation of the extracellular matrix, as well as the transition of benign tissue into solid tumours [102-104]. Recent studies have suggested that the PI3K/AKT signalling cascade may be implicated in tumour angiogenesis [105-107]. In clinical trial studies, high VEGF levels have been negatively correlated with survival of patients. Ovarian cancer cells over-expressing VEGF own a metastatic advantage over those VEGF low expressing [108, 109] and even more higher levels of serum VEGF are found in patients with metastasis if compared to metastasis-free patients [110]. Moreover, down-modulation of VEGF has been shown to inhibit tumour growth and to suppress tumour invasion and metastasis. These findings have laid the basis for the clinical evaluation of agents targeting VEGF signaling pathway in patients with ovarian cancer [101]. Bevacizumab (Avastin) has been the first and most studied anti-VEGF agent in clinical evaluation for ovarian cancer [111]. Bevacizumab showed additive or synergistic effects in combinational therapy with paclitaxel and marked reduction of tumour growth and ascites formation [112]. Using a murine ovarian cancer model a significant antitumour activity of Bevacizumab as a single agent or in combination with cisplatinum was demonstrated [113]. In the meantime Bevacizumab was approved as a treatment in combination with paclitaxel, topotecan, or pegylated liposomal doxorubicin chemotherapy for women with recurrent ovarian cancer that are resistant to platinum-based chemotherapy [114-117].

Furthermore, other agents targeting VEGF receptors have also been evaluated for the use in treatment of ovarian cancer as Ramucirumab, a fully humanized monoclonal antibody, that specifically block VEGFR-2 resulting in reduced tumour growth, increased apoptosis and decreased tumour microvessel proliferation and density [118]. Following a phase I evaluation [119], it is currently being assessed in a phase II trial as monotherapy in patients with platinum-refractory persistent or recurrent epithelial ovarian cancer.

5. Role of AKT expression level in tumour cells in regard to NK killing

Another important aspect in cancer development and progression is the role of the immune system. Since survival is strongly influenced by immunological parameters, immunotherapeutic strategies appear promising and for this reason during the last years the interest in tumour immunology has constantly increased. A necessary prerequisite for immunotherapy in patients is a better understanding of the interaction between ovarian tumour cells and cells of the immune system especially with natural-killer (NK)-cells. NK-cells are a critical component of the innate immune response against infectious pathogens and malignant transformation [120, 121]. NK-cells mediate this activity through the elaboration of various cytokines as well as through direct cytolytic activity. However, unlike adaptive immune cells, which utilize specific clonal recognition receptors, NK-cell activation depends on a complex balance between activating and inhibitory signals [122, 123]. Nevertheless, NK-cells play an important role in immune surveillance and coordinating responses of other immune cells. Most tumour cells express surface molecules that can be recognized by activating receptors on NK-cells [124]. The expression of these receptors make such cells susceptible to endogenous NK-cells, but malignant cells have developed mechanisms to evade these mechanisms of innate immune surveillance [125-127]. In patients with cancer, it is presumed that tumour cells have developed mechanisms to suppress NK-cell activation and resist lysis by endogenous NK-cells, but the molecular basis for target resistance is not well understood. Recent studies have suggested that AKT can regulate the development and functions of innate immune cells [128] thus providing evidence that AKT plays also an important role in immune modulation. However in this chapter will be addressed only the role of activated AKT in tumour cells in regard to NK-cells.

Dysregulated cytokine release can either lead to or be associated with a failure in cell-cell recognition thus allowing cancer cells to evade the killing system. The PI3K/AKT/mTOR pathway regulates multiple cellular processes which underlie immune responses against pathogens or malignant cells [129, 130]. Conversely, there is accumulating evidence that the PI3K/AKT/mTOR pathway is involved in the development of several malignant traits of cancer cells as well as their escape from immunity [131]. In some studies the interactions between cancer cells and natural-killer (NK)-cells have been enlightened [48, 82, 132-134]. Modified FATAL assay was used for determining the killing efficiency of NK-cells in regard to ovarian cancer cell models *in-vitro* (Figure 3).

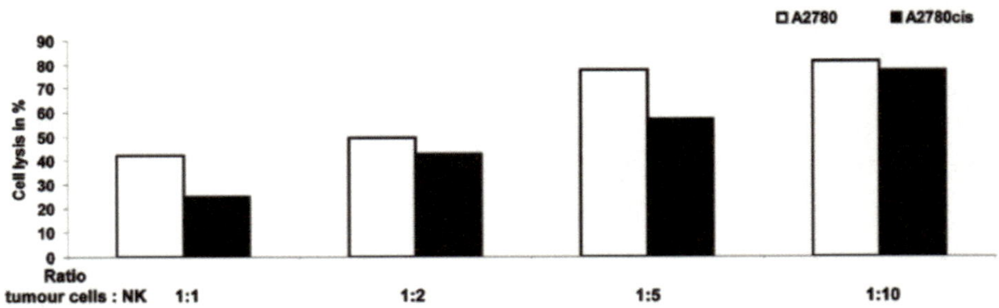

Figure 3. Lytic activity of polyclonal natural-killer (NK)-cells. A2780 and A2780cis cells (10^5 cells/well), respectively, were used as targets in a modified 5 h FATAL assay using various tumour cell : NK-cell ratios. Target cell lysis was determined by flow cytometric analysis. The percentage of tumour cell lysis was determined in relation to a control containing tumour cells with medium alone. A representative of three independent experiments is shown. All data were previously published in "International Journal of Oncology" [48] and is reprinted by permission of Spandidos Publications ©2013.

In this model parental A2780 cells and the cisplatinum resistant A2780cis human ovarian cancer cells have been used. The efficiency of NK-cell mediated cell lysis differs between A2780 cells and the cisplatinum-resistant A2780cis cells. The A2780cis cells are less accessible for NK-cell mediated killing [48, 82] and this findings are in agreement with a report by Bellucci *et al.* [135]. Using a lentiviral shRNA library targeting >1,000 human genes they identified 83 genes that promote target cell resistance to human NK-cell-mediated killing [135]. Many of the genes discovered by this screening belong to common signalling pathways including multiple members of the AKT/PI3K/mTOR pathway as PIK3CA and PIK3CB [135]. The comparison of the cancer cell lines A2780 and A2780cis revealed that the differences observed with regard to NK-cell mediated killing rely mainly on two mechanisms. Firstly, the observed increased expression of anti-apoptotic genes (especially *ciap-1* and *-2*) in A2780cis cells compared to A2780 cells is able to confer resistance to A2780cis cells to apoptosis. Second, the CD112 ligand for NK-cell receptor DNAM-1 was expressed at a lower level in A2780cis cells though ligands for the NK-cell receptor NKG2D, e.g. MICA/B, were more strongly expressed in the platinum-resistant cells than in the parental A2780 cells [48]. Moreover A2780cis cells expressed lower levels of TIMP-3, the inhibitor of MICA/B shedding, whereas specific proteases for shedding were also found expressed and this resulted in a net increase of soluble MICA/B in A2780cis cell lines [48]. It is well known that cleaved MICA/B protects cells against NK mediated cell killing [48, 136, 137]. Therefore, it is reasonable to speculate that the increased amount of soluble MICA/B is responsible for the lower killing rate of platinum-resistant A2780cis cells compared to their parental A2780 cells [48]. It was previously well demonstrated that PI3K/AKT/mTOR pathway is involved in inducing MICA/B expression in breast cancer cells [138]. Overall these findings indicate a more general effect of induced PI3K/AKT/mTOR signal transduction pathway. As well as in breast, in ovarian cancer cells with an increase of phosphorylated AKT-activated, PI3K/AKT/mTOR pathway higher MICA/B expression has been also detected [48]. Recently it has been demonstrated that treatment of tumour cells with JAK inhibitors increased their susceptibility to NK-cell mediated killing [135]. The authors suggested that common signalling pathways can regulate susceptibility of human tumour cells to the surveillance and killing ability of the immunologic effector cells and that small molecules inhibitors of JAK may have promising immunologic effects *in-vivo* [135]. Whether or not inhibition of PI3K/AKT/mTOR pathway might render the platinum-resistant A2780cis cells accessible for NK-cell mediated killing must be evaluated in further studies. Only the few first steps towards the characterization of the molecular basis of resistance mechanisms in ovarian cancer with different AKT expression levels in the context of NK-cell mediated killing are being explored [48, 82].

Author details

Jens C. Hahne[1*], Arnd Honig[2], Jörg B. Engel[3], Andrea Lampis[1] and Nicola Valeri[1]

*Address all correspondence to: jens.hahne@icr.ac.uk

1 Centre for Molecular Pathology, The Institute of Cancer Research, London, UK

2 Gynaecological Hospital, Catholic Clinical Centre Mainz, Germany

3 Department of Obstetrics and Gynaecology, Medical University Gießen, Germany

References

[1] Ferlay J, Soerjomataram I, Dikshit R, Eser S, Mathers C, et al. Cancer incidence and mortality worldwide: Sources, methods and major patterns in GLOBOCAN 2012. Int J Cancer. 2015;136(5): E359-386.10.1002/ijc.29210

[2] Jemal A, Siegel R, Xu J, & Ward E Cancer statistics, 2010. CA Cancer J Clin. 2010;60(5): 277-300.10.3322/caac.20073

[3] Metzger-Filho O, Moulin C, & D'Hondt V First-line systemic treatment of ovarian cancer: a critical review of available evidence and expectations for future directions. Curr Opin Oncol. 2010;22(5): 513-520.10.1097/CCO.0b013e32833ae99c

[4] Stewart DJ Mechanisms of resistance to cisplatin and carboplatin. Crit Rev Oncol Hematol. 2007;63(1): 12-31.10.1016/j.critrevonc.2007.02.001

[5] Vivanco I & Sawyers CL The phosphatidylinositol 3-Kinase AKT pathway in human cancer. Nat Rev Cancer. 2002;2(7): 489-501.10.1038/nrc839

[6] Kondo Y, Kanzawa T, Sawaya R, & Kondo S The role of autophagy in cancer development and response to therapy. Nat Rev Cancer. 2005;5(9): 726-734.10.1038/nrc1692

[7] Roche S, Koegl M, & Courtneidge SA The phosphatidylinositol 3-kinase alpha is required for DNA synthesis induced by some, but not all, growth factors. Proc Natl Acad Sci U S A. 1994;91(19): 9185-9189

[8] Wennstrom S, Hawkins P, Cooke F, Hara K, Yonezawa K, et al. Activation of phosphoinositide 3-kinase is required for PDGF-stimulated membrane ruffling. Curr Biol. 1994;4(5): 385-393

[9] Yao R & Cooper GM Growth factor-dependent survival of rodent fibroblasts requires phosphatidylinositol 3-kinase but is independent of pp70S6K activity. Oncogene. 1996;13(2): 343-351

[10] Toker A & Yoeli-Lerner M Akt signaling and cancer: surviving but not moving on. Cancer Res. 2006;66(8): 3963-3966.10.1158/0008-5472.CAN-06-0743

[11] Kunstle G, Laine J, Pierron G, Kagami Si S, Nakajima H, et al. Identification of Akt association and oligomerization domains of the Akt kinase coactivator TCL1. Mol Cell Biol. 2002;22(5): 1513-1525

[12] Engelman JA Targeting PI3K signalling in cancer: opportunities, challenges and limitations. Nat Rev Cancer. 2009;9(8): 550-562.10.1038/nrc2664

[13] Fresno Vara JA, Casado E, de Castro J, Cejas P, Belda-Iniesta C, et al. PI3K/Akt signalling pathway and cancer. Cancer Treat Rev. 2004;30(2): 193-204.10.1016/j.ctrv.2003.07.007

[14] Shaw RJ & Cantley LC Ras, PI(3)K and mTOR signalling controls tumour cell growth. Nature. 2006;441(7092): 424-430.10.1038/nature04869

[15] Diaz-Padilla I, Duran I, Clarke BA, & Oza AM Biologic rationale and clinical activity of mTOR inhibitors in gynecological cancer. Cancer Treat Rev. 2012;38(6): 767-775.10.1016/j.ctrv.2012.02.001

[16] Jung CH, Ro SH, Cao J, Otto NM, & Kim DH mTOR regulation of autophagy. FEBS Lett. 2010;584(7): 1287-1295.10.1016/j.febslet.2010.01.017

[17] Wang CW & Klionsky DJ The molecular mechanism of autophagy. Mol Med. 2003;9(3-4): 65-76

[18] Santiskulvong C, Konecny GE, Fekete M, Chen KY, Karam A, et al. Dual targeting of phosphoinositide 3-kinase and mammalian target of rapamycin using NVP-BEZ235 as a novel therapeutic approach in human ovarian carcinoma. Clin Cancer Res. 2011;17(8): 2373-2384.10.1158/1078-0432.CCR-10-2289

[19] Shayesteh L, Lu Y, Kuo WL, Baldocchi R, Godfrey T, et al. PIK3CA is implicated as an oncogene in ovarian cancer. Nat Genet. 1999;21(1): 99-102.10.1038/5042

[20] Hennessy BT, Smith DL, Ram PT, Lu Y, & Mills GB Exploiting the PI3K/AKT pathway for cancer drug discovery. Nat Rev Drug Discov. 2005;4(12): 988-1004.10.1038/nrd1902

[21] Bellacosa A, Kumar CC, Di Cristofano A, & Testa JR Activation of AKT kinases in cancer: implications for therapeutic targeting. Adv Cancer Res. 2005;94: 29-86.10.1016/S0065-230X(05)94002-5

[22] Manning BD & Cantley LC AKT/PKB signaling: navigating downstream. Cell. 2007;129(7): 1261-1274.10.1016/j.cell.2007.06.009

[23] Engelman JA, Luo J, & Cantley LC The evolution of phosphatidylinositol 3-kinases as regulators of growth and metabolism. Nat Rev Genet. 2006;7(8): 606-619.10.1038/nrg1879

[24] Kong D, Suzuki A, Zou TT, Sakurada A, Kemp LW, et al. PTEN1 is frequently mutated in primary endometrial carcinomas. Nat Genet. 1997;17(2): 143-144.10.1038/ng1097-143

[25] Minaguchi T, Yoshikawa H, Oda K, Ishino T, Yasugi T, et al. PTEN mutation located only outside exons 5, 6, and 7 is an independent predictor of favorable survival in endometrial carcinomas. Clin Cancer Res. 2001;7(9): 2636-2642

[26] Samuels Y & Velculescu VE Oncogenic mutations of PIK3CA in human cancers. Cell Cycle. 2004;3(10): 1221-1224

[27] Kurman RJ & Shih Ie M Molecular pathogenesis and extraovarian origin of epithelial ovarian cancer--shifting the paradigm. Hum Pathol. 2011;42(7): 918-931.10.1016/j.humpath.2011.03.003

[28] Vazquez F & Sellers WR The PTEN tumor suppressor protein: an antagonist of phosphoinositide 3-kinase signaling. Biochim Biophys Acta. 2000;1470(1): M21-35

[29] Wu X, Senechal K, Neshat MS, Whang YE, & Sawyers CL The PTEN/MMAC1 tumor suppressor phosphatase functions as a negative regulator of the phosphoinositide 3-kinase/Akt pathway. Proc Natl Acad Sci U S A. 1998;95(26): 15587-15591

[30] Leslie NR, Gray A, Pass I, Orchiston EA, & Downes CP Analysis of the cellular functions of PTEN using catalytic domain and C-terminal mutations: differential effects of C-terminal deletion on signalling pathways downstream of phosphoinositide 3-kinase. Biochem J. 2000;346 Pt 3: 827-833

[31] Dahia PL, Aguiar RC, Alberta J, Kum JB, Caron S, et al. PTEN is inversely correlated with the cell survival factor Akt/PKB and is inactivated via multiple mechanismsin haematological malignancies. Hum Mol Genet. 1999;8(2): 185-193

[32] Hashiguchi Y, Tsuda H, Inoue T, Berkowitz RS, & Mok SC PTEN expression in clear cell adenocarcinoma of the ovary. Gynecol Oncol. 2006;101(1): 71-75.10.1016/j.ygyno.2005.09.047

[33] Carpten JD, Faber AL, Horn C, Donoho GP, Briggs SL, et al. A transforming mutation in the pleckstrin homology domain of AKT1 in cancer. Nature. 2007;448(7152): 439-444.10.1038/nature05933

[34] McCubrey JA, Steelman LS, Chappell WH, Abrams SL, Montalto G, et al. Mutations and deregulation of Ras/Raf/MEK/ERK and PI3K/PTEN/Akt/mTOR cascades which alter therapy response. Oncotarget. 2012;3(9): 954-987

[35] Ulku AS, Schafer R, & Der CJ Essential role of Raf in Ras transformation and deregulation of matrix metalloproteinase expression in ovarian epithelial cells. Mol Cancer Res. 2003;1(14): 1077-1088

[36] Taylor V, Wong M, Brandts C, Reilly L, Dean NM, et al. 5' phospholipid phosphatase SHIP-2 causes protein kinase B inactivation and cell cycle arrest in glioblastoma cells. Mol Cell Biol. 2000;20(18): 6860-6871

[37] Fan Y, Wang L, Han X, Liu X, & Ma H Rab25 is responsible for phosphoinositide 3-kinase/AKTmediated cisplatin resistance in human epithelial ovarian cancer cells. Mol Med Rep. 2015;11(3): 2173-2178.10.3892/mmr.2014.2963

[38] Wang T, Li Y, Tuerhanjiang A, Wang W, Wu Z, et al. Twist2 contributes to cisplatin-resistance of ovarian cancer through the AKT/GSK-3beta signaling pathway. Oncol Lett. 2014;7(4): 1102-1108.10.3892/ol.2014.1816

[39] Wang Y, Tu Q, Yan W, Xiao D, Zeng Z, et al. CXC195 suppresses proliferation and inflammatory response in LPS-induced human hepatocellular carcinoma cells via regulating TLR4-MyD88-TAK1-mediated NF-kappaB and MAPK pathway. Biochem Biophys Res Commun. 2015;456(1): 373-379.10.1016/j.bbrc.2014.11.090

[40] Levine DA, Bogomolniy F, Yee CJ, Lash A, Barakat RR, et al. Frequent mutation of the PIK3CA gene in ovarian and breast cancers. Clin Cancer Res. 2005;11(8): 2875-2878.10.1158/1078-0432.CCR-04-2142

[41] Chen R, Yang Q, & Lee JD BMK1 kinase suppresses epithelial-mesenchymal transition through the Akt/GSK3beta signaling pathway. Cancer Res. 2012;72(6): 1579-1587.10.1158/0008-5472.CAN-11-2055

[42] Lee S, Choi EJ, Jin C, & Kim DH Activation of PI3K/Akt pathway by PTEN reduction and PIK3CA mRNA amplification contributes to cisplatin resistance in an ovarian cancer cell line. Gynecol Oncol. 2005;97(1): 26-34.10.1016/j.ygyno.2004.11.051

[43] Gagnon V, Mathieu I, Sexton E, Leblanc K, & Asselin E AKT involvement in cisplatin chemoresistance of human uterine cancer cells. Gynecol Oncol. 2004;94(3): 785-795.10.1016/j.ygyno.2004.06.023

[44] Mondesire WH, Jian W, Zhang H, Ensor J, Hung MC, et al. Targeting mammalian target of rapamycin synergistically enhances chemotherapy-induced cytotoxicity in breast cancer cells. Clin Cancer Res. 2004;10(20): 7031-7042.10.1158/1078-0432.CCR-04-0361

[45] Engel JB, Schonhals T, Hausler S, Krockenberger M, Schmidt M, et al. Induction of programmed cell death by inhibition of AKT with the alkylphosphocholine perifosine in in vitro models of platinum sensitive and resistant ovarian cancers. Arch Gynecol Obstet. 2011;283(3): 603-610.10.1007/s00404-010-1457-6

[46] Benedetti V, Perego P, Luca Beretta G, Corna E, Tinelli S, et al. Modulation of survival pathways in ovarian carcinoma cell lines resistant to platinum compounds. Mol Cancer Ther. 2008;7(3): 679-687.10.1158/1535-7163.MCT-07-0450

[47] Hahne JC, Honig A, Meyer SR, Gambaryan S, Walter U, et al. Downregulation of AKT reverses platinum resistance of human ovarian cancers in vitro. Oncol Rep. 2012;28(6): 2023-2028.10.3892/or.2012.2041

[48] Hahne JC, Meyer SR, Gambaryan S, Walter U, Dietl J, et al. Immune escape of AKT overexpressing ovarian cancer cells. Int J Oncol. 2013;42(5): 1630-1635.10.3892/ijo.2013.1846

[49] Honig A, Hahne JC, Meyer S, Kranke P, Hausler S, et al. PI3K inhibitor D-116883 is effective in in vitro models of ovarian cancer. Anticancer Res. 2012;32(5): 2035-2041

[50] Eckstein N Platinum resistance in breast and ovarian cancer cell lines. J Exp Clin Cancer Res. 2011;30: 91.10.1186/1756-9966-30-91

[51] Cheng JQ, Lindsley CW, Cheng GZ, Yang H, & Nicosia SV The Akt/PKB pathway: molecular target for cancer drug discovery. Oncogene. 2005;24(50): 7482-7492.10.1038/sj.onc.1209088

[52] Hovelmann S, Beckers TL, & Schmidt M Molecular alterations in apoptotic pathways after PKB/Akt-mediated chemoresistance in NCI H460 cells. Br J Cancer. 2004;90(12): 2370-2377.10.1038/sj.bjc.6601876

[53] Westfall SD & Skinner MK Inhibition of phosphatidylinositol 3-kinase sensitizes ovarian cancer cells to carboplatin and allows adjunct chemotherapy treatment. Mol Cancer Ther. 2005;4(11): 1764-1771.10.1158/1535-7163.MCT-05-0192

[54] Testa JR & Bellacosa A AKT plays a central role in tumorigenesis. Proc Natl Acad Sci U S A. 2001;98(20): 10983-10985.10.1073/pnas.211430998

[55] Nicholson KM & Anderson NG The protein kinase B/Akt signalling pathway in human malignancy. Cell Signal. 2002;14(5): 381-395

[56] Dobbin ZC & Landen CN The Importance of the PI3K/AKT/MTOR Pathway in the Progression of Ovarian Cancer. Int J Mol Sci. 2013;14(4): 8213-8227.10.3390/ijms14048213

[57] Chau Q & Stewart DJ Cisplatin efflux, binding and intracellular pH in the HTB56 human lung adenocarcinoma cell line and the E-8/0.7 cisplatin-resistant variant. Cancer Chemother Pharmacol. 1999;44(3): 193-202.10.1007/s002800050967

[58] Andersson A, Hedenmalm H, Elfsson B, & Ehrsson H Determination of the acid dissociation constant for cis-diammineaquachloroplatinum(II) ion. A hydrolysis product of cisplatin. J Pharm Sci. 1994;83(6): 859-862

[59] Perego P, Romanelli S, Carenini N, Magnani I, Leone R, et al. Ovarian cancer cisplatin-resistant cell lines: multiple changes including collateral sensitivity to Taxol. Ann Oncol. 1998;9(4): 423-430

[60] Fokkema E, Groen HJ, Helder MN, de Vries EG, & Meijer C JM216-, JM118-, and cisplatin-induced cytotoxicity in relation to platinum-DNA adduct formation, glutathione levels and p53 status in human tumour cell lines with different sensitivities to cisplatin. Biochem Pharmacol. 2002;63(11): 1989-1996

[61] Byun SS, Kim SW, Choi H, Lee C, & Lee E Augmentation of cisplatin sensitivity in cisplatin-resistant human bladder cancer cells by modulating glutathione concentrations and glutathione-related enzyme activities. BJU Int. 2005;95(7): 1086-1090.10.1111/j.1464-410X.2005.05472.x

[62] Siddik ZH Cisplatin: mode of cytotoxic action and molecular basis of resistance. Oncogene. 2003;22(47): 7265-7279.10.1038/sj.onc.1206933

[63] Richardson A & Kaye SB Drug resistance in ovarian cancer: the emerging importance of gene transcription and spatio-temporal regulation of resistance. Drug Resist Updat. 2005;8(5): 311-321.10.1016/j.drup.2005.09.001

[64] Gonzalez VM, Fuertes MA, Alonso C, & Perez JM Is cisplatin-induced cell death always produced by apoptosis? Mol Pharmacol. 2001;59(4): 657-663

[65] Achanzar WE, Webber MM, & Waalkes MP Altered apoptotic gene expression and acquired apoptotic resistance in cadmium-transformed human prostate epithelial cells. Prostate. 2002;52(3): 236-244.10.1002/pros.10106

[66] Pink RC, Samuel P, Massa D, Caley DP, Brooks SA, et al. The passenger strand, miR-21-3p, plays a role in mediating cisplatin resistance in ovarian cancer cells. Gynecol Oncol. 2015.10.1016/j.ygyno.2014.12.042

[67] Zhou Y, Chen Q, Qin R, Zhang K, & Li H MicroRNA-449a reduces cell survival and enhances cisplatin-induced cytotoxicity via downregulation of NOTCH1 in ovarian cancer cells. Tumour Biol. 2014;35(12): 12369-12378.10.1007/s13277-014-2551-3

[68] Chen S, Chen X, Xiu YL, Sun KX, Zong ZH, et al. microRNA 490-3P enhances the drug-resistance of human ovarian cancer cells. J Ovarian Res. 2014;7: 84.10.1186/s13048-014-0084-4

[69] He J, Yu JJ, Xu Q, Wang L, Zheng JZ, et al. Downregulation of ATG14 by EGR1-MIR152 sensitizes ovarian cancer cells to cisplatin-induced apoptosis by inhibiting cyto-protective autophagy. Autophagy. 2015: 0.10.1080/15548627.2015.1009781

[70] Bae HJ, Noh JH, Kim JK, Eun JW, Jung KH, et al. MicroRNA-29c functions as a tumor suppressor by direct targeting oncogenic SIRT1 in hepatocellular carcinoma. Oncogene. 2014;33(20): 2557-2567.10.1038/onc.2013.216

[71] Yan M, Chen C, Gong W, Yin Z, Zhou L, et al. miR-21-3p regulates cardiac hypertrophic response by targeting histone deacetylase-8. Cardiovasc Res. 2014.10.1093/cvr/cvu254

[72] Osanto S, Qin Y, Buermans HP, Berkers J, Lerut E, et al. Genome-wide microRNA expression analysis of clear cell renal cell carcinoma by next generation deep sequencing. PLoS One. 2012;7(6): e38298.10.1371/journal.pone.0038298

[73] Huang Y, Dai Y, Yang J, Chen T, Yin Y, et al. Microarray analysis of microRNA expression in renal clear cell carcinoma. Eur J Surg Oncol. 2009;35(10): 1119-1123.10.1016/j.ejso.2009.04.010

[74] Chow TF, Youssef YM, Lianidou E, Romaschin AD, Honey RJ, et al. Differential expression profiling of microRNAs and their potential involvement in renal cell carcinoma pathogenesis. Clin Biochem. 2010;43(1-2): 150-158.10.1016/j.clinbiochem.2009.07.020

[75] Youssef YM, White NM, Grigull J, Krizova A, Samy C, et al. Accurate molecular classification of kidney cancer subtypes using microRNA signature. Eur Urol. 2011;59(5): 721-730.10.1016/j.eururo.2011.01.004

[76] Yao Y, Ma J, Xue Y, Wang P, Li Z, et al. MiR-449a exerts tumor-suppressive functions in human glioblastoma by targeting Myc-associated zinc-finger protein. Mol Oncol. 2014.10.1016/j.molonc.2014.11.003

[77] Hales EC, Taub JW, & Matherly LH New insights into Notch1 regulation of the PI3K-AKT-mTOR1 signaling axis: targeted therapy of gamma-secretase inhibitor resistant T-cell acute lymphoblastic leukemia. Cell Signal. 2014;26(1): 149-161.10.1016/j.cellsig.2013.09.021

[78] Cheng Q, Yi B, Wang A, & Jiang X Exploring and exploiting the fundamental role of microRNAs in tumor pathogenesis. Onco Targets Ther. 2013;6: 1675-1684.10.2147/OTT.S52730

[79] Liu X, Gao Y, Lu Y, Zhang J, Li L, et al. Oncogenes associated with drug resistance in ovarian cancer. J Cancer Res Clin Oncol. 2015;141(3): 381-395.10.1007/s00432-014-1765-5

[80] Beaufort CM, Helmijr JC, Piskorz AM, Hoogstraat M, Ruigrok-Ritstier K, et al. Ovarian cancer cell line panel (OCCP): clinical importance of in vitro morphological subtypes. PLoS One. 2014;9(9): e103988.10.1371/journal.pone.0103988

[81] Behrens BC, Hamilton TC, Masuda H, Grotzinger KR, Whang-Peng J, et al. Characterization of a cis-diamminedichloroplatinum(II)-resistant human ovarian cancer cell line and its use in evaluation of platinum analogues. Cancer Res. 1987;47(2): 414-418

[82] Hahne JC, Kurz A, Meyer SR, Dietl J, Engel JB, et al. Anti-tumour activity of phosphoinositide-3-kinase antagonist AEZS-126 in models of ovarian cancer. Arch Gynecol Obstet. 2015;291(1): 131-141.10.1007/s00404-014-3389-z

[83] Ali AY, Kim JY, Pelletier JF, Vanderhyden BC, Bachvarov DR, et al. Akt confers cisplatin chemoresistance in human gynecological carcinoma cells by modulating PPM1D stability. Mol Carcinog. 2014.10.1002/mc.22205

[84] Bao L, Jaramillo MC, Zhang Z, Zheng Y, Yao M, et al. Induction of autophagy contributes to cisplatin resistance in human ovarian cancer cells. Mol Med Rep. 2015;11(1): 91-98.10.3892/mmr.2014.2671

[85] Zhao JX, Liu H, Lv J, & Yang XJ Wortmannin enhances cisplatin-induced apoptosis in human ovarian cancer cells in vitro. Eur Rev Med Pharmacol Sci. 2014;18(17): 2428-2434

[86] Liu G, Du P, & Zhang Z Myeloid Differentiation Factor 88 Promotes Cisplatin Chemoresistance in Ovarian Cancer. Cell Biochem Biophys. 2014.10.1007/s12013-014-0294-9

[87] He G, Kuang J, Khokhar AR, & Siddik ZH The impact of S- and G2-checkpoint response on the fidelity of G1-arrest by cisplatin and its comparison to a non-cross-resistant platinum(IV) analog. Gynecol Oncol. 2011;122(2): 402-409.10.1016/j.ygyno.2011.04.034

[88] Hayakawa J, Ohmichi M, Kurachi H, Kanda Y, Hisamoto K, et al. Inhibition of BAD phosphorylation either at serine 112 via extracellular signal-regulated protein kinase cascade or at serine 136 via Akt cascade sensitizes human ovarian cancer cells to cisplatin. Cancer Res. 2000;60(21): 5988-5994

[89] Betito S & Cuvillier O Regulation by sphingosine 1-phosphate of Bax and Bad activities during apoptosis in a MEK-dependent manner. Biochem Biophys Res Commun. 2006;340(4): 1273-1277.10.1016/j.bbrc.2005.12.138

[90] Yang X, Fraser M, Moll UM, Basak A, & Tsang BK Akt-mediated cisplatin resistance in ovarian cancer: modulation of p53 action on caspase-dependent mitochondrial death pathway. Cancer Res. 2006;66(6): 3126-3136.10.1158/0008-5472.CAN-05-0425

[91] Fraser M, Bai T, & Tsang BK Akt promotes cisplatin resistance in human ovarian cancer cells through inhibition of p53 phosphorylation and nuclear function. Int J Cancer. 2008;122(3): 534-546.10.1002/ijc.23086

[92] Sasano T, Mabuchi S, Kuroda H, Kawano M, Matsumoto Y, et al. Preclinical Efficacy for AKT Targeting in Clear Cell Carcinoma of the Ovary. Mol Cancer Res. 2014.10.1158/1541-7786.MCR-14-0314

[93] Marsh Rde W, Rocha Lima CM, Levy DE, Mitchell EP, Rowland KM, Jr., et al. A phase II trial of perifosine in locally advanced, unresectable, or metastatic pancreatic adenocarcinoma. Am J Clin Oncol. 2007;30(1): 26-31.10.1097/01.coc. 0000251235.46149.43

[94] Leighl NB, Dent S, Clemons M, Vandenberg TA, Tozer R, et al. A Phase 2 study of perifosine in advanced or metastatic breast cancer. Breast Cancer Res Treat. 2008;108(1): 87-92.10.1007/s10549-007-9584-x

[95] Snyder EL, Bailey D, Shipitsin M, Polyak K, & Loda M Identification of CD44v6(+)/ CD24- breast carcinoma cells in primary human tumors by quantum dot-conjugated antibodies. Lab Invest. 2009;89(8): 857-866.10.1038/labinvest.2009.54

[96] Argiris A, Cohen E, Karrison T, Esparaz B, Mauer A, et al. A phase II trial of perifosine, an oral alkylphospholipid, in recurrent or metastatic head and neck cancer. Cancer Biol Ther. 2006;5(7): 766-770

[97] Knowling M, Blackstein M, Tozer R, Bramwell V, Dancey J, et al. A phase II study of perifosine (D-21226) in patients with previously untreated metastatic or locally advanced soft tissue sarcoma: A National Cancer Institute of Canada Clinical Trials Group trial. Invest New Drugs. 2006;24(5): 435-439.10.1007/s10637-006-6406-7

[98] Posadas EM, Gulley J, Arlen PM, Trout A, Parnes HL, et al. A phase II study of perifosine in androgen independent prostate cancer. Cancer Biol Ther. 2005;4(10): 1133-1137

[99] Ernst DS, Eisenhauer E, Wainman N, Davis M, Lohmann R, et al. Phase II study of perifosine in previously untreated patients with metastatic melanoma. Invest New Drugs. 2005;23(6): 569-575.10.1007/s10637-005-1157-4

[100] Vink SR, Schellens JH, Beijnen JH, Sindermann H, Engel J, et al. Phase I and pharmacokinetic study of combined treatment with perifosine and radiation in patients with advanced solid tumours. Radiother Oncol. 2006;80(2): 207-213.10.1016/j.radonc. 2006.07.032

[101] Masoumi Moghaddam S, Amini A, Morris DL, & Pourgholami MH Significance of vascular endothelial growth factor in growth and peritoneal dissemination of ovarian cancer. Cancer Metastasis Rev. 2012;31(1-2): 143-162.10.1007/s10555-011-9337-5

[102] Hahne JC, Okuducu AF, Sahin A, Fafeur V, Kiriakidis S, et al. The transcription factor ETS-1: its role in tumour development and strategies for its inhibition. Mini Rev Med Chem. 2008;8(11): 1095-1105

[103] Folkman J & Shing Y Angiogenesis. J Biol Chem. 1992;267(16): 10931-10934

[104] Risau W Mechanisms of angiogenesis. Nature. 1997;386(6626): 671-674.10.1038/386671a0

[105] Xia C, Meng Q, Cao Z, Shi X, & Jiang BH Regulation of angiogenesis and tumor growth by p110 alpha and AKT1 via VEGF expression. J Cell Physiol. 2006;209(1): 56-66.10.1002/jcp.20707

[106] Arbiser JL, Kau T, Konar M, Narra K, Ramchandran R, et al. Solenopsin, the alkaloidal component of the fire ant (Solenopsis invicta), is a naturally occurring inhibitor of phosphatidylinositol-3-kinase signaling and angiogenesis. Blood. 2007;109(2): 560-565.10.1182/blood-2006-06-029934

[107] Jiang BH & Liu LZ PI3K/PTEN signaling in tumorigenesis and angiogenesis. Biochim Biophys Acta. 2008;1784(1): 150-158.10.1016/j.bbapap.2007.09.008

[108] Weis S, Cui J, Barnes L, & Cheresh D Endothelial barrier disruption by VEGF-mediated Src activity potentiates tumor cell extravasation and metastasis. J Cell Biol. 2004;167(2): 223-229.10.1083/jcb.200408130

[109] Zhang L, Yang N, Garcia JR, Mohamed A, Benencia F, et al. Generation of a syngeneic mouse model to study the effects of vascular endothelial growth factor in ovarian carcinoma. Am J Pathol. 2002;161(6): 2295-2309

[110] Li L, Wang L, Zhang W, Tang B, Zhang J, et al. Correlation of serum VEGF levels with clinical stage, therapy efficacy, tumor metastasis and patient survival in ovarian cancer. Anticancer Res. 2004;24(3b): 1973-1979

[111] Ferrara N, Hillan KJ, & Novotny W Bevacizumab (Avastin), a humanized anti-VEGF monoclonal antibody for cancer therapy. Biochem Biophys Res Commun. 2005;333(2): 328-335.10.1016/j.bbrc.2005.05.132

[112] Hu L, Hofmann J, Zaloudek C, Ferrara N, Hamilton T, et al. Vascular endothelial growth factor immunoneutralization plus Paclitaxel markedly reduces tumor burden and ascites in athymic mouse model of ovarian cancer. Am J Pathol. 2002;161(5): 1917-1924.10.1016/S0002-9440(10)64467-7

[113] Mabuchi S, Terai Y, Morishige K, Tanabe-Kimura A, Sasaki H, et al. Maintenance treatment with bevacizumab prolongs survival in an in vivo ovarian cancer model. Clin Cancer Res. 2008;14(23): 7781-7789.10.1158/1078-0432.CCR-08-0243

[114] Errico A Breast cancer: combining bevacizumab with chemotherapy--from maintenance to second-line treatment. Nat Rev Clin Oncol. 2014;11(11): 621.10.1038/nrclinonc.2014.179

[115] Burger RA, Brady MF, Bookman MA, Fleming GF, Monk BJ, et al. Incorporation of bevacizumab in the primary treatment of ovarian cancer. N Engl J Med. 2011;365(26): 2473-2483.10.1056/NEJMoa1104390

[116] Perren TJ, Swart AM, Pfisterer J, Ledermann JA, Pujade-Lauraine E, et al. A phase 3 trial of bevacizumab in ovarian cancer. N Engl J Med. 2011;365(26): 2484-2496.10.1056/NEJMoa1103799

[117] Aghajanian C, Blank SV, Goff BA, Judson PL, Teneriello MG, et al. OCEANS: a randomized, double-blind, placebo-controlled phase III trial of chemotherapy with or without bevacizumab in patients with platinum-sensitive recurrent epithelial ovarian, primary peritoneal, or fallopian tube cancer. J Clin Oncol. 2012;30(17): 2039-2045.10.1200/JCO.2012.42.0505

[118] Krupitskaya Y & Wakelee HA Ramucirumab, a fully human mAb to the transmembrane signaling tyrosine kinase VEGFR-2 for the potential treatment of cancer. Curr Opin Investig Drugs. 2009;10(6): 597-605

[119] Spratlin JL, Cohen RB, Eadens M, Gore L, Camidge DR, et al. Phase I pharmacologic and biologic study of ramucirumab (IMC-1121B), a fully human immunoglobulin G1 monoclonal antibody targeting the vascular endothelial growth factor receptor-2. J Clin Oncol. 2010;28(5): 780-787.10.1200/JCO.2009.23.7537

[120] Caligiuri MA Human natural killer cells. Blood. 2008;112(3): 461-469.10.1182/blood-2007-09-077438

[121] Vivier E, Raulet DH, Moretta A, Caligiuri MA, Zitvogel L, et al. Innate or adaptive immunity? The example of natural killer cells. Science. 2011;331(6013): 44-49.10.1126/science.1198687

[122] Lanier LL Up on the tightrope: natural killer cell activation and inhibition. Nat Immunol. 2008;9(5): 495-502.10.1038/ni1581

[123] Moretta L, Biassoni R, Bottino C, Mingari MC, & Moretta A Human NK-cell receptors. Immunol Today. 2000;21(9): 420-422

[124] Lanier LL NK cell recognition. Annu Rev Immunol. 2005;23: 225-274.10.1146/annurev.immunol.23.021704.115526

[125] Dunn GP, Bruce AT, Ikeda H, Old LJ, & Schreiber RD Cancer immunoediting: from immunosurveillance to tumor escape. Nat Immunol. 2002;3(11): 991-998.10.1038/ni1102-991

[126] Orr MT & Lanier LL Natural killer cell education and tolerance. Cell. 2010;142(6): 847-856.10.1016/j.cell.2010.08.031

[127] Smyth MJ, Dunn GP, & Schreiber RD Cancer immunosurveillance and immunoediting: the roles of immunity in suppressing tumor development and shaping tumor immunogenicity. Adv Immunol. 2006;90: 1-50.10.1016/S0065-2776(06)90001-7

[128] Zhang Y, Wang X, Yang H, Liu H, Lu Y, et al. Kinase AKT controls innate immune cell development and function. Immunology. 2013;140(2): 143-152.10.1111/imm.12123

[129] Hawkins PT & Stephens LR PI3K signalling in inflammation. Biochim Biophys Acta. 2014.10.1016/j.bbalip.2014.12.006

[130] Soliman GA The role of mechanistic target of rapamycin (mTOR) complexes signaling in the immune responses. Nutrients. 2013;5(6): 2231-2257.10.3390/nu5062231

[131] Dituri F, Mazzocca A, Giannelli G, & Antonaci S PI3K functions in cancer progression, anticancer immunity and immune evasion by tumors. Clin Dev Immunol. 2011;2011: 947858.10.1155/2011/947858

[132] Bhoopathi P, Quinn BA, Gui Q, Shen XN, Grossman SR, et al. Pancreatic cancer-specific cell death induced in vivo by cytoplasmic-delivered polyinosine-polycytidylic acid. Cancer Res. 2014;74(21): 6224-6235.10.1158/0008-5472.CAN-14-0819

[133] Engel JB, Honig A, Kapp M, Hahne JC, Meyer SR, et al. Mechanisms of tumor immune escape in triple-negative breast cancers (TNBC) with and without mutated BRCA 1. Arch Gynecol Obstet. 2014;289(1): 141-147.10.1007/s00404-013-2922-9

[134] Noh KH, Kang TH, Kim JH, Pai SI, Lin KY, et al. Activation of Akt as a mechanism for tumor immune evasion. Mol Ther. 2009;17(3): 439-447.10.1038/mt.2008.255

[135] Bellucci R, Nguyen HN, Martin A, Heinrichs S, Schinzel AC, et al. Tyrosine kinase pathways modulate tumor susceptibility to natural killer cells. J Clin Invest. 2012;122(7): 2369-2383.10.1172/JCI58457

[136] Boutet P, Aguera-Gonzalez S, Atkinson S, Pennington CJ, Edwards DR, et al. Cutting edge: the metalloproteinase ADAM17/TNF-alpha-converting enzyme regulates proteolytic shedding of the MHC class I-related chain B protein. J Immunol. 2009;182(1): 49-53

[137] Waldhauer I, Goehlsdorf D, Gieseke F, Weinschenk T, Wittenbrink M, et al. Tumor-associated MICA is shed by ADAM proteases. Cancer Res. 2008;68(15): 6368-6376.10.1158/0008-5472.CAN-07-6768

[138] Okita R, Mougiakakos D, Ando T, Mao Y, Sarhan D, et al. HER2/HER3 signaling regulates NK cell-mediated cytotoxicity via MHC class I chain-related molecule A and B expression in human breast cancer cell lines. J Immunol. 2012;188(5): 2136-2145.10.4049/jimmunol.1102237

Chapter 8

Recurrent Ovarian Cancer — Basic Knowledge, Current Management, and Future Directions

Bernardo L. Rapoport

Additional information is available at the end of the chapter

http://dx.doi.org/10.5772/60609

Abstract

Recurrent ovarian cancer is incurable. Chemotherapy is indicated to control disease-related symptoms. The benefit from chemotherapy in these patients depends on the platinum-free interval. Patients with platinum-resistant disease (a relapse of less than six months from the completion of platinum treatment) are managed with non-platinum agents. Patients with platinum semi-sensitive relapse (six to 12 months from the completion of treatment) have a response rate of 30% to second-line platinum treatment. In patients with platinum-sensitive relapse (more than 12 months from the completion of treatment), the response rate to platinum is 60–70%. Limited data is available regarding the benefits of secondary cytoreductive surgery. GOG 213 and the AGO Desktop III studies will define the role of this procedure in patients with recurrent disease. Two studies have shown benefit of bevacizumab in the treatment of patients with platinum-sensitive (Oceans) and refractory disease (Aurelia). Additional studies are needed to establish the optimal duration and timing of treatment. Cediranib has shown activity in patients with recurrent platinum-sensitive ovarian cancer (ICON 6 trial). Numerous novel biological agents are being investigated in relapsed ovarian cancer. This chapter focuses on current management and future directions in patients with relapsed ovarian cancer.

Keywords: Ovarian Cancer, relapsed, platinum sensitive, targeted therapy

1. Introduction

The vast majority of patients with advanced ovarian cancer will recur after first-line chemotherapy. [1] A common sign of relapse is a rise in the serum CA-125 level in the absence of symptoms (defined as marker-only relapse) or objective evidence of disease as assessed by physical or radiological examinations. Recurrent disease is not curable, and the majority of patients with recurrent disease will succumb to their disease irrespective of the second-line treatment modality used. As there is no compelling evidence that early treatment with chemotherapy is beneficial in relapsed asymptomatic disease, patients with marker-only-relapse are often observed. The MRC OV05/EORTC 55955 did not show a survival benefit with early treatment of relapse on the basis of a raised CA125 concentration only. [2] Some patients with asymptomatic disease with tumour-marker elevation only may develop symptomatic disease within months, while others may take years. [2] Assessment of the rate of progression by CA 125 is essential and useful for most patients with advanced ovarian cancer in remission. CA 125 is elevated in most patients with documented progressive disease. Serial measurement is a useful marker to assess the response to chemotherapy according to GCIG criteria. [3] Clinicians should keep in mind that CA 125 is not specific for ovarian cancer. Raised CA 125 levels may also be found in non-gynaecological malignancies (breast cancer and lung cancer, as well as colon and pancreatic malignancies). An elevated CA 125 can be found in patients with benign conditions such as endometriosis, pelvic inflammatory disease, and ovarian cysts.

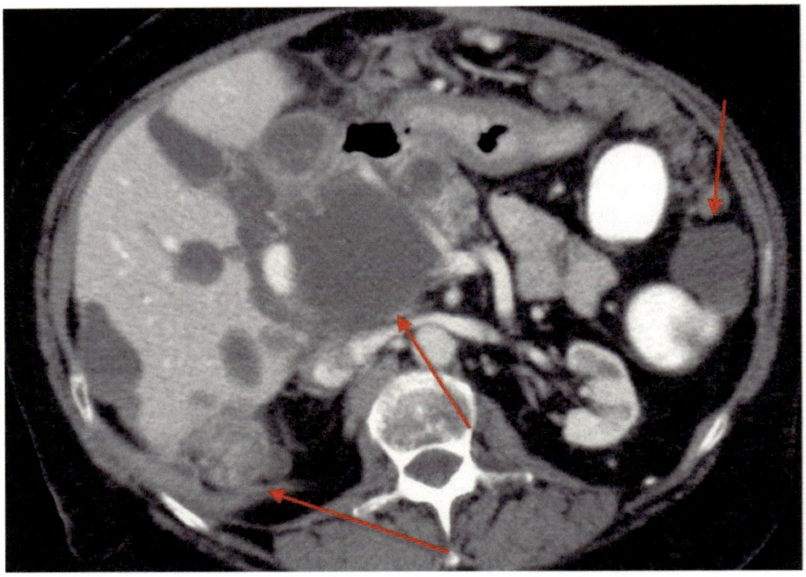

Figure 1. Progressive disease — shows multiple complex cystic/solid peritoneal deposits on the liver's surface (visceral peritoneum) and elsewhere in the peritoneal cavity.

2. Chemotherapy

The role of chemotherapy in the management of recurrent ovarian cancer is palliative and is usually indicated for ovarian cancer-related symptoms, or for patients with objective evidence of significant disease progression on physical or radiological examination.

The likelihood of benefit from chemotherapy treatment in patients with relapsed ovarian cancer depends on the platinum-free interval (PFI). PFI is defined as the interval between the last dose of platinum and the time of relapse. Patients with platinum-resistant disease (PFI of less than six months) are unlikely to respond to second-line platinum agents and are often managed with an alternative agent (see Table 1). Patients with platinum semi-sensitive disease (PFI of between six and 12 months) have a response rate of approximately 30% to second-line platinum treatment. In patients with fully platinum-sensitive disease (PFI more than 12 months with a subset greater than 24 months), the response rate to second-line platinum may be as high as 60–70%. [4]

The role of combination chemotherapy has been assessed in randomized trials in the setting of platinum semi-sensitive and fully sensitive relapses. Patients with fully sensitive disease should be re-challenged with a platinum-based (cisplatin or carboplatin) chemotherapy regime. [5] Patients with platinum semi-sensitive disease should be treated with a platinum-based doublet combination. It has been demonstrated that retreatment results in valuable responses that translate into improvement in quality of life and survival. Patients with a PFI of greater than six months usually receive treatment with a platinum-based regimen either as a single-agent or in combination with agents like paclitaxel [6], gemcitabine [7], or pegylated liposomal doxorubicin (PLD) [8]

Agent	Author	ORR	PFS	OS
(months)	(%)	(months)	(months)	
Liposomal Doxorubicin	Colombo [14]	15	3.9	13.2
Topotecan weekly	Sehouli [18]	19	3.7	9.6
Paclitaxel weekly	Markman [15]	20	5.6	13.5
Paclitaxel 3 weekly	Trimble [16]	22	4.5	8.8
Docetaxel	Francis [17]	40	5.0	8.0
Gemcytabine	Lund [19]	19	2.8	6.2
Pemetrexed	Miller [20]	21	2.9	11.4
Etoposide oral	Rose [22]	26	5.7	10.8
Ixabepilone	De Geest [21]	14	4.4	14.8

Table 1. Platinum refractory.

The International Collaborative Ovarian Neoplasm-4 (ICON-4) trial compared combination chemotherapy with paclitaxel and platinum to single-agent platinum in patients with platinum-sensitive disease. In this study, most patients had a PFI of 12 months or greater. ICON-4 showed a statistically significant improvement in overall survival (OS) in favour of combination chemotherapy for recurrent ovarian cancer, with a 7% absolute increase at two years (P = 0.023). Although the ICON-4 trial showed a positive outcome, the results remain controversial because of methodological limitations. Around, 40% of patients randomized to the platinum single-agent arm never received a taxane during the course of their disease, including first-line therapy and at disease progression, raising the possibility that the sequential use of platinum followed by paclitaxel at disease progression might have conferred the same survival advantage. [6]

Docetaxel has been investigated in the treatment of metastatic ovarian cancer, in both the front-line and relapsed setting. In the front-line setting, docetaxel was shown to be equivalent to paclitaxel. [9] Docetaxel may also be a useful choice for patients at risk of developing peripheral neuropathy. [9–11]

In a subsequent study, the AGO (Arbeitsgemeinschaft Gynaekologische Onkologie) from Germany conducted a randomized Phase III trial in patients with platinum-sensitive relapse to either gemcitabine and carboplatin, or carboplatin alone. [7] PFS was 8.6 months for the combination versus 5.8 months for single-agent carboplatin (P =.0038), with no improvement in OS. Quality of life was similar between the two arms, despite a higher incidence of thrombocytopoenia, neutropoenia, and anaemia with the combination.

Rapoport et al. investigated pegylated liposomal doxorubicin (PLD) in combination with carboplatin in a Phase II trial in patients with relapsed ovarian cancer with semi-sensitive and fully sensitive relapse. Results were encouraging, with a complete response rate of 35% and a partial response rate of 32.5% (overall response, 67.5%). Median time to progression was 11.9 months, and median survival was 30.0 months. Overall responses were higher in the platinum fully sensitive subgroup as opposed to the semi-sensitive group. [12] The GCIG (Gynecologic Cancer Intergroup) conducted a Phase III study (CALYPSO trial) comparing paclitaxel and carboplatin with PLD and carboplatin in patients presenting with platinum-sensitive relapse. There was a significant improvement in median progression-free survival (PFS) (11.3 months vs. 9.4 months; P =.005), with a lower incidence of severe hypersensitivity reactions (5% vs. 18%), in favour of the PLD-containing arm. No difference in OS was noted. Toxicities were similar to the toxicities reported in the Phase II study by Rapoport et al. and included grade 2 or greater alopecia (83.6% vs. 7%) and sensory neuropathy (26.9% vs. 4.9%) in the paclitaxel-containing arm, and with more hand-foot syndrome (grades 2 to 3, 12.0% vs. 2.2%), nausea (35.2% vs. 24.2%), and mucositis (grades 2 to 3, 13.9% vs. 7%) in the PLD containing arm. [8]

As recurrent ovarian cancer is incurable, palliation and symptom control is the goal of second-line treatment. Choosing the most appropriate agent for use in the recurrent disease setting, therefore, involves balancing the need to attain a response to treatment against maintenance of reasonable quality of life. The decision to use platinum-based chemotherapy combinations or single-agent platinum in this setting should be based on a number of factors. These factors include patient age, disease burden, rate of relapse, and patient preference. For elderly patients who require chemotherapy for mild symptomatic and low tumour burden, platinum-sensitive relapse, the usage of single-agent carboplatin is a reasonable approach. PLD is a well-tolerated alternative in patients that develop an allergy to carboplatin during the course of treatment or if further use of carboplatin is contraindicated. Both agents are associated with a good quality of life as well as acceptable toxicity profiles in terms of alopecia or severe myelosuppression. A more aggressive approach is needed for younger patients with rapidly growing cancer and platinum-sensitive relapse. Combination chemotherapy with either paclitaxel and carboplatin, docetaxel and carboplatin [13], gemcitabine and carboplatin [7], or PLD and carboplatin are reasonable [8].

Patients with platinum/taxane-resistant disease (defined by a short PFI of less than six months, or progression during platinum-based chemotherapy) are best treated with agents who lack cross-resistance to platinum compounds or are not susceptible to the common resistance mechanisms.

Potentially non-cross-resistant drugs with activity in the platinum-resistant setting include PLD [14], paclitaxel [15–16], docetaxel [17], topotecan [18], gemcitabine [19], pemetrexed [20], ixabepilone [21], or oral etoposide [22] (Table 1). In the platinum-resistant setting, the overall response rate to any of these agents is approximately 20%. Responses are short, with a median PFS of four to six months. These responses are progressively shorter with each subsequent regimen.

In the setting of platinum-resistant relapse, PLD is well tolerated at doses of 40 mg/m2 given every four weeks. Common toxicities include palmer-plantar erythrodysesthesia (hand-foot syndrome) and mucositis. Topotecan may cause significant myelosuppression and fatigue. A recently reported Phase II randomized multicenter study however showed that weekly topotecan has a favourable toxicity profile compared to the conventional 5-day schedule of topotecan with similar OS. [23]

The Cochrane Gynaecological Cancer Group conducted a meta-analysis of 14 randomized trials evaluating the usefulness of PLD in relapsed epithelial ovarian cancer. Results of this meta-analysis concluded that in patients with platinum-sensitive disease, PLD and carboplatin is more effective than paclitaxel and carboplatin, and is better tolerated. Therefore, PLD and carboplatin should be considered as the first option of treatment in women with platinum-sensitive relapse. PLD alone is also a useful agent for platinum-resistant disease. It remains unclear, however, how it compares with other single agents in this subgroup, and in which order these agents should be used. There is no data available to support the use of PLD in combination with other agents in patients with platinum-resistant relapse. [24]

As a general rule, combination chemotherapy regimens are not superior to single agents in the management of patients with platinum-resistant relapse. Combination regimens are also more toxic and should not be used in this palliative setting.

3. The role of surgery in the treatment of relapsed ovarian cancer

3.1. Secondary cytoreductive surgery

Surgery for the debulking of disease at the time of relapse, referred to as secondary cytoreductive surgery, is performed in selected patients prior to second-line chemotherapy. [25]

Due to a lack of large randomized trials, conclusive data are limited regarding the benefits of secondary cytoreductive surgery. The ability to complete a successful secondary cytoreduction may identify patients presenting with a biologically less aggressive disease or those patients who have a lower tumour burden at the time of relapse. A prospective randomized trial of secondary cytoreduction is required to determine whether this procedure improves survival in these patients. The value of secondary cytoreduction is currently being investigated in two prospective, randomized trials, GOG 213 and the AGO Desktop III study.

The Gynaecologic Oncology group (GOG) currently defines 'optimal' cytoreductive surgery as having residual tumours having a maximum diameter of 1 cm or less. Complete cytoreduction is the ideal surgical outcome in the form of microscopic disease. [26]

Secondary cytoreduction might be considered for the subgroup of patients with a progression-free interval of more than 12 to 18 months from the time of completion of adjuvant chemotherapy, localized recurrence amenable to complete cytoreduction, potentially chemosensitive disease, and good performance status. [27–31]

On the other hand, a patient with a rapid, multifocal recurrence is unlikely to obtain any clinical benefit from surgery. [26]

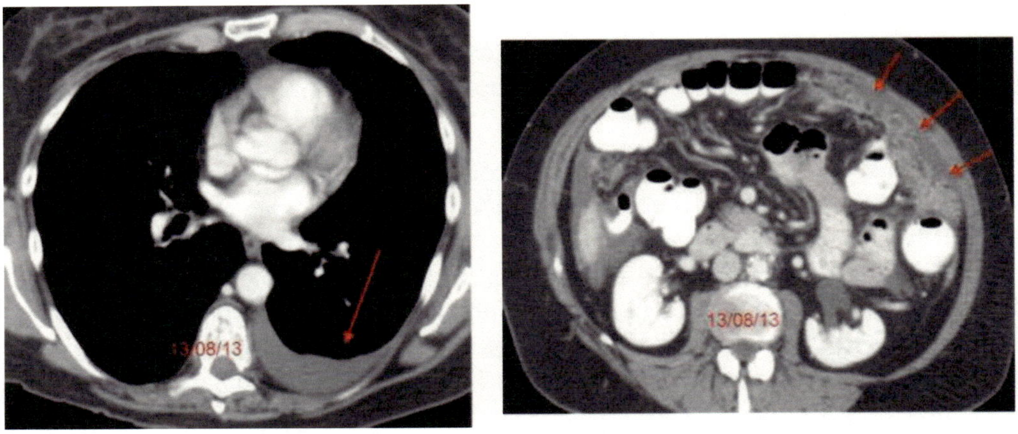

Figure 2. Pleural and peritoneal recurrence.

3.2. Palliative surgery

Palliative surgery may be indicated in patients with recurrent ovarian cancer. Standard operations performed in this setting include colostomy for relief of a large bowel obstruction, treatment of peritoneal adhesions, and management of small bowel obstruction. [32] Surgery to relieve small bowel obstruction should take into account the likelihood of continued responsiveness to chemotherapy postoperatively (platinum-sensitive as opposed to platinum-refractory disease). Women who develop a small bowel obstruction during first-line chemotherapy have aggressive and resistant ovarian cancer, and the procedure is not beneficial in this subset of patients. A palliative gastrostomy tube may be most appropriate in this situation. Best outcomes are seen in women who have had prolonged PFI, usually lasting more than one year.

Surgery is not indicated in the management of patients with a pseudo-obstruction due to an intra-abdominal carcinomatosis and infiltration of the myoenteric plexus of the small bowel. Pharmacological treatment with metoclopramide (an agent that improves motility of the upper gastrointestinal tract without stimulating gastric, biliary, or pancreatic secretions) may be helpful to treat this complication. A palliative colostomy may be indicated for patients developing a large bowel obstruction. This type of surgery can provide significant prolongation of survival and improved quality of life in selected patients.

3.3. Radiation therapy

Radiation therapy may be useful in the palliation of patients with recurrent ovarian cancer. Symptomatic pelvic masses may cause bleeding, pain, and rectal narrowing. Palliative pelvic radiotherapy can offer symptom relief. Cerebral or bone metastases are unusual complications of ovarian cancer and can be successfully palliated with radiotherapy.

4. Investigational Agents

Several investigational agents are being studied in the relapse setting.

4.1. Bevacizumab

4.1.1. Bevacizumab single-agent activity

Bevacizumab is a humanized antibody that recognizes and neutralizes vascular endothelial growth factor (VEGF). VEGF is a pro-angiogenic factor that is secreted by ovarian cancer cells. Randomized data in other metastatic malignant diseases have shown a survival advantage for the use of bevacizumab in combination with chemotherapy [33–35].

Single-agent bevacizumab has been shown by the GOG to induce a response rate of 18% in patients with relapsed ovarian cancer. In this GOG trial, there were two complete and 11 partial responses, with a median response duration of 10 months, and 25 patients (40%) survived progression-free for at least six months. Median PFS was 4.7 months and OS was 17 months. This study did not show a significant association with prior platinum sensitivity, age, number of prior chemotherapeutic regimens, or performance status. [36]

Cannistra et al. reported a risk of life-threatening bowel perforation in patients with ovarian cancer treated with bevacizumab. All patients in this trial were heavily pre-treated, with 50% having received three prior regimens. Partial responses were observed in seven patients (15.9%). Median PFS was 4.4 months (95% CI, 3.1 to 5.5 months), with a median survival duration of 10.7 months at study termination. Bevacizumab-associated grades 3 to 4 events included hypertension (9.1%), proteinuria (15.9%), bleeding (2.3%), and wound-healing complications (2.3%). The incidence of bowel perforation was 11.4%. This was higher than reported in bevacizumab trials of other tumour types. Risk factors for bevacizumab-induced bowel perforation included a higher number of prior chemotherapy regimens, radiographic presence of bowel wall involvement by tumour, or evidence of bowel obstruction. [37]

4.1.2. Bevacizumab in combination with chemotherapy in newly diagnosed ovarian cancer patients

Two randomized studies (GOG-0218 and ICON7) have shown improvement in the PFS in patients with advanced ovarian cancer treated with chemotherapy and bevacizumab. [38–39] In these trials, bevacizumab was evaluated in combination with standard paclitaxel plus carboplatin as part of initial treatment for women with ovarian cancer. Both these trials met their primary endpoints and demonstrated an improvement in PFS.

In the GOG-0218 trial, 1,873 women with newly diagnosed stage III (incompletely resectable) or stage IV epithelial ovarian cancer which had undergone debulking surgery were randomized to receive one of three treatments in a double-blind, placebo-controlled trial. Each of the three study regimens comprised 22 3-week cycles of intravenous infusions on day one, with the first six cycles consisting of standard chemotherapy with carboplatin and paclitaxel. [38]

Arm 1 — Control: chemotherapy with a placebo added in cycles 2 to 22.

Arm 2 — Chemotherapy with bevacizumab (15mg per kilogram of body weight) added in cycles 2 to 6, and a placebo from cycles 7 to 22.

Arm 3 — Chemotherapy with bevacizumab added in cycles 2 to 22.

At a median follow-up of 17.4 months, the median PFS was 10.3, 11.2, and 14.1 months in the control group, the bevacizumab-initiation group, and the bevacizumab-throughout group, respectively. No significant difference in OS was reported. The potential to detect a difference in survival is likely to be limited by lack of control for multiple subsequent regimens, including crossover to bevacizumab or other anti-VEGF agents. [38]

Although bevacizumab use resulted in additional toxicity, it was not associated with a decrease in quality of life. Grade 2 or greater hypertension was significantly more frequent with use of bevacizumab than a placebo. [38]

The second trial, ICON 7 was led by the U.K. Medical Research Council Clinical Trials Unit. This trial enrolled 1528 women with histologically confirmed, high-risk, early-stage disease (FIGO stage I or IIA and clear-cell or grade 3 tumours), or advanced (FIGO stage IIB to IV) epithelial ovarian cancer, primary peritoneal cancer, or fallopian-tube cancer. Patients were randomized to receive carboplatin and paclitaxel given every three weeks for six cycles, or to the same regimen plus bevacizumab (7.5mg per kilogram) given concurrently every three weeks for five or six cycles and continued for 12 additional cycles or until disease progression. Complete or partial response rates were reported in 67% of patients in the bevacizumab group and 48% in the control group ($p = 0.001$). With a median follow-up of 19.4 months, the data provide clear evidence of the biologic activity of bevacizumab with a median PFS of 19 months compared to 17.4 months in the standard therapy group (HR 0.81, CI, 0.70 to 0.94; $p = 004$). Final survival data are expected soon. Bevacizumab treatment did not affect the delivery of chemotherapy; it was, however, associated with a significant increase in side effects, including grade 2 or greater hypertension and bowel perforation. [39]

4.1.3. Bevacizumab in combination with chemotherapy in patients with recurrent platinum-sensitive disease

The OCEANS (Carboplatin and Gemcitabine plus Bevacizumab in Patients with Ovary, Peritoneal, or Fallopian Tube Carcinoma) study showed a benefit for the addition of bevacizumab to platinum-based chemotherapy in terms of PFS and a trend towards a benefit in OS.

Updated data by Aghajanian et al. indicate a median PFS advantage of four months (12.4 vs. 8.4 months) (hazard ratio 0.484) and overall response rate by RECIST of 21% (response rate 78.5% vs. 57.4%) were seen when bevacizumab was added to carboplatin and gemcitabine chemotherapy. Nevertheless, no benefit in OS was seen, but the data is still immature. [40]

Agent	Target	Phase	Clinical Setting
Cediranib	VEGFR1 VEGFR2 VEGFR3 Lymphangenesis C-Kit	Phase III	Concurrent carboplatin and paclitaxel for platinum sensitive relapse
Aflibercept	VEGF Placental Growth Factor	Phase II	In combination with docetaxel
AMG 386 (Trebananib)	TIE-2 receptor Angiopoietin-1 Angiopoietin-2	Phase III	TRINOVA-1 paclitaxel combination and maintenance in platinum sensitive and refractory relapse
		Phase III	TRINOVA-2 PLD combination and maintenance in platinum refractory relapse
		Phase III	TRINOVA-3 paclitaxel and carboplatin combination and maintenance in newly diagnosed metastatic disease
BIBF-1120	VEGFR PDGFR FGFR	Phase II	Maintenance of relapsed ovarian cancer
Pazopanib	VEGFR-1 VEGFR-2 VEGFR-3 PDGFR-α PDGFR-β FGFR-1 FGFR-3 C-Kit	Phase III	Maintenance of advanced ovarian cancer in the front-line setting
Olaparib	PARP	Phase III	Maintenance in inhibitor platinum-sensitive relapsed

VEGFR: Vascular endothelial growth factor receptor
PDGFR: platelet-derived growth factor receptor
FGFR: fibroblast growth factor receptor
PARP: poly-adenosine diphosphate [ADP]-ribose polymerase
TIE-2 receptor: receptor tyrosine kinase expressed predominantly on endothelial cells
c-Kit: trans-membrane receptor tyrosine kinase KIT, which is defined by the CD117 antigen

Table 2. Antiangiogenesis agents under investigation for the treatment of relapsed ovarian cancer.

4.1.4. Bevacizumab in combination with chemotherapy in patients with platinum-resistant disease

The AURELIA randomized Phase III study showed that addition of bevacizumab to standard chemotherapy with either PLD, topotecan, or weekly paclitaxel was associated with an improvement in PFS of 3.3 months and overall response rate by RECIST of 18%. OS and quality of life data from this study are still immature. [41]

Bevacizumab is an active agent in advanced and recurrent ovarian cancer. Large clinical trials are needed to improve the knowledge of the safety and effectiveness of bevacizumab, the duration and timing of treatment, and activity of this agent when given in combination with other chemotherapeutic agents. There is also an urgent need to identify biologic predictive factors of efficacy. When to start and end anti-angiogenesis therapy remain controversial questions, and further evaluation of personalized novel angiogenesis-based therapy is needed.

4.2. Cediranib

Cediranib (AZD2171) is a highly potent, small-molecule, oral tyrosine kinase inhibitor of VEGFR-1, -2, and -3, and c-Kit, which compete for the ATP-binding site within the receptor kinase domain. [42–43] It is postulated that cediranib is useful in the prevention of tumour progression, by inhibiting VEGFR-2 activity and angiogenesis, and also by concomitantly inhibiting VEGFR-3 activity and lymphangiogenesis.

Cediranib has been shown to be an active drug in recurrent ovarian cancer, fallopian tube, and peritoneal cancer with the predictable toxicities observed with other tyrosine kinase inhibitors. In a Phase II trial, partial responses were seen in eight of the 46 treated patients (17.4%). [44] The original dose was 45 mg/d, but the dose was lowered to 30 mg because of toxicity observed in the first 11 patients. Major grade 3 toxicities included hypertension (46%), fatigue (24%), and diarrhoea (13%). Grade 4 toxicities included central nervous system haemorrhage (n = 1), hypertriglyceridaemia/hypercholesterolaemia/elevated lipase (n = 1), and dehydration/elevated creatinine (n = 1). No GI perforations or fistulas occurred. [44]

Initial results of the international three-arm Phase III randomized trial (ICON 6) showed that the addition of cediranib to chemotherapy (carboplatin and paclitaxel) increased PFS by about three months in women with recurrent platinum-sensitive ovarian cancer. Additional benefit was obtained when cediranib was used as maintenance therapy, increasing overall PFS over chemotherapy alone. The time to disease progression increased from 9.4 to 12.6 months and OS was extended from 17.6 to 20.3 months over a follow-up period of two years. [45, 46]

5. Other investigational agents

Other anti-angiogenic agents have also been evaluated in recurrent ovarian cancer.

Aflibercept is a potent inhibitor of both VEGF and placental growth factor. Aflibercept has shown anti-tumour activity in combination with docetaxel and is useful as a single agent in the reduction of malignant ascites. The combination was tested in a Phase I/II study in patients with measurable, recurrent, or persistent epithelial ovarian cancer. The confirmed objective response rate was 54% (25 of 46 patients responded to treatment, with 11 patients achieving a complete response and 14 a partial response). [47]

AMG 386 (trebananib) is a peptide-Fc fusion protein that inhibits angiogenesis by neutralizing the interaction between the Tie2 receptor and angiopoietin 1 and 2. Targeting of the angiopoietins/Tie2 pathway as a strategy to overcome bevacizumab resistance and toxicities has gained increasing interest in recent years. A randomized study of 161 patients with recurrent epithelial ovarian, fallopian tube, or primary peritoneal cancer evaluated weekly treatment with paclitaxel plus intravenous AMG 386 at a dose of 10mg/kg week (arm A), weekly paclitaxel plus AMG 386 at a dose of 10mg/kg week (arm B), or weekly paclitaxel plus placebo (arm C). Median PFS was 7.2 months in arm A, 5.7 months in arm B, and 4.6 months in arm C. The study has shown promising anti-cancer activity with a manageable safety profile when combined with weekly paclitaxel and a dose-response effect. [48] A recent publication of 919 enrolled patients, of whom 461 were randomly assigned to the trebananib group and 458 to the placebo group, was associated with a significantly longer median progression-free survival in favour of trebananib compared to placebo (7 2 months vs. 5 4 months; hazard ratio 0.66, p<0 0001). There was no significant increase in the incidence of grade 3 or higher adverse events between treatment groups (244 [54%] of 452 patients) for the placebo group compared to 258 [56%] of 461 patients) in the trebananib group. In this Phase III study, inhibition of angiopoietins 1 and 2 with trebananib resulted in a significant prolongation in progression-free survival. The results of the ongoing TRINOVA-1, -2, and -3 trials will define the role of trebananib in the management of patients with advanced epithelial ovarian cancer. [49]

BIBF-1120 is a triple angiokinase inhibitor of VEGFR, PDGFR, and FGFR. This agent has shown promising activity in a randomized Phase II placebo-controlled trial in relapsed ovarian cancer in the maintenance setting. The study showed a 36 week PFS of 16.3% vs. 5.0% in favour of BIBF 1120 compared to the placebo group with a hazard ratio of 0.65 (95% CI, 0.42 to 1.02; P = 0.06). [50]

5.1. Pazopanib

Pazopanib inhibits this signalling pathway via ATP-competitive inhibition of VEGFR-1, VEGFR-2, and VEGFR-3; platelet-derived growth factor receptor (PDGFR)-α, PDGFR-β; fibroblast growth factor receptor (FGFR)-1, FGFR-3, and c-Kit. [51] Friedlander et al. reported responses to pazopanib in 11 of 36 patients (31%) with advanced ovarian cancer. The median time to response was 29 days and median response duration 113 days. The overall response rate was 18% in patients with measurable disease at baseline. [52]

De Bois et al. reported results of the AGO OVAR16 trial investigating the role of pazopanib as maintenance treatment for patients with advanced ovarian cancer in the front-line setting following induction chemotherapy. A total of 940 patients with stage 3 or 4 disease were randomized. The median time from diagnosis to randomization was 7.1 months in the placebo arm and 7.0 months in the pazopanib arm. At a median follow-up of 24 months, patients in the pazopanib arm had a prolonged PFS compared to a placebo, 17.9 versus 12.3 months, respectively (HR = 0.766; 95% CI: 0.64-0.91; p = 0.0021). Sensitivity and subgroup analyses of

PFS, and analysis of PFS by GCIG criteria, were consistent with the primary analysis. The first interim analysis for OS (only 189 OS events = 20.1% of the population) showed no difference between the arms. Pazopanib treatment was associated with a higher incidence of adverse and serious adverse events (26% vs. 11%). The most common toxicities included hypertension, diarrhoea, nausea, headache, fatigue, and neutropoenia. The AGO investigators concluded that pazopanib maintenance therapy provided a statistically significant and clinically meaningful PFS benefit in patients with advanced ovarian cancer. It is possible that pazopanib will be incorporated into the armamentarium of ovarian cancer drugs in routine practice in the near future. The OS data are not mature. [53–54]

5.2. PARP inhibitors

A new class of agents that inhibit poly-adenosine diphosphate [ADP]-ribose polymerase (PARP) demonstrated significant activity in patients with recurrent disease, especially those with a germline mutation in BRCA1 or BRCA2. Several recent ongoing studies are evaluating the activity of PARP inhibitors in epithelial ovarian cancer, primarily in BRCA-mutation carriers. A proof-of-concept Phase I study of olaparib was conducted in 50 BRCA-carrier patients with relapsed ovarian cancer. This study showed a 40% objective response rate judged by RECIST criteria and/or a CA125 response assessed by a greater than 50% decline in CA125. Patients that were platinum sensitive had a higher chance of achieving a response to olaparib. [55] In an international multicenter Phase II study, 57 BRCA-carriers patients with recurrent ovarian cancer were enrolled in two sequential cohorts of two doses of olaparib (400 mg and 100 mg orally twice daily). The overall response rate as per the RECIST criteria was 33% in the 400 mg and 13% in the 100 mg cohort. These results suggest a possible dose-response effect. [56] Finally, PARP inhibitors may also show activity in patients with sporadic disease without germline BRCA1 or BRCA2 mutations. Gelmon et al. had shown a 24% objective response rate in relapsed ovarian cancer in the absence of BRCA1 or BRCA2 mutations to PARP inhibitors. Olaparib was well tolerated with the most common adverse events being fatigue in 70% of patients, nausea in 66%, vomiting in 39%, and decreased appetite in 36%. [57]

Ledermann et al. studied the role of olaparib maintenance in the subset of patients with relapsed platinum-sensitive high-grade serous ovarian cancer. The study was a double-blind, placebo-controlled, Phase II study. Results showed a significantly higher PFS rate compared to a placebo (median, 8.4 months vs. 4.8 months, with a hazard ratio for progression of 0.35, $P < 0.001$). OS analysis is not yet mature. [58]

Olaparib was also investigated in combination with chemotherapy in patients with advanced ovarian cancer. In a randomized, open-label, Phase II study, adult patients with platinum-sensitive, recurrent, high-grade serous ovarian cancer who had received up to three previous courses of platinum-based chemotherapy and who were progression-free for at least six months before randomization received either olaparib (200 mg capsules twice daily, administered orally on days one to 10 of each 21-day cycle) plus paclitaxel (175 mg/m2, administered intravenously on day one) and carboplatin (area under the curve [AUC] 4 mg/mL per min, according to the Calvert formula, administered intravenously on day one). Subsequently, patients received either olaparib monotherapy (400 mg capsules twice daily, given continuously) until disease progression in the olaparib plus chemotherapy group, or paclitaxel (175 mg/m2 on day one) and carboplatin (AUC 6 mg/mL per min on day one) then no further treatment in the chemotherapy alone group. The progression-free survival was significantly longer in the olaparib plus chemotherapy group (median 12.2 months [95% CI 9.7–15.0]) compared to chemotherapy alone group (median 9.6 months; 95% CI 9.1–9.7 and a HR 0.51; 95% CI 0.34–0.77; p=0.0012) — the difference was more pronounced in patients with BRCA mutations (HR 0.21 [0.08–0.55]; p=0.0015). [59]

Both the U.S. Food and Drug Administration and the EMA granted accelerated approval for olaparib (Lynparza) in the treatment of women with advanced ovarian cancer associated with defective BRCA genes, as detected by an FDA-approved test. [60]

6. Summary

Recurrent ovarian cancer is not curable. The goals of therapy should focus on palliation of cancer-related symptoms, extension of life, and maintenance of quality of life. The outlook has clearly improved over the last decade, due to an increase in options for the management of recurrent disease. Secondary cytoreduction has been advocated, but it remains controversial. For patients with platinum-sensitive disease retreatment with a platinum or a platinum-containing combination, such as carboplatin, should be considered. For patients with platinum-refractory or platinum-resistant disease, clinical trials should be considered. For patients who are not entering a trial, treatment with agents like PLD, paclitaxel, docetaxel, topotecan, gemcitabine, pemetrexed, ixabepilone, or oral etoposide can be considered. Despite the advances made in biological and targeted therapies like bevacizumab and pazopanib in extending disease-free survival in patients with recurrent advanced ovarian cancer, further research is needed to better understand the safety and effectiveness, the optimal duration and timing of treatment, and activity in association with other chemotherapeutic agents.

Author details

Bernardo L. Rapoport

Address all correspondence to: brapoport@rosebankoncology.co.za

The Medical Oncology Center of Rosebank, Saxonwold, Johannesburg, South Africa

References

[1] S. A. Cannistra. Cancer of the ovary. *The New England Journal of Medicine*, vol. 351, no. 24, pp. 2519–2529, 2004.

[2] G. J. Rustin, M. E. van der Burg, C. L. Griffin, et al.; MRC OV05; EORTC 55955 investigators. Early versus delayed treatment of relapsed ovarian cancer (MRC OV05/ EORTC 55955): a randomised trial. *Lancet*, vol. 376, no. 9747, pp. 1155–63, 2010.

[3] G. J. Rustin, I. Vergote, E. Eisenhauer, et al. Definitions for response and progression in ovarian cancer clinical trials incorporating RECIST 1.1 and CA 125 agreed by the Gynecological Cancer Intergroup (GCIG). *International Journal of Gynecological Cancer*, vol. 21, no. 2, pp. 419–423, 2011.

[4] M. Markman, R. Rothman, T. Hakes, et al. Second-line platinum therapy in patients with ovarian cancer previously treated with cisplatin. *Journal of Clinical Oncology*, vol. 9, no. 3, pp. 389–93, 1991.

[5] N. Colombo, J. L. Speyer, M. Green, et al. Phase II study of carboplatin in recurrent ovarian cancer: severe hematologic toxicity in previously treated patients. *Cancer Chemotherapy and Pharmacology*, vol. 23, no. 5, pp. 323–8, 1989.

[6] M. K. Parmar, J. A. Ledermann, N. Colombo, et al.; ICON and AGO Collaborators. Paclitaxel plus platinum-based chemotherapy versus conventional platinum-based chemotherapy in women with relapsed ovarian cancer: the ICON4/AGO-OVAR-2.2 trial. *Lancet*, vol. 361, no. 9375, pp. 2099–106, 2003.

[7] J. Pfisterer, M. Plante, I. Vergote, et al. Gemcitabine plus carboplatin compared with carboplatin in patients with platinum-sensitive recurrent ovarian cancer: an intergroup trial of the AGO-OVAR, the NCIC CTG, and the EORTC GCG. *Journal of Clinical Oncology*, vol. 24, no. 29, pp. 4699–707, 2006.

[8] U. Wagner, C. Marth, R. Largillier, et al. Final overall survival results of phase III GCIG CALYPSO trial of pegylated liposomal doxorubicin and carboplatin vs paclitaxel and carboplatin in platinum-sensitive ovarian cancer patients. *British Journal of Cancer*, vol. 107, no. 4, pp. 588–91, 2012.

[9] P. A. Vasey, G. C. Jayson, A. Gordon, et al. Scottish Gynaecological Cancer Trials Group. Phase III randomized trial of docetaxel-carboplatin versus paclitaxel-carboplatin as first-line chemotherapy for ovarian carcinoma. *Journal of the National Cancer Institute*, vol. 96, no. 22, pp. 1682–91, 2004.

[10] D. A. Vorobiof, B. L. Rapoport, M. R. Chasen, et al. Phase II clinical trial of carboplatin and docetaxel in patients with metastatic ovarian cancer: active combination with low incidence of peripheral neuropathy. *International Journal of Gynecological Cancer*, vol. 13, no. 3, pp. 287–91, 2003.

[11] D. Kudlowitz, F. Muggia. Defining risks of taxane neuropathy: insights from randomized clinical trials. *Clinical Cancer Research*, vol. 19, no. 17, pp. 4570–7, 2013.

[12] B. L. Rapoport, D. A. Vorobiof, C. Slabber, et al. Phase II study of pegylated liposomal doxorubicin and carboplatin in patients with platinum-sensitive and partially

platinum-sensitive metastatic ovarian cancer. *International Journal of Gynecological Cancer*, vol. 19, no. 6, pp. 1137–41, 2009.

[13] A. Alvarez Secord, A. Berchuck, R. V. Higgins, et al. A multicenter, randomized, phase 2 clinical trial to evaluate the efficacy and safety of combination docetaxel and carboplatin and sequential therapy with docetaxel then carboplatin in patients with recurrent platinum-sensitive ovarian cancer. *Cancer,* vol. 118, no. 13, pp. 3283–93, 2012.

[14] N. Colombo, E. Kutarska, M. Dimopoulos, et al. Randomized, open-label, phase III study comparing patupilone (EPO906) with pegylated liposomal doxorubicin in platinum-refractory or -resistant patients with recurrent epithelial ovarian, primary fallopian tube, or primary peritoneal cancer. *Journal of Clinical Oncology,* vol. 30, no. 31, pp. 3841–7, 2012.

[15] M. Markman, J. Hall, D. Spitz, et al. Phase II trial of weekly single-agent paclitaxel in platinum/paclitaxel-refractory ovarian cancer. *Journal of Clinical Oncology,* vol. 20, no. 9, pp. 2365–9, 2002.

[16] E. L. Trimble, J. D. Adams, D. Vena, et al. Paclitaxel for platinum-refractory ovarian cancer: results from the first 1,000 patients registered to National Cancer Institute Treatment Referral Center 9103. *Journal of Clinical Oncology,* vol. 12, pp. 2405-10, 1993.

[17] P. Francis, J. Schneider, L. Hann, et al. Phase II trial of docetaxel in patients with platinum-refractory advanced ovarian cancer. *Journal of Clinical Oncology,* vol. 12, no. 11, pp. 2301–8, 1994.

[18] J. Sehouli, D. Stengel, P. Harter, et al. Topotecan weekly versus conventional 5-day schedule in patients with platinum-resistant ovarian cancer: a randomized multicenter phase II trial of the North-Eastern German Society of Gynecological Oncology Ovarian Cancer Study Group. *Journal of Clinical Oncology* vol. 29, no. 2, pp. 242–8, 2011.

[19] Lund B, Hansen OP, Theilade K, et al. Phase II study of gemcitabine (2',2'-difluorodeoxycytidine) in previously treated ovarian cancer patients. *Journal of the National Cancer Institute,* vol. 86, no. 20, pp. 1530–3, 1994.

[20] D. S. Miller, J. A. Blessing, C. N. Krasner, et al. Phase II evaluation of pemetrexed in the treatment of recurrent or persistent platinum-resistant ovarian or primary peritoneal carcinoma: a study of the Gynecologic Oncology Group. *Journal of Clinical Oncology,* vol. 27, no. 16, pp. 2686–91, 2009.

[21] K. De Geest, J. A. Blessing, R. T. Morris, et al. Phase II clinical trial of ixabepilone in patients with recurrent or persistent platinum- and taxane-resistant ovarian or primary peritoneal cancer: a gynecologic oncology group study. *Journal of Clinical Oncology,* vol. 28, no. 1, pp. 149–53, 2010.

[22] P. G. Rose, J. A. Blessing, A. R. Mayer et al. Prolonged oral etoposide as second-line therapy for platinum-resistant and platinum-sensitive ovarian carcinoma: a Gyneco-

logic Oncology Group study. *Journal of Clinical Oncology*, vol. 16, no. 2, pp. 405–410, 1998.

[23] J. Sehouli, D. Stengel, P. Harter, et al. Topotecan weekly versus conventional 5-day schedule in patients with platinum-resistant ovarian cancer: a randomized multicenter phase II trial of the North-Eastern German Society of Gynecological Oncology Ovarian Cancer Study Group. *Journal of Clinical Oncology*, vol. 29, no. 2, pp. 242–8, 2011.

[24] T. A. Lawrie, A. Bryant, A. Cameron, et al. Pegylated liposomal doxorubicin for relapsed epithelial ovarian cancer. The Cochrane Library (2013).

[25] J. S. Berek, N. F. Hacker, L. D. Lagasse, et al. Survival of patients following secondary cytoreductive surgery in ovarian cancer. *Obstetrics and Gynecology*, vol. 61, no. 2, pp. 189–93, 1983.

[26] . Sehouli, R. Richter, E. I. Braicu, et al. Role of secondary cytoreductive surgery in ovarian cancer relapse: who will benefit? A systematic analysis of 240 consecutive patients. *Journal of Surgical Oncology*, vol. 102 no. 6, pp. 656–62, 2010.

[27] A. R. Munkarah, R. L. Coleman. Critical evaluation of secondary cytoreduction in recurrent ovarian cancer. *Gynecologic Oncology*, vol. 95, no. 2, pp. 273–280, 2004.

[28] M. Güngör, F. Ortaç, M. Arvas et al. The role of secondary cytoreductive surgery for recurrent ovarian cancer. *Gynecologic Oncology*, vol. 97, no. 1, pp. 74–79, 2005.

[29] T. Onda, H. Yoshikawa, T. Yasugi, et al. Secondary cytoreductive surgery for recurrent epithelial ovarian carcinoma: proposal for patients selection. *British Journal of Cancer*, vol. 92, no. 6, pp. 1026–1032, 2005.

[30] R. Salani, A. Santillan, M. L. Zahurak, et al. Secondary cytoreductive surgery for localized, recurrent epithelial ovarian cancer: analysis of prognostic factors and survival outcome. *Cancer*. vol. 109, no. 4, pp. 685–691, 2007.

[31] D. S. Chi, K. McCaughty, J. P. Diaz, et al. Guidelines and selection criteria for secondary cytoreductive surgery in patients with recurrent, platinum sensitive epithelial ovarian carcinoma. *Cancer*, vol. 106, no. 9, pp. 1933–1939, 2006.

[32] D. F. Kolomainen, D. P. Barton. Surgical management of bowel obstruction in gynecological malignancies. *Current Opinion in Supportive and Palliative Care*, vol. 5, no. 1, pp. 55–9, 2011.

[33] J. D. Patel, M. A. Socinski, E. B. Garon, et al. PointBreak: A randomized phase III study of pemetrexed plus carboplatin and bevacizumab followed by maintenance pemetrexed and bevacizumab versus paclitaxel plus carboplatin and bevacizumab followed by maintenance bevacizumab in patients with stage IIIb or IV nonsquamous non-small-cell lung cancer. *Journal of Clinical Oncology*, vol. 31, no. 34, pp. 4349–57, 2013.

[34] D. Cunningham, I. Lang, E. Marcuello, et al. AVEX study investigators. Bevacizumab plus capecitabine versus capecitabine alone in elderly patients with previously untreated metastatic colorectal cancer (AVEX): an open-label, randomised phase 3 trial. *The Lancet Oncology*, vol. 14, no. 11, pp. 1077–85, 2013.

[35] H. I. Hurwitz, N. C. Tebbutt, F. Kabbinavar, et al. Efficacy and safety of bevacizumab in metastatic colorectal cancer: pooled analysis from seven randomized controlled trials. *The Oncologist*, vol. 18, no. 9, pp. 1004–12, 2013.

[36] R. A. Burger, M. W. Sill, B. J. Monk, et al. Phase II trial of bevacizumab in persistent or recurrent epithelial ovarian cancer or primary peritoneal cancer: a Gynecologic Oncology Group Study. *Journal of Clinical Oncology*, vol. 25, no. 33, pp. 5165, 2007.

[37] S. A. Cannistra, U. A. Matulonis, R. T. Penson, et al. Phase II study of bevacizumab in patients with platinum-resistant ovarian cancer or peritoneal serous cancer. *Journal of Clinical Oncology*, vol. 25, no. 33, pp. 5180–6, 2007.

[38] R. A. Burger, M. F. Brady, M. A. Bookman, et al. Gynecologic Oncology Group incorporation of bevacizumab in the primary treatment of ovarian cancer. *The New England Journal of Medicine*, vol. 365, no. 26, pp. 2473–2483, 2011.

[39] T. J. Perren, A. M. Swart, J. Pfisterer, et al.; ICON7 Investigators. A phase 3 trial of bevacizumab in ovarian cancer. *The New England Journal of Medicine*, vol. 365, no. 26, pp. 2484–96, 2011.

[40] C. Aghajanian, S. V. Blank, B. A. Goff, et al. OCEANS: a randomized, double-blind, placebo-controlled phase III trial of chemotherapy with or without bevacizumab in patients with platinum-sensitive recurrent epithelial ovarian, primary peritoneal, or fallopian tube cancer. *Journal of Clinical Oncology*, vol. 30, no. 17, pp. 2039–45, 2012.

[41] E. Pujade-Lauraine, F. Hilpert, B. Weber, et al. Bevacizumab combined with chemotherapy for platinum-resistant recurrent ovarian cancer: the AURELIA open-label randomized phase III trial. *Journal of Clinical Oncology*. vol. 32, no 13, pp. 1302–8, 2014.

[42] C. A. Heckman, T. Holopainen, M. Wirzenius, et al. The tyrosine kinase inhibitor cediranib blocks ligand-induced vascular endothelial growth factor receptor-3 activity and lymphangiogenesis. *Cancer Research*, vol. 68, no. 12, pp. 4754–4762, 2008.

[43] S. R. Wedge, J. Kendrew, L. F. Hennequin, et al. AZD2171: a highly potent, orally bioavailable, vascular endothelial growth factor receptor-2 tyrosine kinase inhibitor for the treatment of cancer. *Cancer Research*, vol. 65, no. 10, pp. 4389–4400, 2005.

[44] U. A. Matulonis, S. Berlin, P. Ivy, et al. Cediranib, an oral inhibitor of vascular endothelial growth factor receptor kinases, is an active drug in recurrent epithelial ovarian, fallopian tube, and peritoneal cancer. *Journal of Clinical Oncology*, vol. 27, no. 33, pp. 5601–6, 2009.

[45] F. A. Raja, C. L. Griffin, W. Qian, et al. Initial toxicity assessment of ICON6: a randomised trial of cediranib plus chemotherapy in platinum-sensitive relapsed ovarian cancer. *British Journal of Cancer*, vol. 105, no. 7, pp. 884–9, 2011.

[46] J. A. Ledermann, T. J. Perren, F. A. Raja, et al. on behalf of the ICON6 Collaborators. Randomised double-blind phase III trial of cediranib (azd 2171) in relapsed platinum sensitive ovarian cancer: results of the icon6 trial. *International Journal of Gynecological Cancer*, vol. 23, no. 8, 2013.

[47] R. L. Coleman, L. R. Duska, P. T. Ramirez, et al. Phase 1–2 study of docetaxel plus aflibercept in patients with recurrent ovarian, primary peritoneal, or fallopian tube cancer. *The Lancet Oncology*, vol. 12, no. 12, pp. 1109–17, 2011.

[48] B. Y. Karlan, A. M. Oza, G. E. Richardson, et al. Randomized, double-blind, placebo-controlled phase II study of AMG 386 combined with weekly paclitaxel in patients with recurrent ovarian cancer. *Journal of Clinical Oncology*, vol. 30, no. 4, pp. 362–71, 2102.

[49] J. Monk, A. Poveda, I. Vergote, et al. Anti-angiopoietin therapy with trebananib for recurrent ovarian cancer (TRINOVA-1): a randomised, multicentre, double-blind, placebo-controlled phase 3 trial. *The Lancet Oncology*, vol. 15, no. 8, pp. 799–808, 2014.

[50] J. A. Ledermann, A. Hackshaw, S. Kaye, et al. Randomized phase II placebo-controlled trial of maintenance therapy using the oral triple angiokinase inhibitor BIBF 1120 after chemotherapy for relapsed ovarian cancer. *Journal of Clinical Oncology*, vol. 29, no. 28, pp. 3798–804, 2011.

[51] G. Sonpavde, T. E. Hutson. Pazopanib: A novel multitargeted tyrosine kinase inhibitor. *Current Oncology Reports*, vol. 9, no 2, pp. 115–119, 2007.

[52] M. Friedlander, K. C. Hancock, D. Rischin, et al. A phase II, open-label study evaluating pazopanib in patients with recurrent ovarian cancer. *Gynecologic Oncology*, vol. 119, no. 1, pp. 32–7, 2010.

[53] A. Floquet, I. Vergote, N. Colombo, et al. Progression-free survival by local investigator versus independent central review: comparative analysis of the AGO-OVAR16 Trial. *Gynecologic Oncology*, vol. 136, no. 1, pp. 37–42, 2015.

[54] A. du Bois, A. Floquet, J. W. Kim, et al. Incorporation of pazopanib in maintenance therapy of ovarian cancer. *Journal of Clinical Oncology*, vol. 32, no. 30, pp. 3374–82, 2014.

[55] P. C. Fong, T. A. Yap, D. S. Boss, et al. Poly ADP-ribose polymerase inhibition: frequent durable responses in BRCA carrier ovarian cancer correlating with platinum-free interval. *Journal of Clinical Oncology*, vol. 28, no. 15, pp. 2512–9, 2010.

[56] M. W. Audeh, J. Carmichael, R. T. Penson, et al. Oral poly ADP-ribose polymerase inhibitor olaparib in patients with BRCA1 or BRCA2 mutations and recurrent ovarian cancer: a proof-of-concept trial. *Lancet*, vol. 376, no. 9737, pp. 245–51, 2010.

[57] K. A. Gelmon, M. Tischkowitz, H. Mackay, et al. Olaparib in patients with recurrent high-grade serous or poorly differentiated ovarian carcinoma or triple-negative breast cancer: a phase 2, multicentre, open-label, non-randomised study. *The Lancet Oncology*, vol. 12, no. 9, pp. 852–61, 2011.

[58] J. Ledermann, P. Harter, C. Gourley, et al. Olaparib maintenance therapy in platinum-sensitive relapsed ovarian cancer. *The New England Journal of Medicine* vol. 366, no. 15, pp.1382–92, 2012.

[59] A. M. Oza, D. Cibula, A. O. Benzaquen, et al. Olaparib combined with chemotherapy for recurrent platinum-sensitive ovarian cancer: a randomised phase 2 trial. *The Lancet Oncology*. vol. 16, no. 1, pp. 87–97, 2015.

[60] E. D. Deeks. Olaparib: first global approval. Drugs. vol. 75, no. 2, pp. 231–40.

Chapter 9

Management of Ovarian Cancer — Is There a Role for Cytoreductive Surgery (CRS) and Hyperthermic Intraperitoneal Chemotherapy (HIPEC)?

Melissa Ching Ching Teo and Grace Hwei Ching Tan

Additional information is available at the end of the chapter

http://dx.doi.org/10.5772/60601

Abstract

Ovarian cancer is one of the commonest malignancy in women worldwide, and is the most lethal of all the gynaecological malignancies. Ovarian cancer often presents at an advanced stage, with the involvement of the peritoneal surface either at the initial diagnosis or at recurrence. Despite the advances made in the surgical techniques and chemotherapeutic options regarding agents, schedule, and route of administration, majority of the patients recur and eventually succumb to their disease. The change in the surgical approach supporting more radical and extensive surgical procedures, in a bid to attain optimal cytoreduction with no gross residual disease, has seen improvement in the survival, as has the use of intraperitoneal chemotherapy in combination with i.v. agents. Although peritoneal carcinomatosis has always been a poor prognostic factor, it ceases to be a factor of much importance if complete cytoreduction can be achieved. Cytoreductive surgery (CRS) and hyperthermic intraperitoneal chemotherapy (HIPEC) provide the combined benefits of surgical eradication and effective chemotherapy, and can be performed with acceptable morbidity and mortality. Further trials are being undertaken to examine its role in the primary, as well as recurrent settings of advanced ovarian cancer and to determine the ideal drug combinations and dosages. We aim to discuss the role of CRS and HIPEC in the treatment of ovarian cancer.

Keywords: Ovarian Cancer, CRS, HIPEC

1. Introduction

Ovarian cancer one of the commonest malignancies in women worldwide, with an annual incidence of 239,000 [1, 2]. It is the most lethal of all the gynaecological malignancies, the fifth leading cause of cancer deaths, and claimed 151,917 lives in [1, 2]. Most patients with ovarian cancer present with ostensibly innocuous symptoms of abdominal bloatedness and discomfort, and hence are often diagnosed at an advanced stage, with 60–70% of patients having stage 3 or 4 disease at diagnosis [3]. The standard approach is optimal debulking and adjuvant chemotherapy with platinum-based and taxol-based chemotherapy. Even with optimal treatment, the median five-year survival is less than 50% [4] and in advanced ovarian cancer, this drops to less than 25% [4]. Up to 70% of all patients diagnosed with ovarian cancer relapse and ultimately succumb to their disease.

2. Optimal debulking

Surgery remains the foundation of the management of ovarian cancers, as it is often required initially to attain a diagnosis, to formally stage the patient, and is the mainstay of treatment in the majority of diagnosed cases [5]. The definition of optimal cytoreduction has evolved over the years, but was originally defined as residual disease less than 2 cm in size. This was further altered with evidence establishing the significantly superior survival of those with residual disease measuring less than 1 cm and subsequently 5 mm in size [6–8]. Even in those with traditionally defined optimal cytoreduction with residual disease measuring less than 1 cm, the risk of death increases considerably when compared with those with no residual disease [9]. Over the years, there has been a glut of data concluding that complete cytoreduction, with no gross residual disease, yields the best results in terms of survival [10]. Patients with no gross residual disease, 0.1–2 cm residual disease, and more than 2 cm residual disease had five-year survivals of 60,35, and less than 20%, respectively [11, 12].

3. What happens after debulking?

In the bulk of patients with ovarian cancer, adjuvant chemotherapy is required [13]. Initially, the chemotherapeutic agents of choice included a platinum-based chemotherapy and a classic alkylating agent, and common agents used were cisplatin and cyclophosphamide [14]. After the Gynaecological Oncology Group (GOG) 111 and OV10 trials, looking specifically at the combinations of cisplatin with either cyclophosphamide or paclitaxel, were performed, the standard of care following surgery for stage 3 and 4 ovarian cancer was a combination of a platinum-based agent and a taxane, with intravenous (i.v.) cisplatin and paclitaxel being the agents of choice. Subsequently, a combination of paclitaxel and carboplatin showed similar results for response and survival rates, but without the toxicity often related to cisplatin treatment, and with a better quality of life. The standard approach is six cycles of paclitaxel 175mg/m2 administered every three weeks, in combination with carboplatin area under the curve (AUC) 5–6 [15].

The response and survival rates vary between the different histological types, with the clear cell and endometrioid subtypes having the worst and best prognoses, respectively, and mucinous and serous subtypes having intermediate prognoses [16, 17]. High-grade features likewise affect the prognosis unfavourably and such diseases often take on a much more aggressive course [16, 17].

In an attempt to improve response rates to chemotherapy, and progression-free and overall survivals, dose intense and dose-dense chemotherapy were introduced. The former refers to the increase of dosages with each drug delivery, whereas the latter implies increasing the frequency of drug administration. It was thought that tumour growth escalated in the initial phase but slowed as the tumour volume increased; hence, delivering higher doses of chemotherapy from the start and at close intervals would increase tumour cell death. This theory was confirmed in a large meta-analysis studying the effects of dose-intense and dose-dense chemotherapy for ovarian cancer [18]. The encouraging results of the JGOG trial, with first-line dose-dense chemotherapy, depict an improvement of median progression-free survival from 17.5 to 28.2 months and an overall survival that was not reached [19].

4. The role of Intraperitoneal (IP) chemotherapy versus Intravenous (IV) chemotherapy

The route of administration of chemotherapy for ovarian cancer has traditionally been intravenous (i.v.). In the1960s, intraperitoneal (i.p.) chemotherapy was introduced with the aim of controlling malignant ascites. It was found that certain drugs such as cisplatin were cleared from the peritoneal cavity gradually, which meant that a high concentration of the drug could be delivered intraperitoneally without resulting in a systemic overdose of the drug.

Drugs that are particularly suited for i.p. delivery have high molecular weights and are water soluble, leading to a delayed peritoneal but high systemic clearance, and so having a pharmacological advantage for treating peritoneal disease.

Ovarian cancer is an ideal cancer for treatment via an i.p. route. The majority of diagnosed cases present with peritoneal disease in the absence of extra-peritoneal metastases [3]. Even in patients who have undergone seemingly curative surgery and adjuvant chemotherapy, up to 70% develop recurrent disease, the majority of which remains confined to the peritoneal cavity. The propensity for peritoneal recurrences as the only site of disease makes this cancer the model candidate for such loco-regional treatment. I.p. chemotherapy has also been used with significant success in mucinous tumours of the appendix and peritoneum [20], colon cancers [21], and has even been shown to provide improved survival in gastric cancers [22].

The underlying principle behind i.p. chemotherapy is the delivery of high concentrations of the appropriate drug to the site that is most likely to develop recurrences, at the opportune moment where tumour burden is at its minimum, i.e., after the performance of complete cytoreduction, with eradication of all macroscopic disease. It is critical that no gross residual disease is present, as penetration of i.p. chemotherapy is up to a depth of 2.5 mm [23–25]; hence, there is an inherent risk that larger volumes of tumour deposits will not be sufficiently treated by the intraperitoneal chemotherapy.

There have been numerous studies examining the results of i.p. chemotherapy in the management of ovarian cancer. Amongst the first few randomized controlled trials (RCTs) was that conducted by the Southwest Oncology Group (SWOG) and GOG 104 trial, in which patients with then-defined optimal cytoreduction of less than 2 cm residual disease were administered i.v. cyclophosphamide and either i.v. or i.p. cisplatin. The patients who received the i.p. chemotherapy had significantly increased median overall survival [26]. The GOG 111 trial that combined i.v. paclitaxel with i.v. or i.p. cisplatin reached similar conclusions, in favour of the i.p. treatment. Other RCTs produced progression-free and overall survivals of 28 and 63–66 months, respectively. In the GOG 172 trial, the median overall survival was 65.6 and 49.7 months for the combination i.p./i.v. and cytoreductive surgery (CRS) and i.v. chemotherapy alone arms, respectively. There were criticisms of these trials as the i.p. arm in GOG 114 and GOG 172 received two cycles of carboplatin at AUC 9 and i.p. paclitaxel on day 8, respectively; hence, we await the results of additional RCTs that aim to study the effect of i.p. chemotherapy and determine the ideal algorithm for the management of ovarian cancer [27].

5. Recurrent ovarian cancer

Despite optimal treatment, up to 70% of all patients diagnosed with ovarian cancer suffer from relapse. In the past, early detection of persistent disease by second-look laparotomies was often performed, but as it was found to make no difference in GOG-0158 it is no longer practiced [28]. Currently, the practice of close follow-up of patients by serial CA-125 levels at intervals of one to three months is practiced. In patients who are in clinical complete remission, an increase in CA-125 from initial levels is the most common method to detect disease relapse. However, the MRC-OV05 trial [29], which examined the consequences of early treatment for recurrence versus treatment delayed until clinical symptoms appeared, showed that there was no benefit in the detection of the early presence of disease by CA-125, with only a 1.4 month benefit in survival for the early treatment group.

In patients with clinically evident relapse, treatment options include secondary cytoreduction with or without hyperthermic intraperitoneal chemotherapy (HIPEC), and systemic chemotherapeutic regimes. Systemic treatment is dependent on the platinum sensitivity of the disease. In platinum-sensitive disease, re-treatment with a platinum or platinum-containing combination is advocated, and in platinum-resistance disease, clinical trials involving topotecan, docataxel, gemcitabine, paclitaxel, pemetrexed and bevacizumab should be considered.

6. The rationale for Cytoreductive Surgery (CRS) and Hyperthermic Intraperitoneal Chemotherapy (HIPEC)

Hyperthermic intraperitoneal chemotherapy (HIPEC) was first introduced in the early 1980s for the treatment of peritoneal carcinomatosis. CRS and HIPEC were popularized for the management of peritoneal surface malignancies by Dr. Sugarbaker in the 1990s [21]. The addition of hyperthermia to the i.p. chemotherapy has been shown to boost penetration of the chemotherapy and improve its absorption into the tumour cells, increasing the intracellular accumulation of the drug [30]. The cytotoxic effect appears to be similarly potentiated, secondary to an impairment of the cells' ability to perform DNA repair, and thus has a greater deleterious effect [30, 31]. The drugs selected must be heat stable, with a high molecular weight and a low water solubility to be optimally used in the process of HIPEC. Cisplatin, mitomycin-C, and doxorubicin are the frequently employed drugs.

HIPEC is performed intraoperatively, while the patient is under general anaesthesia, via a pump that maintains the temperature and circulation of the drug solution. In addition to patient comfort, advantages include an ability to ensure that the entire peritoneal surface is bathed in the chemotherapeutic agent, before the formation of obstructing adhesions that may develop in the postoperative period. If HIPEC is administered in an opened-abdomen fashion, the surgeon would be able to manually swirl the chemotherapy to achieve this target. The most important prognostic factor remains the completeness of cytoreduction, with a 5.5% increase in the median overall survival for every 10% of patients undergoing optimal cytoreduction [5], leading to the inevitable conclusion that the changing surgical paradigm for ovarian cancer embracing radical CRS has resulted in meaningfully better survival results [32].

The combination of CRS and HIPEC has shown promising results, with median overall and progression-free survivals of up to 64 and 57 months, respectively [30, 33, 34]. Optimal cytoreduction yields five-year survivals of 12–66% [34]. These results are compatible with those of the author's institution [35]. A meta-analysis examining i.p. versus i.v. trials also conclusively showed the superiority of the i.p. over the i.v. arms, with hazard ratios of 0.79 for both disease-free and overall survivals [36]. Patients with platinum-sensitive disease have better response rates of 20–77% compared with up to 28% in those with platinum-resistant disease [37].

7. CRS and HIPEC: When to do it?

The time points at which CRS and HIPEC have been used in the management of advanced ovarian cancer include the primary setting, after neoadjuvant chemotherapy, at the point of recurrence, and as a second-line treatment [38]. In the Milan 2006 consensus statement, it was concluded that CRS and HIPEC could be feasible at all of these time points.

The morbidity and mortality for such a procedure range from 0 to 40 and 0 to 10%, respectively [34, 35], and include nausea and vomiting, gastrointestinal disturbances and ileus, anastomotic leaks, perioperative bleeding, pleural effusions and pneumothoraces, intra-abdominal collections/abscesses, and sepsis. The key is in patient selection, and it is imperative that patients with a good ECOG and an ability to tolerate such a radical procedure be chosen. The best candidates have long disease-free intervals and low volume disease that can be confidently optimally debulked. Many of the studies included in the review of CRS and HIPEC for advanced ovarian cancer show the usage of this modality of treatment in the recurrent setting. However, evidence supporting the use of i.p. chemotherapy in the initial setting of advanced ovarian cancer [39] suggests that there is sound rationale behind CRS and HIPEC, even in the primary setting. There are more than 40 studies that have reported on the role of HIPEC in the management of ovarian cancer, but many of these studies are small in number and heterogeneous in their design. Further trials such as the Italian HORSE study (available at http://clinicaltrials.gov/show/ NCT01539785) that randomizes patients with platinum-sensitive disease to CRS and HIPEC with cisplatin 75mg/m2 and CRS alone, and the French CHIPOR study (available at http://clinicaltrials.gov/show/NCT01376752) that randomizes patients with recurrent platinum-sensitive disease (relapse beyond six months) after they have received platinum-based chemotherapy and optimal cytoreduction (less than 2.5 mm residual disease) to HIPEC with i.p. cisplatin 75mg/m2 and no HIPEC [37] will provide answers about the role of HIPEC in patients with platinum-sensitive disease. There is a need for phase 3 randomized trials to elucidate which timing and cohort of patients would be most beneficial for CRS and HIPEC.

8. Future directions

8.1. CRS and HIPEC

It is evident that complete cytoreduction, with no residual disease, yields the best clinical outcome. However, in a significant proportion of patients recurrence in the peritoneal cavity occurs, and CRS and HIPEC are considered. Perhaps the role of CRS and HIPEC as an adjuvant treatment should be considered an upfront treatment option for primary ovarian cancers, especially with improved morbidity results for this treatment modality. A randomized trial examining the overall and disease-free survivals of patients managed with CRS and adjuvant i.v. chemotherapy and those who undergo CRS and HIPEC, with adjuvant i.v. chemotherapy, for ovarian cancer in the primary setting would enable this questions to be addressed.

8.2. Intraperitoneal bevacizumab

The role of vascular endothelial growth factor (VEGF) in ovarian cancer has received much attention because VEGF increases vascular permeability and enhances angiogenesis [40]. Overexpression of VEGF has been reported in ovarian cancer [41-43] and several studies have indicated that VEGF-regulated angiogenesis is an important component of ovarian cancer growth [44, 45]. Microvessel density and level of VEGF expression in ovarian cancer directly correlate with poor prognosis, suggesting that angiogenesis, possibly mediated at least in part by VEGF, influences disease progression [44, 45]. Currently, vascular endothelial growth factor receptor (VEGFR) antibody, bevacizumab, is given intravenously for select patients with ovarian cancer.

The role of intraperitoneal VEGF inhibition using bevacizumab has been explored for the treatment of malignant ascites [46]. In a mouse peritoneal model of human ovarian cancer, the author demonstrated that the administration of i.p. bevacizumab and rapamycin not only reduced ascites, but was also able to suppress the development of peritoneal carcinomatosis [47]. This is an indication that this therapy may potentially be useful for the treatment of peritoneal carcinomatosis and may also be a novel, efficient strategy for reducing recurrence of ovarian cancers.

9. Conclusion

Ovarian cancer often presents at an advanced stage, with the involvement of the peritoneal surface either at initial diagnosis or at recurrence. Despite the advances made in surgical techniques and chemotherapeutic options regarding agents, schedule, and route of administration, the majority of the patients relapse and eventually succumb to their disease. A change in the surgical approach, supporting more radical and extensive surgical procedures in a bid to attain optimal cytoreduction with no gross residual disease, has seen an improvement in survival, as has the use of intraperitoneal chemotherapy in combination with i.v. agents. Although peritoneal carcinomatosis has always been a poor prognostic factor, it ceases to be a factor of much importance if complete CRS can be achieved [31, 48]. CRS and HIPEC provide the combined benefits of surgical eradication and effective chemotherapy, and can be performed with acceptable morbidity and mortality [49]. Further trials are being undertaken to examine its role in the primary as well as recurrent settings of advanced ovarian cancer, and to determine the ideal drug combinations and dosages [50–52].

Author details

Melissa Ching Ching Teo* and Grace Hwei Ching Tan

*Address all correspondence to: melissa.teo.c.c@nccs.com.sg

Department of Surgical Oncology, National Cancer Centre Singapore, Singapore

References

[1] Ferlay J, Soerjomataram I, Ervik M, et al. GLOBOCAN 2012 v1.0, Cancer incidence and mortality worldwide: IARC CancerBase No. 11 [Internet]. Lyon, France: International Agency for Research on Cancer; 2013. Available from: http://globocan.iarc.fr

[2] Bernard W. Stewart and Christopher P. Wild. World cancer report 2014. IARC publication; 2014.

[3] Coleman RL, Monk BJ, Sood AK, et al. Latest research and treatment of advanced-stage epithelial ovarian cancer. Nat Rev Clin Oncol 2013; 10: 211–224. doi: 10.1038/nrclinonc.2013.5.

[4] Horner MJ, Ries LA, Kracho M, et al. SEER cancer statistics review, 1975-2006. Bethesda, MD: National Cancer Institute; 2009. http://seer.cancer.- AQ5 gov/csr/1975_2006/.

[5] Kang S, Park SY. To predict or not to predict? The dilemma of predicting the risk of suboptimal cytoreduction in ovarian cancer. Ann Oncol 2011; 22 (Suppl. 8): viii23–viii28. doi: 10.1093/annonc/mdr530.

[6] Bookman MA, Brady MF, McGuire WP, et al. Evaluation of new platinum based treatment regimens in advanced-stage ovarian cancer: a Phase III Trial of the Gynecologic Cancer Intergroup. J Clin Oncol 2009; 27: 1419–1425.

[7] Chang SJ, Bristow RE. Evolution of surgical treatment paradigms for advanced-stage ovarian cancer: redefining 'optimal' residual disease. Gynecol Oncol 2012; 125: 483–492. doi: 10.1016/j.ygyno.2012.02.024.

[8] Chang SJ, Bristow RE, Ryu HS. Impact of complete cytoreduction leaving no gross residual disease associated with radical cytoreductive surgical procedures on survival in advanced ovarian cancer. Ann Surg Oncol 2012; 19: 4059–4067.

[9] Elattar A, Bryant A, Winter-Roach BA, et al. Optimal primary surgical treatment for advanced epithelial ovarian cancer. Cochrane Database Syst Rev 2011; CD007565.

[10] Gavin S, Henry K, Monica B, et al., on behalf of the participants of the 4th Gynaecological Ovarian Cancer Consensus Conference (OCCC) 2010. Gynaecologic Cancer Intergroup (GCIC) consensus statement on clinical trials in ovarian cancer: report from the Fourth Ovarian Cancer Consensus Conference. Int J Gynaecol Cancer 2011; 21: 750–755.

[11] Fotopoulou C, Savvatis K, Kosian P, et al. Quaternary cytoreductive surgery in ovarian cancer: does surgical effort still matter? Br J Cancer 2013; 108: 32–38

[12] Chang SJ, Hodeib M, Chang J, Bristow RE. Survival impact of complete cytoreduction to no gross residual disease for advanced-stage ovarian cancer: a meta-analysis. Gynecol Oncol 2013; 130: 493–498.

[13] NCCN Practice Guidelines in Oncology (NCCN Guidelines). http://www.nccn.org/professionals/physician_gls/pdf/ovarian.pdf. [Accessed 6 September 2013].

[14] Kroep JR. Advances in epithelial ovarian cancer. Curr Pharmaceut Des 2012; 250: 3735–3740.

[15] Thigpen T, duBois A, McAlpine J, et al. First-line therapy in ovarian cancer trials. Int J Gynaecol Cancer 2011; 21: 756–762.

[16] Mackay HJ, Brady MF, Oza AM, et al. Prognostic relevance of uncommon ovarian histology in women with stage III/IV epithelial ovarian cancer. Int J Gynecol Cancer 2010; 20: 945–952.

[17] Landrum LM, Java J, Mathews CA, et al. Prognostic factors for stage III epithelial ovarian cancer treated with intraperitoneal chemotherapy: a Gynecologic Oncology Group study. Gynecol Oncol 2013; 130: 12–18.

[18] Boere IA, van der Burg ME. Review of dose-intense platinum and/or paclitaxel containing chemotherapy in advanced and recurrent epithelial ovarian cancer. Curr Pharmaceut Des 2012; 18: 3741–3753.

[19] Katsumata N, Yasuda M, Isonishi S, et al. Long-term results of dose-dense paclitaxel and carboplatin versus conventional paclitaxel and carboplatin for treatment of advanced epithelial ovarian, fallopian tube, or primary peritoneal cancer (JGOG 3016): a randomised, controlled, open-label trial. Lancet Oncol 2013; 14: 1020–1026.

[20] Schomas DA, Miller RC, Donohue JH et al. Intraperitoneal treatment for peritoneal mucinous carcinomatosis of appendiceal origin after operative management: long-term follow-up of the Mayo Clinic experience. Ann Surg. 2009 Apr; 249(4): 588-95.

[21] Mohamed F, Cecil T, Moran B, Sugarbaker P. A new standard of care for the management of peritoneal surface malignancy. Curr Oncol 2011; 18: e84–e96.

[22] Sun J, Song Y, Wang Z. Benefits of hyperthermic intraperitoneal chemotherapy for patients with serosal invasion in gastric cancer: a meta-analysis of the randomized controlled trials. BMC Cancer 2012; 12: 526.

[23] Van der Speeten K, Govaerts K, Stuart OA, Sugarbaker PH. Pharmacokinetics of the perioperative use of cancer chemotherapy in peritoneal surface malignancy patients. Gastroenterol Res Pract 2012; 2012: 378064.

[24] De Bree E, Helm CW. Hyperthermic intraperitoneal chemotherapy in ovarian cancer: rationale and clinical data. Expert Rev Anticancer Ther 2012; 12: 895–911.

[25] Dedrick RL, Flessner MF. Pharmacokinetic problems in peritoneal drug administration: tissue penetration and surface exposure. J Natl Cancer Inst 1997; 89: 480–487.

[26] Echarri Gonzalez MJ, Green R, Muggia FM. Intraperitoneal drug delivery for ovarian cancer: why, how, who, what, and when? Oncology (Williston Park) 2011; 25: 156–165, 170.

[27] Gujiwara K, Nagao S, Aotani E, et al. Principle and evolving role of intraperitoneal chemotherapy in ovarian cancer. Expert Opin Pharmacother 2013; 14: 1797–1806.

[28] Ozols RF, Bundy BN, Greer BE, et al. Phase III trial of carboplatin and paclitaxel compared with cisplatin and paclitaxel in patients with optimally resected stage III ovarian cancer: a Gynecologic Oncology Group study. J Clin Oncol 2003; 21 (17): 3194-3200

[29] Rustin GJ1, van der Burg ME, Griffin CL et al. Early versus delayed treatment of relapsed ovarian cancer (MRC OV05/EORTC 55955): a randomised trial. Lancet. 2010 Oct 2; 376 (9747): 1155-1163.

[30] Saladino E, Flere F, Irato S, et al. The role of cytoreductive surgery and hyperthermic intraperitoneal chemotherapy in the treatment of ovarian cancer relapse. Updates Surg 2013. AQ7.

[31] Deraco M, Baratti D, Laterza B, et al. Advanced cytoreduction as surgical standard of care and hyperthermic intraperitoneal chemotherapy as promising treatment in epithelial ovarian cancer. Eur J Surg Oncol 2011; 37: 4–9.

[32] Chi DS, Eisenhauer EL, Zivanovic O, et al. Improved progression-free and overall survival in advanced ovarian cancer as a result of a change in surgical paradigm. Gynaecol Oncol 2009; 114: 26–31.

[33] Biliatis I, Haidopoulos D, Rodolakis A, et al. Survival after secondary cytoreduction for recurrent ovarian cancer: which are the prognostic factors? J Surg Oncol 2010; 102: 671–675. doi: 10.1002/jso.21686.

[34] Chua TC, Robertson G, Liauw W, et al. Intraoperative hyperthermic intraperitoneal chemotherapy after cytoreductive surgery in EOC peritoneal carcinomatosis: systematic review of current results. J Cancer Res Clin Oncol 2009; 135: 1637–1645.

[35] Teo MC, Tan GH, Tham CK, et al. Cytoreductive surgery and hyperthermic intraperitoneal chemotherapy in Asian patients: 100 consecutive patients in a single institution. Ann Surg Oncol 2013; 20: 2968–2974.

[36] Cascales Campos P. Morbidity and mortality outcomes of cytoreductive surgery and hyperthermic intraperitoneal chemotherapy in patients with primary and recurrent advanced ovarian cancer. Eur J Surg Oncol 2013. S0748-7983(13)00752-X.

[37] Furet E, Che′ reau E, Lambaudie E, et al. Feasibility, morbidity and survival of surgery combined with HIPEC in the management of recurrent ovarian cancer. Gynecol Obstet Fertil 2013; 41: 493–498. 2013.07.011.

[38] Mulier S, Claes JP, Dierieck V, et al. Survival benefit of adding hyperthermic intraperitoneal chemotherapy (HIPEC) at the different time points of treatment of ovarian cancer: review of evidence. Curr Pharmaceut Des 2012; 18: 3793–3803.

[39] Rowan K. Intraperitoneal chemotherapy for ovarian cancer: why has it not become standard? J Natl Cancer Inst 2009; 101: 775–777.

[40] Mutch DG, Williams S. Biology of epithelial ovarian cancer. Clin Obstet Gynecol 1994; 37: 406–422.

[41] Boocock CA, Charnock-Jones DS, Sharkey AM, et al. Expression of vascular endothelial growth factor and its receptors flt and KDR in ovarian carcinoma. J Natl Cancer Inst 1995; 87: 506–516.

[42] Dvorak HF, Brown LF, Detmar M, Dvorak AM. Vascular permeability factor/vascular endothelial growth factor, microvascular hyperpermeability, and angiogenesis. Am J Pathol 1995; 146: 1029–1039.

[43] Paley PJ, Staskus KA, Gebhard K, et al. Vascular endothelial growth factor expression in early stage ovarian carcinoma. Cancer 1997; 80: 98–106.

[44] Hu L, Hofmann J, Jaffe RB. Phosphatidylinositol 3-kinase mediates angiogenesis and vascular permeability associated with ovarian carcinoma. Clin Cancer Res 2005; 11: 8208–8212.

[45] Pourgholami MH, Yan CZ, Lu Y, Wang L, Morris DL. Albendazole: a potent inhibitor of vascular endothelial growth factor and malignant ascites formation in OVCAR-3 tumor-bearing nude mice. Clin Cancer Res 2006; 12: 1928–1935.

[46] Kobolda S, Hegewisch-Beckerb S, Oechsle K et. al. Intraperitoneal VEGF inhibition using bevacizumab: a potential approach for the symptomatic treatment of malignant ascites? The Oncologist 2009; 14(12): 1242–1251.

[47] Huynh H, Teo M, Soo KC. Bevacizumab and rapamycin inhibit tumor growth in peritoneal model of human ovarian cancer. Mol Cancer Ther 2007; 6(11): 2959–2966

[48] Herter P, Hahmann M, Lueck HJ, et al. Surgery for recurrent ovarian cancer: role of peritoneal carcinomatosis: exploratory analysis of the DESKTOP 1 trial about risk factors, surgical implications, and prognostic value of peritoneal carcinomatosis. Ann Surg Oncol 2009; 16: 1324–1330.

[49] Chan DL, Morris DL, Rao A, Chua TC. Intraperitoneal chemotherapy in ovarian cancer: a review of tolerance and efficacy. Cancer Manag Res 2012; 4: 413–422.

[50] Chia TC, Liauw W, Robertson G, et al. Towards randomized trials of cytoreductive surgery using peritonectomy and hyperthermic intraperitoneal chemotherapy for ovarian cancer peritoneal carcinomatosis. Gynaecol Oncol 2009; 114: 137–139.

[51] Classe JM, Muller M, Frenel JS, et al. Intraperitoneal chemotherapy in the treatment of advanced ovarian cancer. Mem A′ cad Nat Chir 2009; 8: 86–90.

[52] OVHIPEC trial. ClinicalTrials.gov identifier. NCT0042657. http://clinicaltrials.gov/ct2/show/nct0042657.

Chapter 10

Anti-Angiogenic and Anti-Cancer Effects by Targeting the Protein Kinase G Type-Iα (PKG-Iα) Signaling Pathway and its Downstream Effects on Expression of Inhibitor of Apoptosis Proteins, C-IAP1, Livin and Survivin

Janica C. Wong, Priyatham Gorjala,
Benjamin Costantino and Ronald R. Fiscus

Additional information is available at the end of the chapter

http://dx.doi.org/10.5772/60774

Abstract

Ovarian cancer is often difficult to treat because of the development of resistance to many of the currently-used therapeutic agents (i.e. chemoresistance). The progression and chemoresistance of ovarian cancer can involve tumor angiogenesis, the development of new blood vessels bringing more blood and nutrients to the growing tumor. Tumor angiogenesis also involves the vascular endothelium-induced stimulation of cancer cell growth (1) and the higher expression levels of certain "cell survival proteins", such as the Inhibitor of Apoptosis Proteins (IAPs, including c-IAP1, Livin and Survivin), which are expressed in both the proliferating cancer cells (2, 3) and the vascular endothelial cells involved in tumor angiogenesis (4).

Keywords: Anti-angiogenesis, cancer treatment, protein kinase G (PKG), chemoresistance, cIAP-1, Livin, Survivin, Inhibitor of Apoptosis Proteins (IAPs)

1. Introduction

Ovarian cancer is often difficult to treat because of the development of resistance to many of the currently-used therapeutic agents (i.e. chemoresistance). The progression and chemoresistance of ovarian cancer can involve tumor angiogenesis, the development of new blood vessels bringing more blood and nutrients to the growing tumor. Tumor angiogenesis also involves the vascular endothelium-induced stimulation of cancer cell growth [1] and the higher expression levels of certain "cell survival proteins", such as the Inhibitor of Apoptosis Proteins (IAPs, including c-IAP1, Livin and Survivin), which are expressed in both the proliferating cancer cells [2, 3] and the vascular endothelial cells involved in tumor angiogenesis [4].

Although there are a number of cell signaling pathways that are known to promote angiogenesis and the higher levels of expression of the IAPs, one pathway that has become recognized as an important pro-growth and pro-survival mechanism within both ovarian cancer cells and vascular endothelial cells is the nitric oxide (NO)/cyclic GMP (cGMP)/protein kinase G type-1α (PKG-Iα) signaling pathway. Originally, the NO/cGMP/PKG signaling pathway was recognized to be a key cellular mechanism in regulating the cardiovascular system, specifically involved in promoting vasodilation (relaxation of vascular smooth muscle cells) and in preventing the onset of hypertension and other cardiovascular diseases [5-12]. More recent data from our laboratory have shown that the NO/cGMP/PKG signaling pathway, mediated via one of the isoforms of PKG, i.e. the PKG-Iα splice variant of PKG-I, is involved in promoting cell proliferation and enhanced cell survival (inhibiting the onset of apoptosis) in many types of mammalian cells, including neural cells [3, 6, 10, 13-15], uterine epithelial cells [16], OP9 bone marrow-derived mesenchymal (stromal) stem cells [17], and a number of different type of cancer cells, including ovarian cancer cells [18-22], neuroblastoma cells [15] and lung cancer cells [22].

Our studies have shown that the catalytic/kinase activity of PKG-Iα plays a key role in the phosphorylation of four proteins, BAD, CREB, c-Src and VASP, within mammalian cells, promoting DNA synthesis/cell proliferation and inhibiting the onset of apoptotic cell death, thus enhancing cell survival [22]. We have found that PKG-Iα is hyperactivated in several types of cancer cells, including ovarian cancer cells and lung cancer cells, resulting in abnormally high levels of phosphorylation of BAD, CREB, c-Src and VASP, which contributes to the exaggerated cell proliferation and resistance to certain chemotherapy, such as cisplatin (i.e. platinum resistance) [21]. The key role played by PKG-Iα in promoting DNA synthesis/cell proliferation and chemoresistance has been established by both pharmacological inhibitors and gene knockdown techniques using siRNA and shRNA that target PKG-Iα [21, 22].

Figure 1 shows a cellular model illustrating our findings about the role of NO at low physiological levels, i.e. 10 picomolar (pM) to 1 nanomolar (nM), and its downstream activation of PKG-Iα in promoting increased tumor growth and chemoresistance in cancer cells of epithelial origin, including human ovarian cancer cells [3, 19-22]. The model highlights the recent finding from our laboratory regarding the substrate proteins that can be directly phosphorylated by PKG-Iα, including the apoptosis-regulating protein BAD at serine-155 [15], the transcription factor CREB at serine-133 [3, 6, 22, 23] and the oncogenic tyrosine kinase c-Src at serine-17 [22, 23]. The enhanced phosphorylation of CREB caused by the hyperactivation of PKG-Iα in non-small cell lung cancer (NSCLC) cells was found to be responsible for the maintenance of high levels of expression of several "cell survival proteins", including Mcl-1 and three of the IAPs (c-IAP1, Livin and Survivin) [3]. Gene knockdown of PKG-Iα expression using siRNA targeting this PKG isoform clearly showed that PKG-Iα plays a critical role in promoting the high-level expression of Mcl-1, c-IAP1, Livin and Survivin in lung cancer cells. Ongoing experiments in the Fiscus Lab in the College of Medicine at Roseman University of Health Sciences are currently determining if a similar relationship between PKG-Iα hyperactivation and the high-level expression of "cell survival protein", such as Mcl-1, c-IAP1, Livin and Survivin, also occurs in human ovarian cancer cells, like in lung cancer cells.

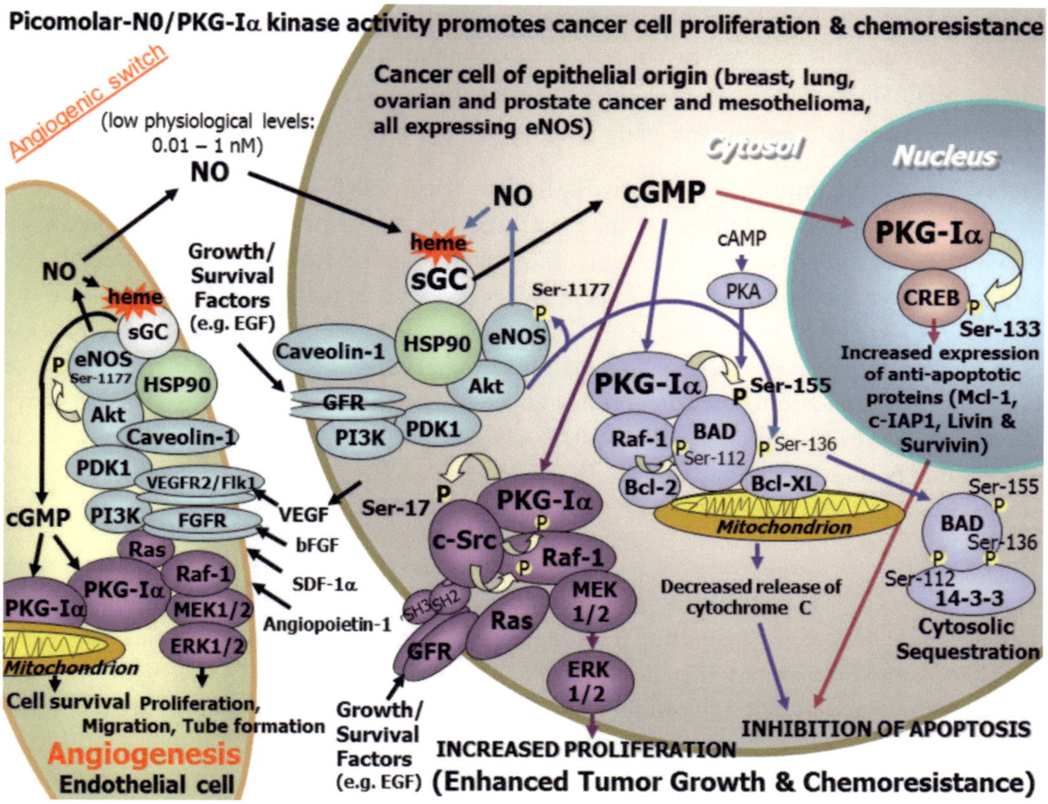

Figure 1. Involvement of picomolar levels of NO and downstream activation of PKG-Iα on promoting tumor angiogenesis and the proliferation and chemoresistance of cancer cells.

Figure 1 also illustrates the role of physiological-level NO and PKG-Iα in mediating the pro-tumor-angiogenesis effects of Vascular Endothelial Growth Factor (VEGF). VEGF is a pro-angiogenesis factor known to be released from many types of cancer cells, including human ovarian cancer cells, and is secreted in especially high amount by higher grade malignancies of the ovary [24]. Interestingly, higher VEGF expression by the ovarian cancer cells of patients was shown to be an independent predictor of poor prognosis of the disease [25].

The model of tumor angiogenesis shown in Figure 1 incorporates the early finding of Hood and Granger published in 1998, showing that VEGF stimulates cell proliferation and tube formation in human umbilical vein endothelial cells (HUVECs), a model of tumor angiogenesis, in a manner that was completely dependent on endogenous PKG [26]. Their study did not determined which isoform of PKG was expressed in the HUVECs, however, our laboratory has recently shown that HUVECs express both of the two PKG-I splice variants (i.e. both PKG-Iα and PKG-Iβ) [4], which has been confirmed in the data illustrated below in Figure 3. We have proposed that it is likely that the PKG-Iα isoform is the splice variant that mediates the enhanced cell proliferation of HUVECs, based on our many studies with other cells (e.g. N1E-115 and NG108-15 neural cells) that express exclusively the PKG-Iα splice variant of PKG-I [3, 4, 15, 17, 21-23]. Two key findings by Hood and Granger was that PKG directly interacted with Raf-1 (c-Raf), as assessed by co-immunoprecipitation, and that PKG activity was necessary for VEGF-induced activation of Raf-1 and the subsequent downstream activations of MEK and ERK1/2, regulating in enhanced endothelial cell proliferation [26].

Figure 2 shows a comparison of the two splice variants of PKG-I, illustrating how two very similar protein kinases, identical in their catalytic and regulatory domains, can have very different biological effects. The key difference between these two splice variants is the N-terminal region, the first 100 amino acids, which is encoded by the unique first exon, Iα in the case of PKG-Iα and Iβ in the case of PKG-Iβ. The first 100 amino acids provide the leucine zipper/protein-protein interaction domain, which determines the subcellular localization of these two isoforms and further determines which downstream target protein is phosphorylated by the two PKG-I isoforms within cells. Because of phosphorylating very different subsets of substrate proteins, PKG-Iα and PKG-Iβ are involved in mediating very different biological effects, in some cases, even opposite effects.

The PKG-Iα splice variant promotes cell proliferation and cell survival in both normal non-transformed cells (e.g. neural cells and OP9 bone marrow-derived mesenchymal stem cells) as well as malignant cells (contributing to exaggerated cell proliferation and chemoresistance in lung cancer and ovarian cancer cells) [3, 4, 15, 17, 20-23]. In contrast, the PKG-Iβ splice variant, at least when there is chemically-induced hyperactivation (e.g. using Exisulind to cause large increases in the intracellular cGMP levels) or forced overexpression (e.g. Deguchi et al., 2004), promotes effects that are just opposite of those mediated by PKG-Iα, i.e. inhibition of cell proliferation and induction of cell death mediated by PKG-Iβ [22, 23, 27]. This has led to confusion over the real function of PKG in regulating cell proliferation and cell survival, where PKG appears to have opposite effects in different experiments and/or different laboratories. Our studies have shown that it is critically important to differentiate between the actions of the different splice variants of PKG-I to avoid this confusion and the misunderstanding regarding the functions of PKG.

Recently, NO has been shown to be a positive regulator of the Warburg effect in ovarian cancer cells, promoting a metabolic switch toward increased glycolysis, with increased glucose consumption, enhanced uptake of glutamine and increased release of lactate [28]. The downstream signaling pathway mediating these metabolic effects of NO in ovarian cancer cells was not reported, but likely involves a mediator role for the different PKG isoforms that are downstream from the NO exposure.

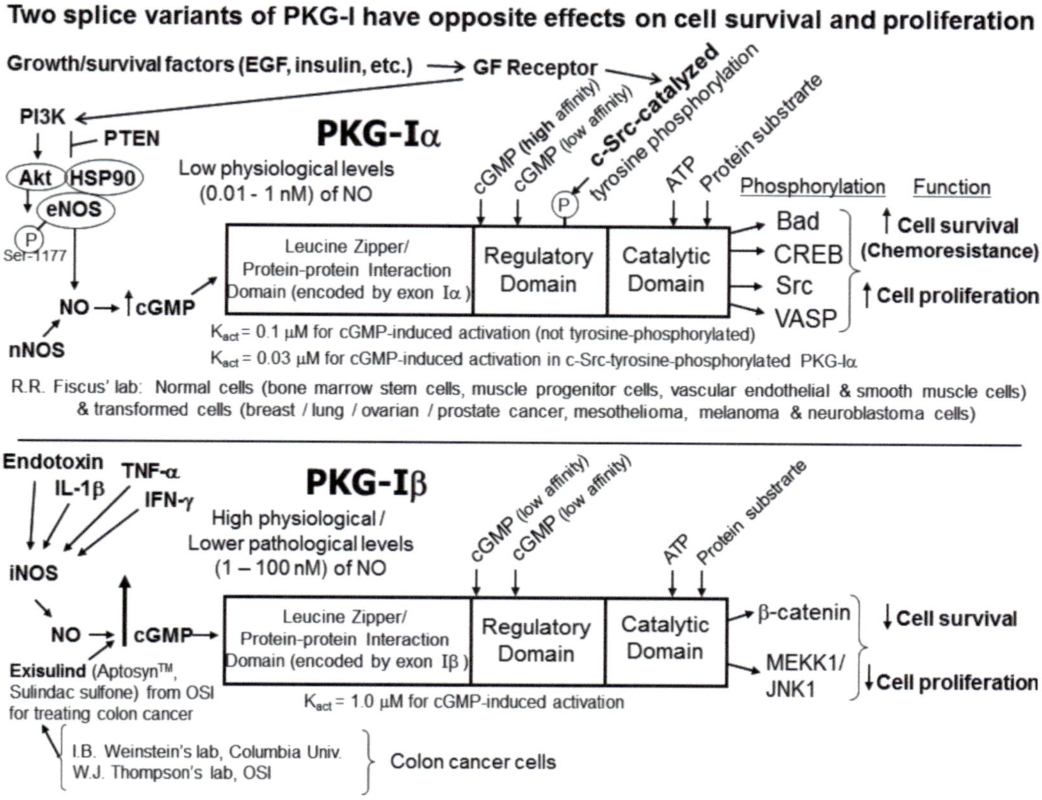

Figure 2. Opposite effects on cell proliferation and cell survival mediated by the two splice variants of PKG-I. The different biological effects of PKG-Iα and PKG-Iβ likely result from the different subcellular distributions of these to isoform (determined by the unique exon, Iα versus Iβ, of the two splice variants), resulting in the phosphorylation and activation of very different downstream substrates proteins, as depicted in the models. Modified from the original model in R.R. Fiscus, E.L. Leung, J.C. Wong and M.G. Johlfs, 2012 [22].

2. Hyeractivation of PKG-Iα kinase activity in cancer cells contributes to the higher expression levels of Mcl-1 and certain Inhibitor of Apoptosis Proteins (IAPs), including c-IAP1, Livin and Survivin

Downstream from PKG-Iα hyperactivity in cancer cells is the high levels of expression of "cell survival proteins", including Mcl-1 and certain IAPs, such as c-IAP1, Livin and Survivin [22]. These IAPs have been shown to regulate apoptosis and tumorigenesis [29]. Eight human IAPs have been identified [30] and are known to suppress apoptotic cell death, thus promoting cell survival and, in cancer cells, chemoresistance [31]. c-IAP1 and c-IAP2 possess a caspase recruitment domain [32], and c-IAP1, c-IAP2 and XIAP are known to directly inhibit caspase-3 and caspase-7 activity [33, 34]. Elevated expression of IAP proteins has been shown in almost all types of human cancers and has been implicated as therapeutic targets [35]. Particularly, XIAP was shown to play a predominant role in the inactivation of apoptosome in non-small cell lung cancer NCI-H460 cells [36]. Survivin-specific siRNA was shown to increase apoptosis and inhibit cell proliferation in A549 lung cancer cells associated with activation of caspase-9 [37].

Although the NF-κB transcription factor is traditionally thought to regulate the expression of the IAPs, another transcription factor, CREB, has also been implicated in regulating some IAPs. For example, CREB phosphorylation at serine-133 and its subsequent activation are thought to be key events in the induction of c-IAP2 and Livin expression, potentially mediated by multiple protein kinases, including PKA, ERK1/2 and p38 MAPK, in colon cancer cells [38, 39].

Recent data from our laboratory have shown that the expression of three of the IAPs, c-IAP1, Livin and Survivin, are dependent on the NO/cGMP/PKG-Iα signaling pathway in non-small cell lung cancer (NSCLC) cells, which appears to involve the exaggerated phosphorylation of CREB at serine-133 catalyzed by the hyperactivated PKG-Iα [3]. We have also shown that some of these same signaling proteins, especially PKG-Iα and downstream elevation of the protein expression of c-IAP1and Livin as well as two other IAPs (c-IAP2 and XIAP) are involved in angiogenesis, using human endothelial cells (the HUVECs) as a model of tumor angiogenesis [4]. Interestingly, we found that resveratrol, a polyphenol from red wine, grapes, berries and peanuts known for its protection against cancers, when added at anti-angiogenesis and anti-cancer concentrations, inhibits the intracellular catalytic/kinase activity of PKG-Iα in the HUVECs, dramatically decreasing protein expression levels of c-IAP1, c-IAP2, Livin and XIAP [4]. Our data suggest that certain naturally-occurring anti-cancer agents, such as resveratrol, may prevent cancers by suppressing the PKG-Iα signaling pathway and lowering the expression levels of the IAPs in the vascular endothelial cells of tumors, thus suppressing tumor angiogenesis.

3. Identification of PKG-I splice variants expressed in human ovarian cancer cells by using a new ultrasensitive advanced nano-proteomics technology, the NanoPro 1000 system

Recent studies from our laboratory have used an ultrasensitive "advanced nano-proteomics" technology, called NanoPro 1000 (ProteinSimple, San Jose, CA, USA), to determine expression and phosphorylation levels of PKG-Iα as well as other protein kinases (especially Akt and c-Src, which interact with PKG-Iα and co-mediate the enhanced cell survival and resistance to apoptosis), and the various IAPs. This technology uses a robotic system for collecting samples and analyzing the samples, involving capillary isoelectricfocusing (cIEF) for separating proteins based on pI values, rather than molecular weight. This has a clear advantage over Western blot analysis when attempting to separate and identify proteins with similar molecular weight, such as isoforms of proteins.

This new NanoPro 1000 technology provides a sensitivity that is >500-times better than conventional Western blot analysis, thus allowing discovery of new signaling proteins that can be used for developing new therapeutic agents. This new technology allows for accurate measurements of lower abundance proteins (undetectable by conventional Western blot analysis), often using fewer than 1,000 mammalian cells for the analysis.

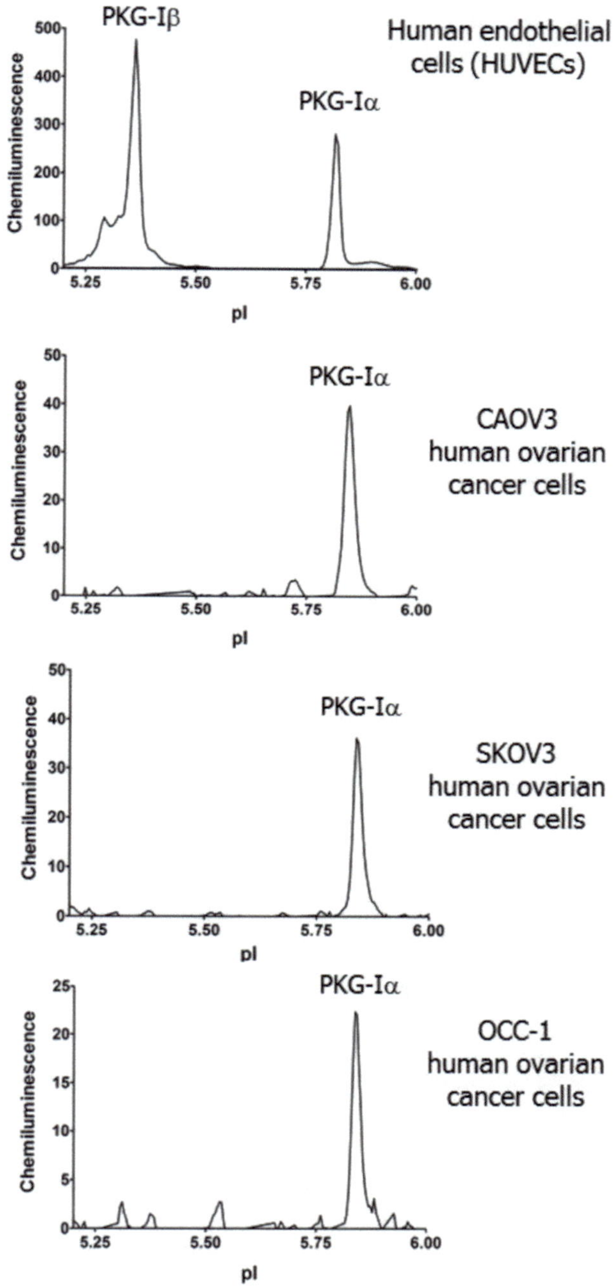

Figure 3. Electropherograms generated by the new technology of NanoPro 1000 system, a capillary isoelectrofocusing (cIEF) instrument for quantifying protein expression levels and phosphorylations levels, with a sensitive >500-times greater than traditional Western blot analysis. The HUVECs are used as positive controls for illustrating the expression of both splice variants of PKG-I in the same cell population. All three of the human ovarian cancer cell lines express only the PKG-Iα splice variant.

Figure 3 illustrates recent experiments showing the expression of PKG-I splice variants in three different ovarian cancer cell lines, CAOV3, SKOV3 and OCC-1 cells, determined by using the NanoPro 1000 technology. The top electropherogram shows that the HUVECs, human endothelial cells, express both PKG-I splice variants, confirming our previous studies of HUVECs using the older, related technology, the NanoPro 100 system, recently published by our laboratory in *Anticancer Research* [4].

Note that all three of the ovarian cancer cell lines shown in Figure 3 express exclusively the PKG-Iα splice variant, in contrast to the expression pattern shown in the human endothelial cells expressing both splice variants of PKG-I. The protein expression levels of PKG-Iα in all of these human ovarian cancer cell lines are typically below the detection limits when analyzed by traditional Western blot analysis, as shown in our previous book chapter on ovarian cancer cells [22]. Thus, the advanced nano-proteomic technology of the robotic cIEF-based NanoPro 1000 system provides a valuable new research tool for studying the expression levels of lower abundance proteins that are undetectable by the 30-year-old technique of Western blot analysis (500-times less sensitive compared to the NanoPro 1000 system).

4. Human ovarian cancer cells have hyperactivated PKG-Iα, as quantified by a newly- developed ultrasensitive near-infrared-fluorescence (NIRF)-based kinase assay for measuring PKG catalytic/kinase activity in tissue samples and cell lysates

Recently, our laboratory has successfully development a new, ultrasensitive methodology for accurately measuring the catalytic/kinase activity of any protein kinase within biological samples (cell lysates and tissue homogenates) using NIRF-labeled peptide substrates rather than the old technique of using radioactive (^{32}P- or ^{33}P-labeled) ATP. The radioactive protein kinase assays were originally developed in the 1970s and 1980s for measuring the catalytic activity of protein kinase A (PKA) and PKG in freshly-prepared tissue homogenates [5-10, 22, 23]. The new NIRF-based protein kinase assays were developed for improving safety and for lowering the cost of analysis.

Figure 4 illustrates the use of this new methodology, showing that four different ovarian cancer cell lines, CAOV3, OCC1, SKOV3 and A2780cp cells, all possess measureable levels of endogenous PKG-Iα catalytic/kinase activity and that this kinase activity is indeed hyperactivated in all of the ovarian cancer cell lines. The NIRF-labeled peptide substrate used in this assay can also be phosphorylated by eight of the most common isoforms of protein kinase C (PKC), but not by other related protein kinases, such as Akt1, Akt2, p70S6-kinase and RSK2. Thus, the catalytic activities of both PKG and PKC can be measured simultaneously in the same biological sample. To define the component of kinase activity contributed by endogenous PKC, we used a combination of four PKC inhibitors (AEB071, Gö 6976, Gö 6983 and LY333,531), which selectively inhibit the eight isoforms of PKC capable of phosphorylating the NIRF-peptide substrate. This defines the PKC catalytic activity from PKG catalytic activity in complex mixtures of protein kinases, such as tissue homogenates and cell lysates. The kinase catalytic activity remaining in the presence of the four PKC inhibitors represents only PKG catalytic activity, show in Figure 4.

The percent activation of PKG-Iα in the four human ovarian cancer cell lines was all above 90%, indicating that PKG-Iα is indeed hyperactivated (Figure 4) in these malignant cells. For comparison, homogenates of two normal tissues, vascular smooth muscle (V.S.M.) from rat aorta and human pancreatic islets, were also analyzed. The % activation of PKG in smooth muscle tissue was 21%, similar to the % activation measured by the ^{32}P-ATP-based methodology developed and used by Dr. R.R. Fiscus in the early and mid-1980s [5, 7-9], and the PKG activation in pancreatic islets was 31%. Thus, compared to normal tissues, all of the ovarian cancer cell lines have highly-activated PKG. This hyperactivation of PKG-Iα in the ovarian cancer cells would result in downstream (hyper)activation of c-Src and CREB, resulting in an exaggerated expression of "cell survival proteins", such as Mcl-1 and certain IAPs, e.g. c-IAP1, Livin and Survivin, likely contributing to the aggressive nature of this form of cancer.

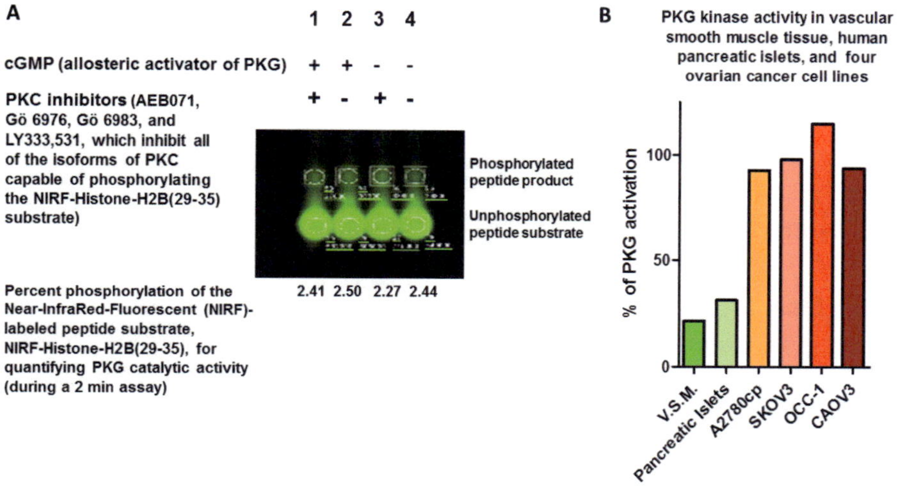

Figure 4. Hyperactivation of PKG catalytic/kinase activity in four ovarian cancer cell lines. A, picture representative of the near infrared-fluorescence (NIRF)-based kinase assay, using the CAOV3 ovarian cancer cells as an example. The % of phosphorylation was calculated based on the fluorescence signal measured by LI-COR Odyssey CLx scanner. The activity ratio, activity –cGMP divided by activity +cGMP (i.e. kinase activity with versus without the addition of exogenous cGMP (10 μM), an allosteric activator of PKG). All measurements were done in the presence of a combination of select PKC inhibitors (to remove kinase activity contributed by PKC isoforms). The remaining kinase activity reflects the PKG catalytic activity in these cell lines. The data in A., i.e. 2.41, 2.50, 2.27 and 2.44, represent the percent phosphorylation of the NIRF-labeled peptide substrate during a 2-min reaction. B, The % of PKG activation (i.e. 100 X the activity ratio) for each sample analyzed is shown in a bar graph. Data was obtained by measuring kinase activity by the new NIRF-based kinase assay method. The four ovarian cancer cell lines, A2780cp, SKOV3, OCC-1 and CAOV3, had % of PKG activation of 93%, 98%, 115% and 94%, respectively, showing that PKG is clearly hyperactivated in all of the ovarian cancer cells tested. For comparison, tissue samples of freshly-isolated vascular smooth muscle (V.S.M.) from rat aorta and human pancreatic islets (purchased from Lonza) were used to show PKG catalytic/kinase activity in normal non-cancerous tissues. Note that the % activation of PKG is considerably lower in normal tissue, showing 21% activation of PKG in vascular smooth muscle cells (V.S.M.) and 31% activation of PKG in human pancreatic islets.

5. Future experiments

Our future studies will focus on: 1) determining the expression of PKG isoform and its various phospho-forms in human ovarian cancer cell lines and clinical samples of ovarian tumors using the NanoPro 1000 system, 2) determining the PKG kinase activity of other ovarian cancer cell lines and clinical samples of ovarian tumors using our patented NIRF-based kinase assay, and 3) studying the phosphorylation/activation of the transcription factor CREB and the expression profile of the IAPs using our advanced nano-proteomics technology, with special focus on c-IAP1, c-IAP2, Livin, Survivin and XIAP, in ovarian cancer cells and vascular endothelial cells. The goal of our future experiments is to ultimately develop new therapeutic agents that can target these novel signaling pathways in order to effectively treat chemoresistant ovarian cancer and tumor angiogenesis.

The NanoPro 1000 system is especially useful for studying the multiple phospho-forms of proteins, because of its ability to separate proteins based on pI values rather than molecular weight. Each addition of a phosphate molecule to a protein typically causes a measurable (and resolvable) shift in the pI value, which can be used to determine intracellular activation and/or the catalytic function of a protein kinase within cells. Likewise, our patented technology using NIRF-based kinase assays will be used to determine the effectiveness and potency of protein kinase inhibitors that could potentially be used to treat cancer.

6. Conclusions

Our studies of human ovarian cancer cells as well as other types of cancer cells (e.g. breast cancer, lung cancer, mesothelioma, neuroblastoma and prostate cancer) have identified the NO/cGMP/PKG-Iα signaling pathway as a key cellular mechanism involved in mediating the exaggerated cell proliferation and chemoresistance of these cancers [3, 15, 19-22]. We have shown that the PKG-Iα splice variant of PKG-I, which is expressed in all of these cancer cells, directly phosphorylates important intracellular proteins, including BAD, CREB and c-Src, leading to enahanced cell survival (i.e. chemoresistance) and exaggerated cell proliferation. Specifically, phosphorylation of CREB at serine-133 following activation of PKG-Iα results in increased gene expression of several "cell survival proteins", including Mcl-1 and some of the the IAPs.

In human lung cancer cells, the NO/PKG-Iα signaling pathway represents a major mechanism for the enhanced gene expression of three IAPs, c-IAP1, Livin and Survivin, which corresponds with exaggerated cell proliferation and resistance to cisplatin-induced apoptosis [3]. Blocking the PKG-Iα catalytic activity or knocking-down the gene expression of PKG-Iα using siRNA dramatically sensitizes these chemoresistant cells to the cancer-killing effects of cisplatin. We anticipate that our future studies with ovarian cancer cells will show similar results.

In HUVECs, human endothelial cells used as a model of tumor angiogenesis, the eNOS/NO/cGMP/PKG signaling pathway is now recognized to mediate the pro-angiogenesis effects of

VEGF [4]. VEGF is a factor that is released in large amounts from cancer cells, including human ovarian cancer cells. Our studies with HUVECs show that four IAPs, c-IAP1, c-IAP2, Livin and XIAP, are all downregulated by resveratrol, a polyphenol from grapes, berries, peanuts and red wine, and that this response corresponds to the inhibition of PKG catalytic activity in the HUVECs.

Figure 5 shows a model representing the involvement of the NO/cGMP/PKG-Iα signaling pathway in mediating the pro-angiogenesis effects of VEGF within vascular endothelial cells, promoting the increased expression of the IAPs, c-IAP1, c-IAP2, Livin and XIAP, based on our recent publication [4]. Also shown is the inhibitory action of resveratrol, at anti-angiogenic and anti-cancer concentrations, on the PKG-Iα catalytic actions and downstream expression of c-IAP1, c-IAP-2, Livin and XIAP. We have proposed that the ability of resveratrol to prevent cancers may relate to its ability to inhibit PKG-Iα catalytic activity selectively in tumor endothelial cells involved in tumor angiogenesis, thus suppressing the expression of IAPs in the endothelial cells and the tumor angiogenesis.

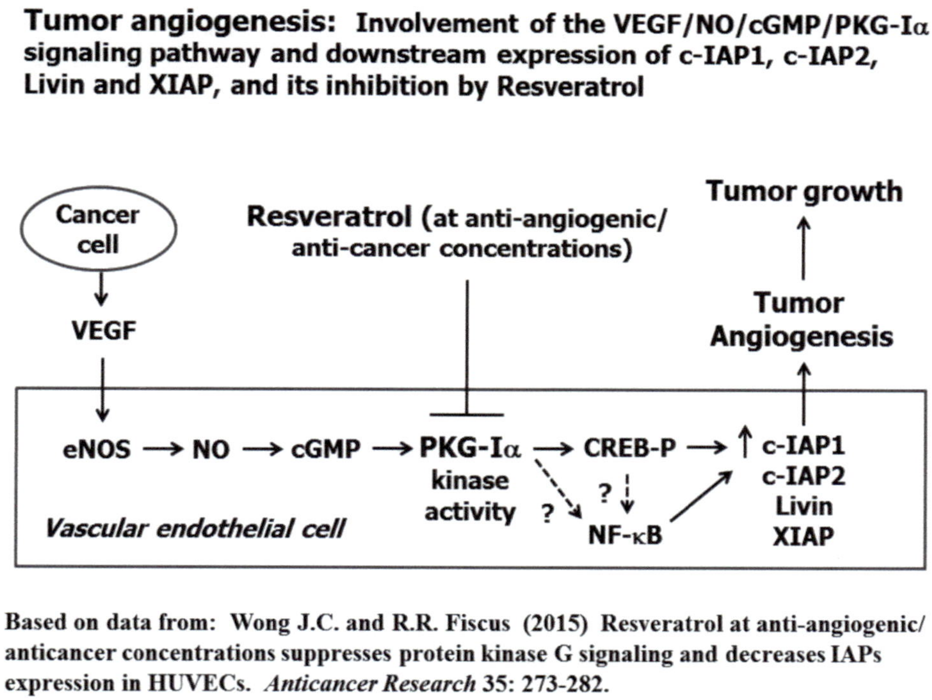

Figure 5. Involvement of eNOS, NO, cGMP and PKG-Iα in the pro-angiogenesis actions of VEGF in vascular endothelial cells. Enhanced PKG-Iα catalytic activity induced by VEGF can increase CREB phosphorylation and activation, increasing expression of certain IAPs. The traditional transcription factor thought to be involved in promoting the gene expression of the IAPs, i.e. NF-κB, is also shown, although its role in PKG-Iα-mediated increases in the IAPs and tumor angiogenesis is not yet known.

Acknowledgements

Financial support for the research and the preparation of this book chapter was provided by Internal Funding from Roseman University of Health Sciences (formerly named the University of Southern Nevada and the Nevada College of Pharmacy), Henderson, Nevada, USA, from a grant from the U.S. Department of Defense (DOD), grant # W81XWH-07-1-0543, and from Start-up Funding from the Nevada Cancer Institute, Las Vegas, Nevada, USA, all awarded to Dr. Fiscus.

Author details

Janica C. Wong[1,2,3], Priyatham Gorjala[1], Benjamin Costantino[1] and Ronald R. Fiscus[1,3,4*]

*Address all correspondence to: rfiscus@roseman.edu

1 Roseman University of Health Sciences, College of Medicine, Department of Biomedical Sciences, the Diabetes & Obesity Research Center and the Cancer Research Center, Roseman Medical Education & Research Building at Summerlin Campus, Las Vegas, Nevada, USA

2 Stanford University, School of Medicine, Department of Pediatrics, Stanford, California, USA

3 Nevada Cancer Institute, Cancer Molecular Biology Section, Las Vegas, Nevada, USA

4 Roseman University of Health Sciences, College of Pharmacy, Henderson, Nevada, USA

References

[1] Teoh DG, Secord AA. Antiangiogenic therapies in epithelial ovarian cancer. Cancer Control. 2011 Jan;18(1):31-43.

[2] Chen L, Liang L, Yan X, Liu N, Gong L, Pan S, et al. Survivin status affects prognosis and chemosensitivity in epithelial ovarian cancer. Int J Gynecol Cancer. 2013 Feb; 23(2):256-63.

[3] Wong JC, Bathina M, Fiscus RR. Cyclic GMP/protein kinase G type-Iα (PKG-Iα) signaling pathway promotes CREB phosphorylation and maintains higher c-IAP1, livin, survivin, and Mcl-1 expression and the inhibition of PKG-Iα kinase activity synergizes with cisplatin in non-small cell lung cancer cells. J Cell Biochem. 2012 Nov;113(11): 3587-98.

[4] Wong JC, Fiscus RR. Resveratrol at anti-angiogenesis/anticancer concentrations suppresses protein kinase G signaling and decreases IAPs expression in HUVECs. Anticancer Research. 2015;35:273-82.

[5] Fiscus RR. Molecular mechanisms of endothelium-mediated vasodilation. Semin Thromb Hemost. 1988;14 Suppl:12-22.

[6] Fiscus RR. Involvement of cyclic GMP and protein kinase G in the regulation of apoptosis and survival in neural cells. Neurosignals. 2002 Jul-Aug;11(4):175-90.

[7] Fiscus RR, Murad F. cGMP-dependent protein kinase activation in intact tissues. Methods Enzymol. 1988;159:150-9.

[8] Fiscus RR, Rapoport RM, Murad F. Endothelium-dependent and nitrovasodilator-induced activation of cyclic GMP-dependent protein kinase in rat aorta. J Cyclic Nucleotide Protein Phosphor Res. 1983;9(6):415-25.

[9] Fiscus RR, Rapoport RM, Waldman SA, Murad F. Atriopeptin II elevates cyclic GMP, activates cyclic GMP-dependent protein kinase and causes relaxation in rat thoracic aorta. Biochim Biophys Acta. 1985 Jul 30;846(1):179-84.

[10] Fiscus RR, Yuen JP, Chan SL, Kwong JH, Chew SB. Nitric oxide and cyclic GMP as pro- and anti-apoptotic agents. J Card Surg. 2002 Jul-Aug;17(4):336-9.

[11] Murad F, Rapoport RM, Fiscus R. Role of cyclic-GMP in relaxations of vascular smooth muscle. J Cardiovasc Pharmacol. 1985;7 Suppl 3:S111-8.

[12] Murad F, Waldman SA, Fiscus RR, Rapoport RM. Regulation of cyclic GMP synthesis and the interactions with calcium. J Cardiovasc Pharmacol. 1986;8 Suppl 8:S57-60.

[13] Barger SW, Fiscus RR, Ruth P, Hofmann F, Mattson MP. Role of cyclic GMP in the regulation of neuronal calcium and survival by secreted forms of beta-amyloid precursor. J Neurochem. 1995 May;64(5):2087-96.

[14] Cheng Chew SB, Leung PY, Fiscus RR. Preincubation with atrial natriuretic peptide protects NG108-15 cells against the toxic/proapoptotic effects of the nitric oxide donor S-nitroso- N-acetylpenicillamine. Histochem Cell Biol. 2003 Sep;120(3):163-71.

[15] Johlfs MG, Fiscus RR. Protein kinase G type-Iα phosphorylates the apoptosis-regulating protein Bad at serine 155 and protects against apoptosis in N1E-115 cells. Neurochem Int. 2010 Mar;56(4):546-53.

[16] Chan SL, Fiscus RR. Guanylyl cyclase inhibitors NS2028 and ODQ and protein kinase G (PKG) inhibitor KT5823 trigger apoptotic DNA fragmentation in immortalized uterine epithelial cells: anti-apoptotic effects of basal cGMP/PKG. Mol Hum Reprod. 2003 Dec;9(12):775-83.

[17] Wong JC, Fiscus RR. Essential roles of the nitric oxide (NO)/cGMP/protein kinase G type-Iα (PKG-Iα) signaling pathway and the atrial natriuretic peptide (ANP)/cGMP/

PKG-Iα autocrine loop in promoting proliferation and cell survival of OP9 bone marrow stromal cells. J Cell Biochem. 2011 Mar;112(3):829-39.

[18] Fraser M, Chan SL, Chan SS, Fiscus RR, Tsang BK. Regulation of p53 and suppression of apoptosis by the soluble guanylyl cyclase/cGMP pathway in human ovarian cancer cells. Oncogene. 2006 Apr 6;25(15):2203-12.

[19] Leung EL, Fraser M, Fiscus RR, Tsang BK. Cisplatin alters nitric oxide synthase levels in human ovarian cancer cells: involvement in p53 regulation and cisplatin resistance. Br J Cancer. 2008 Jun 3;98(11):1803-9.

[20] Leung EL, Wong JC, Johlfs MG, Tsang BK, Fiscus RR. Protein kinase G type Ialpha activity in human ovarian cancer cells significantly contributes to enhanced Src activation and DNA synthesis/cell proliferation. Mol Cancer Res. 2010 Apr;8(4):578-91.

[21] Wong JC, Fiscus RR. Protein kinase G-Iα hyperactivation and VASP phosphorylation in promoting ovarian cancer cell migration and platinum resistance. In: Diaz-Padilla I, editor. Ovarian Cancer - A Clinical and Translational Update: INTECH; 2013. p. 251-73.

[22] Fiscus RR, Leung EL, Wong JC, Johlfs MG. Nitric oxide/protein kinase G-Iα promote c-Src activation, proliferation and chemoresistance in ovarian cancer. In: Farghaly S, editor. Ovarian Cancer - Basic Science Perspective: Intech Open Access Publisher; 2012. p. 315-34.

[23] Fiscus RR, Johlfs MG. Protein kinase G (PKG): Involvement in promoting neural cell survival, proliferation, synaptogenesis and synaptic plasticity and the use of new ultrasensitive capillary-electrophoresis-based methodologies for measuring PKG expression and molecular actions. In: Mukai H, editor. Protein Kinase Technologies - Neuromethods: Springer; 2012. p. 319-48.

[24] Santin AD, Hermonat PL, Ravaggi A, Cannon MJ, Pecorelli S, Parham GP. Secretion of vascular endothelial growth factor in ovarian cancer. Eur J Gynaecol Oncol. 1999;20(3):177-81.

[25] Duncan TJ, Al-Attar A, Rolland P, Scott IV, Deen S, Liu DT, et al. Vascular endothelial growth factor expression in ovarian cancer: a model for targeted use of novel therapies? Clin Cancer Res. 2008 May 15;14(10):3030-5.

[26] Hood J, Granger HJ. Protein kinase G mediates vascular endothelial growth factor-induced Raf-1 activation and proliferation in human endothelial cells. J Biol Chem. 1998 Sep 4;273(36):23504-8.

[27] Deguchi A, Thompson WJ, Weinstein IB. Activation of protein kinase G is sufficient to induce apoptosis and inhibit cell migration in colon cancer cells. Cancer Res. 2004 Jun 1;64(11):3966-73.

http://dx.doi.org/10.5772/60774

[28] Caneba CA, Yang L, Baddour J, Curtis R, Win J, Hartig S, et al. Nitric oxide is a positive regulator of the Warburg effect in ovarian cancer cells. Cell Death Dis. 2014;5:e1302.

[29] Deveraux QL, Reed JC. IAP family proteins--suppressors of apoptosis. Genes Dev. 1999 Feb 1;13(3):239-52.

[30] Salvesen GS, Duckett CS. IAP proteins: blocking the road to death's door. Nat Rev Mol Cell Biol. 2002 Jun;3(6):401-10.

[31] LaCasse EC, Baird S, Korneluk RG, MacKenzie AE. The inhibitors of apoptosis (IAPs) and their emerging role in cancer. Oncogene. 1998 Dec 24;17(25):3247-59.

[32] Hofmann K, Bucher P, Tschopp J. The CARD domain: a new apoptotic signalling motif. Trends Biochem Sci. 1997 May;22(5):155-6.

[33] Roy N, Deveraux QL, Takahashi R, Salvesen GS, Reed JC. The c-IAP-1 and c-IAP-2 proteins are direct inhibitors of specific caspases. EMBO J. 1997 Dec 1;16(23):6914-25.

[34] Eckelman BP, Salvesen GS, Scott FL. Human inhibitor of apoptosis proteins: why XIAP is the black sheep of the family. EMBO Rep. 2006 Oct;7(10):988-94.

[35] Vucic D, Fairbrother WJ. The inhibitor of apoptosis proteins as therapeutic targets in cancer. Clin Cancer Res. 2007 Oct 15;13(20):5995-6000.

[36] Yang L, Mashima T, Sato S, Mochizuki M, Sakamoto H, Yamori T, et al. Predominant suppression of apoptosome by inhibitor of apoptosis protein in non-small cell lung cancer H460 cells: therapeutic effect of a novel polyarginine-conjugated Smac peptide. Cancer Res. 2003 Feb 15;63(4):831-7.

[37] Chen XQ, Yang S, Li ZY, Lu HS, Kang MQ, Lin TY. Effects and mechanism of downregulation of survivin expression by RNA interference on proliferation and apoptosis of lung cancer cells. Mol Med Report. 2012 Apr;5(4):917-22.

[38] Nishihara H, Hwang M, Kizaka-Kondoh S, Eckmann L, Insel PA. Cyclic AMP promotes cAMP-responsive element-binding protein-dependent induction of cellular inhibitor of apoptosis protein-2 and suppresses apoptosis of colon cancer cells through ERK1/2 and p38 MAPK. J Biol Chem. 2004 Jun 18;279(25):26176-83.

[39] Nishihara H, Kizaka-Kondoh S, Insel PA, Eckmann L. Inhibition of apoptosis in normal and transformed intestinal epithelial cells by cAMP through induction of inhibitor of apoptosis protein (IAP)-2. Proc Natl Acad Sci U S A. 2003 Jul 22;100(15):8921-6.

Chapter 11

Cancer of the Vulva — A Review

Fernando Anschau and Manoel Afonso Guimarães Gonçalves

Additional information is available at the end of the chapter

http://dx.doi.org/10.5772/61579

Abstract

Cancer of the Vulva: a review In reporting on cancer of the vulva, we should keep in mind some important aspects of its epidemiology and its early detection. Most of the papers on the subject refer to vulvar cancer as a rare disease, accounting for 4 to 5% of all malignant neoplasms of the female genital tract and less than 1% of women's cancers. The incidence varies from 1 to 3.6 cases per 100,000 women, with peak incidence at ages 70-79 years. Even though the incidence increases with age, the proportion of young patients with vulvar cancer has greatly increased due to its association with infection with human papillomavirus (HPV). The risk of developing cancer of the vulva is related to behavioral, reproductive, hormonal and genetic aspects. Factors that increase risk include other genital cancers, chronic inflammatory diseases of the vulva, smoking, history of genital warts and vulvar intraepithelial neoplasia (VIN). We can consider that, given the epidemiological evidence, there are two etiologic pathways for vulvar cancer: one related to older patients, in the seventh or eighth decades of life, associated with mutations in TP53 and non-neoplastic epithelial disorders such as chronic inflammation or vulvar lichen, shows precursor lesions of differentiated VIN; the other is more common in young patients, accounts for approximately 43-60% of squamous carcinoma of the vulva, is associated with HPV infection, and is a common precursor lesion of VIN. Eighty-five to ninety percent of vulvar cancers are squamous in origin (squamous cell carcinoma); however, when considering the embryological origin of the vulva - the three germ layers - different histologic types can compose neoplasms affecting the region.

Keywords: Vulvar cancer, clinical presentation, staging, treatment, prognostic factor, review, signs and symptoms, therapy, innovations

1. Introduction

In reporting on cancer of the vulva, we should keep in mind some important aspects of its epidemiology and its early detection. Most of the papers on the subject refer to vulvar cancer as a rare disease, accounting for 4–5% of all malignant neoplasms of the female genital tract and less than 1% of women's cancers. The incidence varies from 1 to 3.6 cases per 100,000 women, with peak incidence at ages 70–79 years. [1, 2, 3, 4] Even though the incidence increases with age, the proportion of young patients with vulvar cancer has greatly increased due to its association with infection with human papillomavirus (HPV). 5 The risk of developing cancer of the vulva is related to behavioral, reproductive, hormonal, and genetic aspects. Factors that increase risk include other genital cancers, chronic inflammatory diseases of the vulva, smoking, history of genital warts, and vulvar intraepithelial neoplasia (VIN).

We can consider that, given the epidemiological evidence, there are two etiologic pathways for vulvar cancer: one is related to older patients, in the seventh or eighth decades of life, associated with mutations in TP53 and non-neoplastic epithelial disorders such as chronic inflammation or vulvar lichen, and shows precursor lesions of differentiated VIN; the other is more common in young patients, accounts for approximately 43–60% of squamous carcinoma of the vulva, is associated with HPV infection, and is a common precursor lesion of VIN. [6, 7, 8, 9]

Eighty-five to ninety percent of vulvar cancers are squamous in origin (squamous cell carcinoma); however, when considering the embryological origin of the vulva – the three germ layers – different histologic types can compose neoplasms affecting the region. Melanoma is the second most common and should be discussed separately because of its peculiar characteristics.

Prognosis is strongly related to lymph node status and the stage of disease, reaching 90% survival for early stages without lymph node involvement.[1, 10]

Various important advances in the treatment of vulvar cancer were made in recent decades toward more conservative surgery without compromising survival and toward reduction of comorbidities, such as: (1) conservation of the vulva in patients with unifocal tumors, and normal vulva in other aspects; (2) omission of inguinal lymphadenectomy in patients with T1 tumors and stromal invasion <1 mm; (3) elimination of routine pelvic lymphadenectomy; (4) use separate incisions for inguinal dissection; (5) use of preoperative radiotherapy in selected cases; and (6) postoperative radiotherapy to reduce inguinal recurrence in patients with multiple compromised inguinal lymph nodes.

2. Clinical presentation

The diagnosis is often delayed, since vulvar cancer does not show specific signs and symptoms, and older patients do not usually examine their vulva preventively and report their symptoms. Vulvar cancer may be asymptomatic, but the majority of patients present with nodules or vulvar ulcer. Such signs may be accompanied by pain, but it may also be absent. The long-standing pruritus is frequent and may be associated with vulvar dystrophy. Secretions and bleeding are symptoms that are occasionally present, as well as dyspareunia and burning sensation. Putrid odor due to tissue necrosis may also be diagnostic. Enlarged lymph nodes, especially in the inguinal region, denote disease in later stages.[1, 10, 11] A study of delayed diagnosis showed that in 88% of patients, symptoms were already present for about 6 months and in 28% for more than 5 years. In the same study, emphasis was placed on clinical suspicion in view of symptoms, since 31% of patients had office visits three or more times, but only 25% of cases had undergone biopsy. [12]

As previously mentioned, vulvar melanoma will be addressed separately, but any pigmentation of the vulva deserves attention for diagnosis.

3. Screening

There is no standard procedure for screening for vulvar cancer. However, we must maintain a level of suspicion when seeing patients with signs and symptoms related to the vulvar region and to be attentive to the examination of the female genitalia at check-ups. Patients with history of vaginal and cervical cancer should have the vulva inspected, with or without colposcopy (vulvoscopy), as part of a regular follow-up. Similarly, those with lichen sclerosus or VIN history deserve regular monitoring.

4. Gynecological examination

The vulvar cancer can arise in any region of the vulva, but the most common locations are labia (80%), clitoris (10%), and frenulum region (10%). Most tumors are unilateral, but may present as bilateral or multicentric (Figures 1, 2, and 3). Any malignant neoplastic lesion involving the vagina and the vulva should be classified as vulvar cancer.

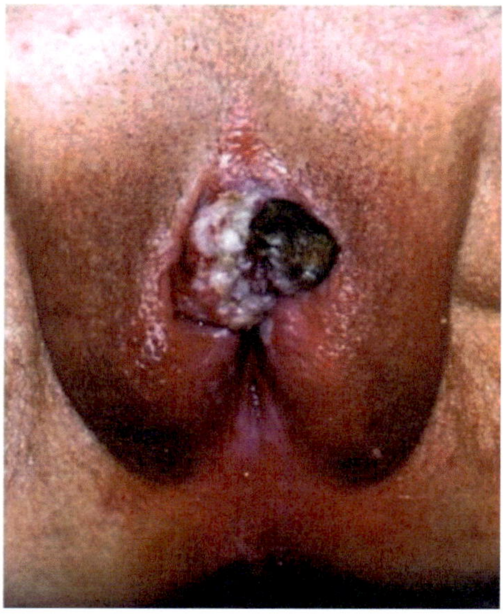

Figure 1. Squamous cell carcinoma of the vulva – clitoral region with involvement of labia minora and majora.

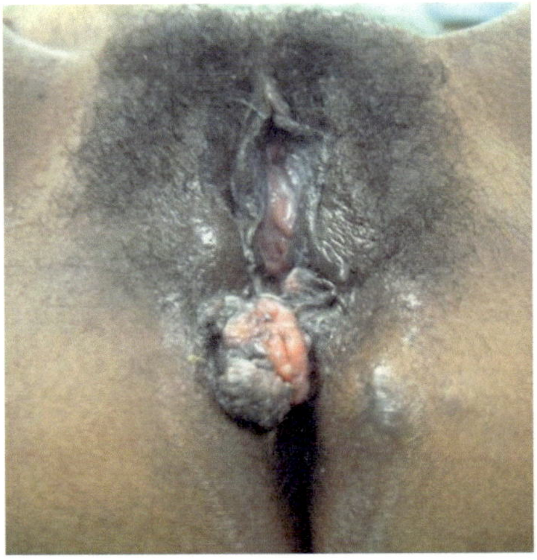

Figure 2. Adenocarcinoma of the vulva – frenulum region extending to the top of the right thigh.

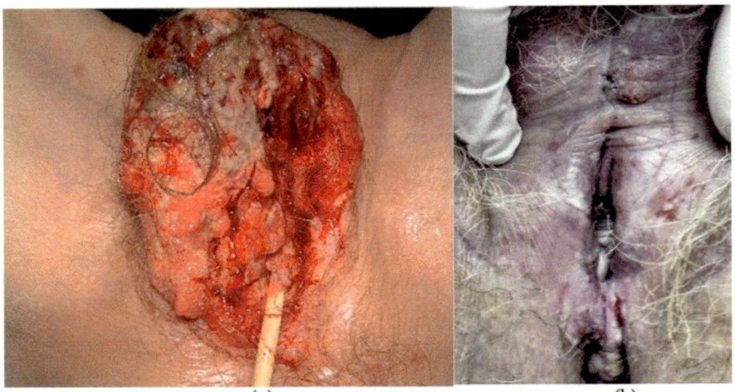

(a) (b)

Figure 3. (a) Squamous cell carcinoma of the vulva with destruction of vulvar anatomy. (b) Carcinoma of the vulva associated with lichen sclerosus Presence of white areas, cracks, macules, plaques, thin and hypochromic skin, and tumor infiltrating next to the clitoris.

On the basis of this knowledge, a careful inspection of the vulva and vagina are important points in the gynecological examination and may include vulvoscopy and colposcopy. Suspicious areas with color changes, redness, ulcers, papules, macules, erosions, thickening of skin, bumps, and cracks must be observed carefully. The lesions may grow and form infiltrating endophytic or exophytic tissue with the formation of visible tumors. When identifying suspicious areas, a histological examination should be performed by biopsy that includes not only the skin but also the subepithelial stroma. Multifocal lesions require multiple biopsies for the investigation of histological changes (Figure 3.1).

Considering that a significant proportion of vulvar cancers are related to HPV infection, especially in younger patients, the vagina (again) and the cervix should be examined. The cytological examination of the cervix should be carried out according to the current screening parameters. Cytology of the vulva – depending on its collection and proper laboratory analysis – achieves a sensitivity of 95% and specificity of 64% 13; although there is no clear reason to recommend it, it would make the biopsy much more effective. In addition to the inspection, palpation of the genitals, anal/rectal region, pelvic walls, and inguinal regions should be performed. 14 Collins' test (based on toluidine blue staining) was used to demonstrate nuclear changes reacting with toluidine blue; however, the method is non-specific and has not been used in the diagnosis of cancer. The use of acetic acid can highlight lesions and their dimensions, but does not adequately differentiate benign from malignant lesions (Figures 4 and 5).

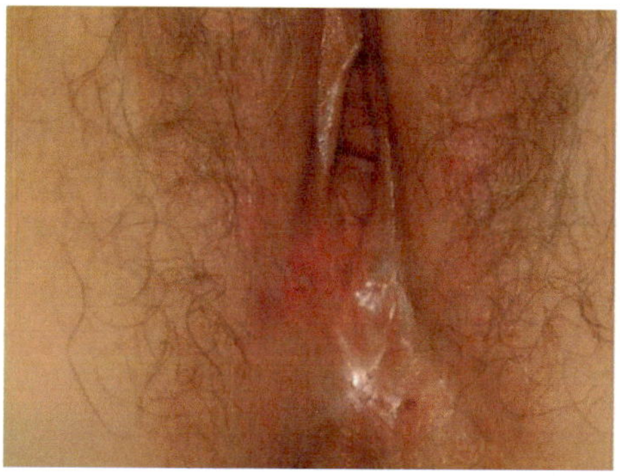

Figure 4. Macula next to right labium majora

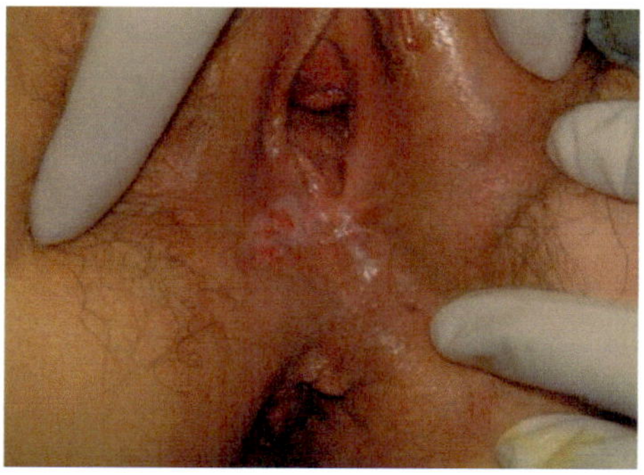

Figure 5. After application of 2% acetic acid – acetowhite lesion with more defined edges (biopsy-confirmed VIN)

5. Staging

The staging system of cancer of the vulva has changed in recent years and since 1988 has become surgical. The final diagnosis and therefore the stage classification depends on the histopathological evaluation of the surgical specimen (vulva and lymph nodes). The classification of the International Federation of Gynecology and Obstetrics (FIGO) was last changed in 2009 by the FIGO Committee on Gynecologic Oncology and provides a good discrimination between prognosis and stages (Table 1). [15] The International Union for Cancer Control (UICC) provides a classification for tumor (T), lymph nodes (N), and metastasis (M) (TNM classification), which is shown in the following text compared to the FIGO classification (Table 2). [16]

FIGO Stage		Description
I	Tumor confined to the vulva	
	IA	Lesions ≤2 cm in size, confined the vulva or perineum and with stromal invasion ≤1.0mm[a], no nodal metastasis
	IB	Lesions >2 cm in size or with stromal invasion >1.0mm[a], confined to the vulva or perineum, with negative lymph nodes
II	Tumor of any size with extension to adjacent perineal structures (lower third of urethra, lower third of vagina, anus) with negative nodes	
III	Tumor of any size with or without extension to adjacent perineal structures (lower third of urethra, lower third of vagina, anus) with positive inguinofemoral lymph nodes	
	IIIA	(i) with 1 lymph node metastasis (≥5 mm), or (ii) with 1–2 lymph node metastasis(es) (<5 mm)
	IIIB	(i) with 2 lymph node metastasis (≥5 mm), or (ii) with 3 lymph node metastasis(es) (<5 mm)
	IIIC	With positive nodes with extracapsular spread
IV	Tumor invades other regional (upper 2/3 urethra, upper 2/3 vagina), or distant structures	
	IVA	Tumor invades any of the following: (i) upper urethral and/or vaginal mucosa, bladder mucosa, rectal mucosa, or fixed to pelvic bone (ii) fixed or ulcerated inguinofemoral lymph nodes
	IVB	Any distant metastasis including pelvic lymph nodes

[a] The depth of invasion is defined as the measurement of the tumor from the epithelial-stromal junction of the adjacent most superficial dermal papilla to the deepest point of invasion.

Table 1. FIGO classification of cancer of the vulva

TNM	Description
T1	Tumor confined to vulva and/or perineum
T1a	<2 cm with stromal invasion <1.0 mm
T1b	>2 cm with stromal invasion >1.0 mm
T2	Tumor with invasion of the lower part of urethra/vagina/anus
T3	Invasion of the upper part of urethra/vagina, bladder, rectal mucosa, bone, fixation in pelvic bones

TNM	Description
N1a	One or two nodules <5mm
N1b	One nodule >5mm
N2a	Three or more nodules <5mm
N2b	Two or more nodules >5mm
N2c	Extracapsular invasion
N3	Fixed, ulcerated
M0	Absence of distant metastases
M1	Distant metastases
FIGO	**TNM**
FIGO I	T1 N0 M0
FIGO IA	T1a N0 M0
FIGO IB	T1b N0 M0
FIGO II	T2 N0 M0
FIGO IIIA	T1, T2 N1a, N1b M0
FIGO IIIB	T1, T2 N2a, N2b M0
FIGO IIIC	T1, T2 N2c M0
FIGO IVA	T1, T2 N3 M0 T3 any N M0
FIGO IVB	Any T any N M1

Table 2. Staging of cancer of the vulva (FIGO and UICC (TNM))

6. Principles of staging

Cancer of the vulva can spread from the original site by the following: local invasion of adjacent tissues; embolization to regional lymph nodes, usually to the superficial and deep inguinal ones and eventually to the pelvic ones (Figure 6); and via blood, rarely reaching the lungs, liver, and bones. Lymph node involvement is the most important prognostic factor, and lymphatic embolization is the major route of spread.[14] The evaluation of patients with vulvar cancer begins with the physical examination, palpation of inguinal and supraclavicular lymph nodes, vaginal examination, and digital rectal examination. Oncologic cervical cytology, colposcopy of the cervix and vagina (because of the association with squamous intraepithelial lesions), hematological/biochemical tests, and chest X-ray are routine. Cystoscopy and sigmoidoscopy are indicated in suspected cases of bladder or rectal invasion. Pelvic computed tomography

(CT), magnetic resonance imaging (MRI), and intravenous urography can be used to evaluate the possibility of metastatic disease in pelvic lymph nodes or surgical planning.[1, 17]

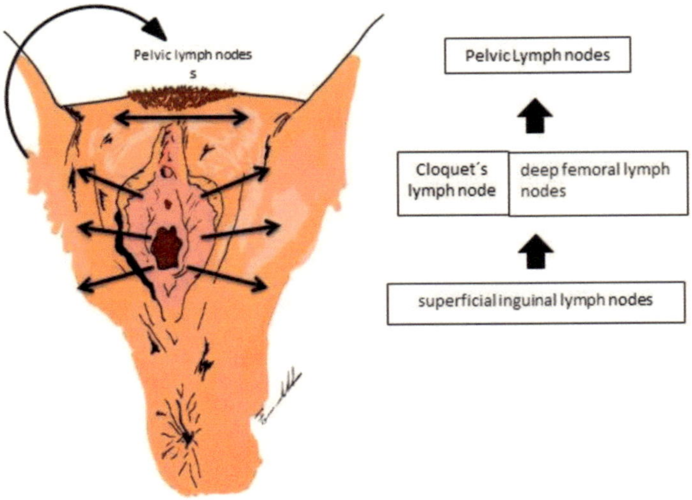

Figure 6. Lymphatic dissemination of vulva

7. Histopathological classification

As mentioned, squamous cell carcinoma is the most common cancer of the vulva, and it is associated with HPV infection especially in younger patients. Melanoma is the second most common vulvar cancer, with approximately 4.8% of these patients; this will be reviewed separately. The other histopathological types of vulvar cancer are verrucous carcinoma, Paget's disease, adenocarcinoma not otherwise specified (NOS), basal cell carcinoma NOS, Bartholin gland carcinoma, and sarcoma.[1]

The three-grade system (G1, well differentiated, G2, moderately differentiated, G3, poorly differentiated or undifferentiated, Gx, grade cannot be accessed) can be used to grade the tumor pathology. In the same aspect, from knowledge of the histopathology, it is important to determine the depth of stromal invasion. The depth of invasion is defined as the measurement of the tumor from the epithelial-stromal junction of the adjacent most superficial dermal papilla to the deepest point of invasion.[11, 15, 18]

8. Prognostic and recurrence factors

As already discussed, prognosis is strongly related to lymph node status and stage of disease. Positive lymph nodes show a direct correlation with the depth and extent of the invasion. FIGO staging indicates 5-year survival rates of 90.4% for stage I, 77.1% for stage II, 51.3% for stage III, and 18% for stage IV. Another study of the Gynecologic Oncology Group (GOG) pointed to a 5-year survival rate of 97.9% for tumors with a diameter <2 cm with negative lymph nodes. In this paper, the authors classified patients with vulvar cancer into 4 groups according to histopathological surgical findings (tumor size and extent of lymph node metastases) (Table 3).[19] Other factors with the histological type and the disease-free interval, although they have been considered possible prognostic factors, do not have great clinical relevance. The free surgical margins are the most important predictive factor for local recurrence. Some studies have indicated recurrence rates of 22.5–50% when the disease-free margins are ≤8 mm.[20, 21] In these same studies, the authors demonstrated that in 50% of cases with margins ≤8 mm in histological specimens, margins on macroscopic examination were 1 cm. Thus, a macroscopic tumor-free margin of 1 cm increased to 2 cm for a positive prognosis.[22, 23]

Risk classification	Tumor size/lymph nodes	5-year survival rate (%)
Minimal	Tumor ≤2 cm and negative lymph nodes	97.9
Low	Tumor 2.1–8cm and negative lymph nodes Tumor ≤2 cm and one positive lymph node	87.4
Intermediate	Tumor >8 cm and negative lymph nodes Tumor >2 cm and one positive lymph node Tumor ≤8 cm and two unilateral positive lymph nodes	74.8
High	Tumor >8 cm and two unilateral positive lymph nodes Three or more positive lymph nodes Bilateral positive lymph nodes	29.0

Table 3. Risk groups and survival (GOG)

Women over 50 years of age have a higher risk of vulvar cancer mortality and this risk increases with age. Likewise, a racial disparity in survival has been shown for vulvar cancer, with a poorer prognosis among white patients.

9. Treatment

Surgery is the treatment of choice for patients with vulvar cancer; however, treatment needs to be individualized. Currently, there is no standard surgery, and the emphasis is on finding the most conservative treatment associated with possible cure of the disease. Aimed at decreasing psychosexual morbidity, where possible, a more conservative surgery is sought, such as local excision of the tumor, with tumor-free margin, rather than radical vulvectomy. Surgical removal, to be effective in controlling the disease locally, needs to have lateral margins of at least 1 cm (histologically) and the deep margin should be inferior fascia of the urogenital diaphragm.[1, 24, 25]

With the introduction of radical vulvectomy with en bloc bilateral inguinofemoral lymphadenectomy (butterfly incision), overall survival for vulva cancer went from 20% to 60%, when compared with the simple excision of the tumor. Thus, for a long period, it was the default operation for the treatment of vulvar cancer.[26, 27] Even in the early stages, all patients underwent inguinofemoral lymphadenectomy; although only 20–30% of these showed lymph node metastases. In case of metastasis in inguinofemoral lymph nodes, the best treatment option was pelvic radiotherapy instead of pelvic lymphadenectomy.[28]

En bloc resection (radical vulvectomy with bilateral inguinofemoral lymphadenectomy) is no longer done these days, except in tumors located in the upper regions of the vulva, near the inguinal incisions. This butterfly incision was replaced by triple incision (Figures 7 and 8), which involves the complete excision of the tumor by radical vulvectomy or local excision (with safety margin) and removal of the lymph nodes by two separate inguinal incisions but without the additional skin removal.[1, 23, 25, 29] The triple incision surgery involves less morbidity, with less risk of seroma and lymphedema, as well as lower rate of dehiscence and pain, without increasing the risk of recurrence or mortality compared with en bloc resection.

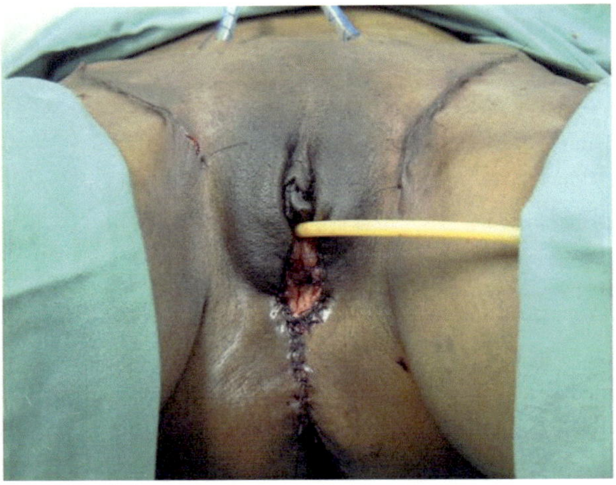

Figure 7. Triple incision (immediate postoperative period) with preservation of the upper part of vulva and clitoris

Patients in stage IA with microinvasive vulvar cancer can be managed with a wide local excision, without the need for inguinal dissection.[30, 31] There is indication of at least ipsilateral inguinal lymphadenectomy in patients with stage IB, II, or any tumor with more than 1 mm stromal invasion.[1] Patients with lateral tumors (in labia majora or minora) without involvement of the midline can be subjected to radical hemivulvectomy, instead of radical vulvectomy, with inguinofemoral lymphadenectomy.

Bilateral inguinal dissection must be performed in patients with tumors in medial regions for those involving the anterior portion of the labia minora and for those with large lateral tumors (>2 cm in diameter, >5 mm of invasion), as well as for patients with positive ipsilateral lymph nodes.[32]

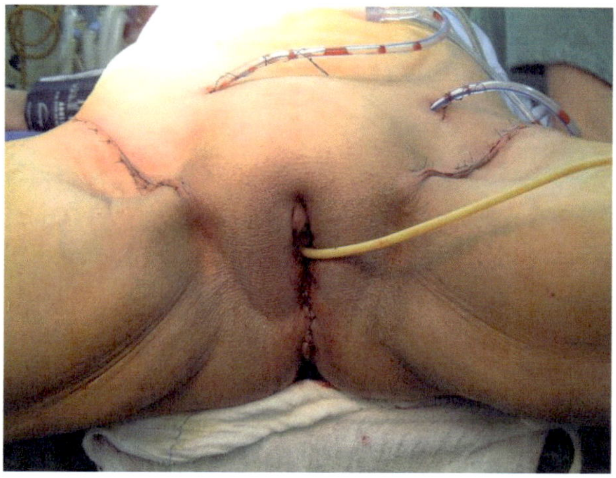

Figure 8. Triple incision (immediate post-operative period) with preservation of clitoris

Patients with FIGO stage III or IV or with extensive involvement of inguinal lymph nodes are considered having advanced disease, for which a multimodal treatment plan should be proposed. Radical vulvectomy combined with partial or total pelvic exenteration is an option for patients with locally advanced disease with clinically resectable lesions.[33, 34]

10. Sentinel lymph nodes

Since only 25–35% of patients with vulvar cancer present with metastasis to lymph nodes, only a small number of patients show a real benefit from inguinofemoral lymphadenectomy. It is therefore evident that alternatives to lymphadenectomy are needed. A sentinel lymph node biopsy has been shown to be a reasonable alternative to complete inguinal and femoral lymphadenectomy in selected patients. In a study of patients with stage I and II with tumor <4 cm, stromal invasion less than 1 mm and clinically negative lymph nodes, sentinel lymph nodes have been shown to have a sensitivity of 94.1% and a negative predictive value of 97.1%.[35] Other studies also demonstrated a sensitivity of 92% and negative predictive value of 97–98%, making sentinel lymph node evaluation an accurate way to stage vulvar cancer.[36, 37] When disease is found in sentinel lymph nodes, or when sentinel lymph node assessment is not possible, bilateral inguinofemoral lymphadenectomy must be performed.

11. Radiotherapy/chemotherapy

Patients undergoing inguinal lymphadenectomy with subsequent identification of a macrometastasis (>5 mm in diameter), extracapsular metastatic spread, or ≥2 micrometastases (<5 mm) should receive bilateral inguinal and pelvic radiotherapy. If the lymph nodes are clinically positive, one should not proceed with full lymphadenectomy, since the inguinal dissection with postoperative irradiation has the potential to cause severe lymphedema. In these cases, where possible, only the largest lymph nodes should be surgically removed before the patient is subjected to postoperative radiotherapy.[28, 38]

Radiotherapy has also been used preoperatively in patients with advanced disease aimed at providing a more complete surgery. Adjuvant radiotherapy has been added in some studies to decrease local recurrence in patients with positive or slim surgical margins; however, other authors are not of the same opinion.[39, 40]

The use of chemotherapy combined with radiotherapy in the primary treatment of locally advanced carcinoma of the vulva shows better results (regarding clinical response and recurrence) compared to radiotherapy alone. If the primary surgery has the potential to result in an intestinal or urinary tract stoma, it is preferable to employ primary chemoradiotherapy, followed by a more limited resection of the tumor bed, or any residual tumor lesion.[41, 42]

Chemotherapy alone is not a common treatment in primary cancer of the vulva. However, studies have already pointed to the characterization of vulvar cancer as chemosensitive, making chemotherapy a valid alternative for the management of these tumors; but data are still insufficient.[43, 44]

12. Melanoma

Vulvar melanomas occur more frequently in postmenopausal white women. Most patients are asymptomatic except for the pigmented lesion. Most lesions of vulvar melanoma occur on the clitoris or labia minora; it is not unusual for them to extend to the urethra and vagina. FIGO staging for melanoma does not apply, since the lesions are smaller and prognosis is related to the depth of tumor invasion. The system of levels created by Clark or that defined by Breslow may be used to stage melanoma. These systems measure the depth of invasion of the skin. A detailed histological analysis of the surgical specimen is required to carry out these micro-stagings. The staging of melanoma is defined by the system of the American Joint Committee on Cancer (AJCC), which includes other prognostic factors such as primary ulceration of the tumor, number of metastatic lymph nodes, micrometastatic disease based on sentinel lymph node biopsy, sites of distant metastatic disease, and serum levels of lactate dehydrogenase (LDH). Any pigmented vulvar lesions should be biopsied, except when known that there has been no change for several years.[45, 46, 47]

There is a tendency for more conservative treatment of vulvar melanoma. Lesions with less than 1 mm invasion can be simply treated with radical local excision. More invasive lesions require resection of the primary tumor and inguinofemoral lymph nodes. Currently, there is controversy as to the benefit of inguinofemoral lymphadenectomy. [1]

http://dx.doi.org/10.5772/61579

Author details

Fernando Anschau[1,2,3,4] and Manoel Afonso Guimarães Gonçalves[2,3,5*]

*Address all correspondence to: mafonsog@terra.com.br

1 Pontifícia Universidade Católica do Rio Grande do Sul, PUCRS, Brazil

2 Faculty of Medicine at the Pontifical Catholic University of Rio Grande do Sul, Brazil

3 Gynecologic Oncology Sector of Gynecology Service at São Lucas Hospital, Rio Grande do Sul, Brazil

4 Conceição Hospital Group - board member, Brazil

5 Universidade Federal de São Paulo, UNIFESP, Brazil

References

[1] Hacker NF, Eifel PJ, Van der Velden J. Cancer of the vulva. Int J GynecolObstet 2012; 119(Suppl 2): S90-6.

[2] Sturgeon SR, Briton LA, Devea SS, Kurman RJ. In situ and invasive vulvar cancer incidence trends. Am J ObstetGynecol 1992; 166:1482-5.

[3] Siegel R, Naishadham D, Jemal A. Cancer Statistics, 2013. CA Cancer J Clin 2013; 63:11-30.

[4] Olsen J, Jørgensen TR, Kofoed K, Kiellberg Larsen H.Incidence and cost of anal, penile, vaginal andvulvar cancer in Denmark.BMC Public Health 2012; 12:1082-9.

[5] Olsen J, Jørgensen TR, Kofoed K, Kiellberg Larsen H.Incidence and cost of anal, penile, vaginal andvulvar cancer in Denmark.BMC Public Health 2012; 12:1082-9.

[6] Stroup AM, Harlan LC, Trimble EL. Demographic, clinical, and treatment trends among women diagnosed with vulvar cancer in the United States. GynecolOncol 2008; 108:577-83.

[7] Rolfe KJ, MacLean AB, Crow JC, Benjamin E, Reid WM, Perrett CW. TP53 mutations in vulvar lichen sclerosus adjacent to squamous cell carcinoma of the vulva. Br J Cancer 2003; 89:2249-53.

[8] Choschzick M, Hantaredja W, Tennstedt P, Gieseking F, Wolber L, Simon R. Role of TP53 mutations in vulvar carcinomas. Int J GynecolPathol 2011; 30:497-504.

[9] Forman D, De Martel C, Larsey CJ, et al. Global burden of human papillomavirus and related diseas. Vaccine 2012; 30(suppl 5): F12-F13.

[10] Duong TH, Flowers LC. Vulvo-vaginal cancers: risks, evaluation, prevention and early detection. ObstetGynecolClin North Am 2007; 34:783-802.

[11] Deppe G, Mert I, WinerIS.Management of squamous cell vulvar cancer: A review. J ObstetGynaecol Res 2014; 40(5):1217-25.

[12] Jones RW, Joura EA. Analysing prior clinical events at presentation in 102 women with vulvar carcinoma: Evidence of diagnostic delays. J Reprod Med 1999; 44:766-8.

[13] Nauth HF. Vulva-Zytologie. Makroskopie, Histologie und Zytologie der normalen und erkranten Vulva. Lehrbuch und Atlas. Thieme, Stuttgart. 1986.

[14] Dittmer C, Fischer D, Diedrich K, Thill M. Diagnosis and treatment options of vulvar cancer: a review. Arch GynecolObstet 2012; 285:183-193.

[15] FIGO Committee on Gynecologic Oncologic. Revised FIGO staging for carcinoma of the vulva, cervix, and endometrium. Int J GynecolObstet 2009; 105(2):103-4.

[16] Sobin LH, Gospodarowicz MK, Wittekind CH. UICC: TNM classification of malignant tumors, 7th ed. Wiley-Black-well, Oxford, ISBN 978-1-4443-3241-4. 2009.

[17] Hawnaur JM, Reynolds K, Wilson G, Hillier V, Kitchener HC. Identification of inguinal lymph node metastases from vulvar carcinoma by magnetic resonance imaging: an initial report. ClinRadiol 2002; 57:995-1000.

[18] Edge SB, Compton CC. The American Joint Committe on Cancer: The 7th edition of the AJCC câncer staging manual and the future of TNM. Ann SurgOncol 2010; 17:1471-4.

[19] Landrum LM, Lanneau GS, Skaggs VJ, Gould N, Walker JL, McMeekin DS, Gold MA. Gynecologic oncology group risk groups for vulvar carcinoma: improvement in survival in the modern era. GynecolOncol 2007; 106(3):521-5.

[20] Heaps JM, Fu YS, Montz FJ, Hacker NF, Berek JS. Surgical-pathologic variables predictive of local recurrence in squamous cell carcinoma of the vulva. GynecolOncol 1990; 38:309-14.

[21] De Hullu JA, Hollema H, Lolkema S, et al. Vulvar carcinoma. The price of less radical surgery. Cancer 2002; 95:2331-8.

[22] Heaps JM, Fu YS, Montz FJ, Hacker NF, Berek JS. Surgical-pathologic variables predictive of local recurrence in squamous cell carcinoma of the vulva. GynecolOncol 1990; 38:309-14.

[23] De Hullu JA, Hollema H, Lolkema S, et al. Vulvar carcinoma. The price of less radical surgery. Cancer 2002; 95:2331-8.

[24] Chan JK, Sugiyama V, Pham H, Gu M, Rutgers J, Osann K, et al. Margin distance and other clinico-pathological prognostic factors in vulvar carcinoma: a multivariate analysis. GynecolOncol 2007; 104(3):636-41

[25] De Hullu JA, Van der Avoort IAM, Oonk MHM, Van der Zee AGJ. Management of vulvar cancers. EJSO 2006; 32:825-31.

[26] Way S. Carcinoma of the vulva. Am J ObstetGynecol 1960; 79:692-7.

[27] Taussig FJ. Cancerof the vulva: an analysis of 155 cases. Am J ObstetGynecol 1940; 40:764-9.

[28] Homesley HD, Bundy BN, Sedlis A, Adcock L. Radiation therapy versus pelvic node resection for carcinoma of the vulva with positive groin nodes. ObstetGynecol 1986; 68:733-40.

[29] Gotlieb WH. The assessment and surgical management of early-stage vulvar cancer. Best Pract Res ClinObstetGynaecol 2003; 17: 557-69.

[30] Iversen T, Abeler V, Aalders J. Individualized treatment of stage I carcinoma of the vulva. ObstetGynecol 1981; 57(1):85-90.

[31] Hacker NF, Berek JS, Lagasse LD, Nieberg RK, Leuchter RS. Individualization of treatment for stage I squamous cell vulvar carcinoma. ObstetGynecol 1984; 63(4): 155-62.

[32] Iversen T, Aas M. Lymph drainage from the vulva. GynecolOncol 1983; 16(2):179-89.

[33] Lataifeh I, Nascimento MC, Nicklin JL, Perrin LC, Crandon AJ, Obermair A. Patterns of recurrence and disease-free survival in advanced squamous cell carcinoma of the vulva. GynecolOncol 2004; 95:701-5.

[34] Hoffman MS. Squamous-cell carcinoma of the vulva: Locally advanced disease. Best Pract Res ClinObstetGynaecol 2003; 17:635-47.

[35] Van der Zee AG, Oonk MH, De Hullu JÁ, et al. Sentinel node dissection is safe in the treatment of early-stage vulvar câncer. J ClinOncol 2008; 26:884-9.

[36] Levenback CF, Van der Zee AG, Rob L, et al. Sentinel Lymph node biopsy in patients with gynecologic cancers Expert panel statement from the International Sentinel Node Society Meeting, February 21. GynecolOncol 2008; 114:151-6.

[37] Hassanzade M, Attaran M, Treglia G, Yousefi Z, Sadeghi R. Lymphatic mapping and sentinela node biopsy in squamous cell carcinoma of the vulva: Systematic review and meta-analysis of the literature. GynecolOncol 2013; 130:237-45.

[38] Hyde SE, Valmadre S, Hacker NF, Schilthuis MS, Van der Velden J. Squamous cell carcinoma of the vulva with bulky positive groin nodes – nodal debulking versus full groin dissection prior to radiation therapy. Int J Gynecol Cancer 2007; 17(1):154-8.

[39] Faul CM, Mirmow D, Huang Q, Gerszten K, Day R, Jones MW. Adjuvant radiation for vulvar carcinoma: Improved local control. Int J RadiatOncolBiolPhys 1997; 38:381-9.

[40] Groenen SM, Timmers PJ, Burger CW. Recurrence rate in vulvar carcinoma in relation to pathological margin distance. Int J Gynecol Cancer 2010; 20: 869-73.

[41] Hacker NF, Berek JS, Juillard GJF, Lagasse LD. Preopeative radiation therapy for locally advanced vulvar cancer. Cancer 1984; 54(10): 2056-60.

[42] Boronow RC, Hickman BT, Reagan MT, Smith RA, Steadham RE. Combined therapy as an alternative to exenteration for locally advanced vulvovaginal cancer. Results, complications and dosimetric and surgical considerations. Am J ClinOncol 1987;10(2):171-81.

[43] Tomao F, Di Tucci C, Marchetti C, Perniola G, Bellati F, Panici PB. Role of chemotherapy in the management of vulvar carcinoma. Crit Rev OncolHematol 2012; 82:25-39.

[44] Deppe G, Mert I, Belotte J, Winer IS. Chemotherapy of vulvar cancer: a review. Wien KlinWochenschr 2013; 125:119-28.

[45] Clark WH, From L, Bernardino EA, et al. The histogenesis and biologic behavior of primary human malignant melanomas of the skin. Cancer Res 1969; 29:705-27.

[46] Breslow A. Thickness, cross-sectional área and depth of invasion in the prognosis of cutaneous melanoma. Ann Surg 1970; 172:902-8.

[47] Kim CJ, Reintgen DS, Balch CM for the AJCC Melanoma Staging Committee. The new melanoma staging system. Cancer Control 2002; 9:9-15.

Chapter 12

Robotic Surgery in the Management of Endometrial Cancer

Mark Williams, John Villeneuve and
Bernice Robinson-Bennett

Additional information is available at the end of the chapter

http://dx.doi.org/10.5772/60835

Abstract

Endometrial cancer remains the most common gynecologic malignancy in the Unites States and Western Europe. It has been estimated that in 2014, about 52, 630 new cases of endometrial cancer was diagnosed and about 8,590 died from the disease. Prior to 1988, endometrial cancer was staged clinically. Since that time surgical staging has been adopted. With the advancement in technology, the vast majority of cases are being staged and treated surgically via minimally invasive approaches. Conventional laparoscopy has been a major advancement in staging and treatment of uterine cancers. However, technical challenges such as 2–D imaging, rigid instruments, and lack of precision and surgeon fatigue did not translate into widespread adoption of this technique. With the advent of computer–enhanced robotic telesurgery, this has dramatically changed the surgical management and staging of endometrial cancer.

Keywords: Endometrial cancer, robotic surgery, oncology, surgical techniques, outcomes

1. Introduction

Endometrial cancer is a general definition that often includes all cancers that develop in the uterus, the most common being endometrioid cancer, or cancers arising in the lining of the uterus or endometrium.[1-3] In the United States, endometrial cancer is the fourth most common cancer among women and also the most common gynecological cancer, with on average about 6% of all female cancers.[4] In the United States, the number of new cases estimated to be diagnosed in 2015 is about 55,000 based on data from the American Cancer Society. Of note, the number of deaths based on these data is expected to be roughly 10,000, with death rates rising between 0.8% and 1.9% per year within the last 5 years.[2] However, there is quite a notable variation in worldwide incidence. For example, the highest incidence is observed in Western Europe, United States, and Canada, while in comparison, Africa and Asia are shown to have the lowest rates of incidence.[5] The overall increase in the incidence of this disease during the last decades is mainly related to higher life expectancy within the developed world.[5]

Endometrial cancer is often described as principally a menopausal state disease, since the majority of the cases occur in advanced age.[4, 5, 6, 8] The risk of endometrial cancer increases with the age of the woman. The median age of diagnosis is around 61 years, with the peak incidence happening between 55 and 70 years old. Data from the research community show that most cases, about 95%, occur in patients over 40 years of age with only up to 5% of disease development occurring in women younger than 40.[9-11] Interestingly, the median age of death is around 73 years.[11] The majority of cases are postulated to be of a sporadic etiology, although there is a minority with evidence of a hereditary basis. A number of research articles have been published detailing the correlation of increased risk of endometrial cancer occurrence in women from families with the autosomal dominant hereditary non-polyposis colorectal cancer (HNPCC) gene. Importantly, endometrial carcinoma is the most common extra-colonic cancer seen in this condition referred to as Lynch syndrome.[6, 12] The lifetime risk in these women is about 40% to 60%, and they have a risk of about 40% of developing endometrial cancer by 70 years old.[6, 11, 13]

A unifying theme among the risk factors is that of increased estrogen exposure.[92] The gradual growth in incidence especially within the last decade also has some correlation with dietary and hormonal factors.[14] Obesity, along with increased abdominal girth, is a known risk factor.[2, 15, 72-73] There has been a notable worldwide increased prevalence of obesity. It appears from some data that developed countries are more disproportionately affected by this phenomenon. Increased body mass index (BMI) is also suggested to result in a higher all–cause mortality and endometrial cancer–specific mortality in endometrial cancer survivors.[16-17] By contrast, Park et al looked at the relation of pre-treatment BMI on known prognostic factors, the impact of disease–free survival, and the cause–specific survival in a recent Korean study of women with endometrial cancer. The study population results, however, found that BMI was not a significant factor for both disease-free and cause-specific survival.[18] Of note, endometrial cancer is the third most common gynecological cancer in Korea. A Swedish cohort study of 11659 women evaluated various lifestyle factors including diet and physical activity and possible association of risk of endometrial cancer. Overall, 133 cases of endometrial cancer were observed. The data suggested that an increased risk was noted with very low intake of fruits and vegetables and statistically significant decreased risk ($p < 0.01$) with increased physical activity.[19] Increased weight in early adult life as well as middle age also increased the risk. The management of peri– and postmenopausal symptoms by unopposed exogenous estrogen is yet another risk factor.[20-21]

http://dx.doi.org/10.5772/60835

Risk factors often associated with decreased risk of endometrial cancer are those that help to decrease the amount of circulating estrogen. These include oral contraceptive (OCP) use, intrauterine device (IUD) use, and cigarette smoking. OCPs have been shown to lower the risk by up to 40%, with protection still noted up to 15 years after last use. A proportional correlation is seen with protection and length of use.

Although the exact etiology still remains elusive, it is known that most cases arise from atypical hyperplasia of the lining of the uterus.[72-76] Epithelial cancers of the uterus are generally divided into two groups. Type I endometrial cancers make up 75% – 90% of endometrial cancers and are usually low grade, diagnosed in early stages with good prognosis and of endometrioid histology. They are estrogen–dependent and tend to develop in an environment of hyperplasia or unopposed estrogen exposure, whether physiological or pharmacological. In addition, this subset may have phosphatase and tensin homologue mutations. Type II endometrial cancers, however, are estrogen–independent, usually high grade, have a poor prognosis, often diagnosed at later stages and are usually of papillary serous, clear cell, or even high-grade endometrioid pathology. Type II cancers may have a link with P53 tumor suppression mutation and the endometrial milieu of Type II cancers is often associated with polyps or simply atrophic in nature.

At diagnosis, the malignancy is frequently found to be localized or within the borders of the uterine corpus in 72-75% of instances, especially since they present early with abnormal uterine bleeding.[11, 15] As mentioned earlier, the chance that postmenopausal bleeding is a result of cancer substantially escalates with a woman's age. Endometrial cancer is usually diagnosed in early stages, although up to 20% of patients with clinical stage I may have indications of extrauterine spread at time of surgical intervention.[22] The relative estimated survival rates at the 5- and 10-year mark are approximately 82% and 79%, respectively.[2]

2. Surgical management

Although not the focus of this chapter, initial evaluation and workup is usually achieved via endometrial biopsy and ultrasound. Abnormal uterine bleeding is often the most common presentation that is seen. Current recommendations from the American College of Obstetricians and Gynecologists and other governing bodies still recommend the evaluation of all patients with postmenopausal bleeding for likelihood of endometrial cancer. In addition, any female over the age of 40 years with abnormal bleeding should also be evaluated. This evaluation consists of obtaining tissue either by an endometrial biopsy or dilatation and curettage.

After histologically confirmed diagnosis, additional evaluation to rule out metastasis may be considered. A chest radiograph may be helpful to note any simultaneous pulmonary disease or involvement and to rule out possible metastases to the lung.[13] In some cases, the measurement of CA-125 is also obtained because in some women with advanced stage disease at time of diagnosis, CA-125 usually may be elevated. These elevated levels can help in determining adequate response to treatment or recurrence of disease during post–treatment surveillance.[23-24] However, for the typical histology of Type I, endometrioid Grade 1 and clinical stage 1 patient, a physical examination and chest X-ray is usually only required.

In the majority of cases, the subsequent step involves surgery for definitive treatment, staging to determine the extent of the disease, and to reduce tumor burden in advanced stages with extrauterine disease. In 1971, the International Federation of Gynecology and Obstetrics (FIGO) put forth a comprehensive clinical staging system, which was used worldwide.[25] This initial step helped to standardize to some degree the diagnosing and relevant treatment of the disease. However, since 1988, clinical staging has mainly been replaced by surgical staging especially since it does not fully evaluate significant histopathological features. [22, 76-78] The Gynecologic Oncology Group (GOG) carried out two large–scale prospective trials looking at surgical staging in 1984 and 1987.[22, 26] The results from these studies aided in determining the important prognostic factors along with indicated treatment goal. Along with age, race, and endocrine status, it was shown that prognosis is related to the presence or absence of certain uterine and extrauterine risk factors. Uterine factors include histologic type, grade, depth of invasion into the myometrium, isthmus-cervix extension, and lymphovascular space invasion. Extrauterine factors include adnexal metastasis, intraperitoneal spread, positive peritoneal cytology, pelvic and aortic node metastasis, and estrogen/progesterone receptor activity. [27] FIGO stage is often considered to be the single strongest predictor regarding outcome in endometrial cancer based on results from various multivariate analyses.[28]

Current staging is based on the FIGO 2009 staging criteria.[25-26, 29-31] The procedure of surgical staging includes an adequate evaluation of the peritoneal contents, peritoneal cytologic washings, hysterectomy, bilateral salpingo-oophorectomy, cytoreduction of all visible disease, and bilateral pelvic and para-aortic lymph node dissection.[11, 13] Ideally, the procedure should entail the same components whether done via a laparotomy or by minimally invasive surgery (MIS). In the instance where a patient is unable to undergo surgery, whole pelvic and intracavitary radiation may be used as definitive treatment. However, some data have shown a notable decrease in 5-year survival times for clinical stage 1 disease treated in this maner (67%) compared to surgery alone (87%).[11]

3. History of laparoscopy in management and staging of endometrial cancer

The introduction and involvement of laparoscopy has become truly integral and beneficial in management of endometrial cancer. For more than 30 years, gynecologic surgeons have used laparoscopy for many procedures, including oophorectomies, ovarian cystectomies, and bilateral tubal ligations. Earlier research studies published information on both the feasibility and technique of radical hysterectomy with pelvic and para-aortic lymphadenectomy.[32-35] These helped set the foundation for the possibility of full and comprehensive surgical staging using an MIS approach. Of note, laparoscopic intervention would not get its introduction into the field of gynecologic endometrial cancer until the earlier part of the 1990s. A 1992 publication by Childers et al.[36] was the first to report on laparoscopically–assisted vaginal hysterectomy (LAVH) for management of endometrial cancer based on two cases. The case report also mentioned techniques such as port placement, insufflation methods, and lymphadenectomy involving pelvic and para-aortic nodes. In a subsequent study series, Childers et al. published data involving the first use of laparoscopy in surgical staging of endometrial cancer.[37] The data showed a total of two conversions to laparotomy in their population (n= 59), with most common indications being complications such as transected ureter and incidental cystotomy. Interestingly, additional deductions from this study were that this new technique appeared to have similar operating times to conventional laparotomy, however, with an increased degree and length of learning curve for surgeons. Another study looked at the utility of LAVH and laparoscopic lymph node dissection with supporting results of association of decreased postoperative pain and blood loss with increased lymph node yield. Yet this study did show increased operating time compared to open surgery.

Since the initial case reports and other similar retrospective studies done around that time, the development and advancement of minimally invasive laparoscopic methodologies to the surgical staging of endometrial cancer has continued. Later studies have included multiple variables such as description of feasibility reports of the standard laparoscopic method, outcome analysis of open surgical versus laparoscopic techniques, analysis of cost-effectiveness, and even development of laparoendoscopic single-site surgery (LESS).[37-46]

4. History of robotics in gynecologic surgery

The natural progression in medicine, and science and technology, tends to show that with new research comes novel breakthroughs. This is evidenced in a wide variety of procedures, algorithms, medications and in this case equipment. More often than not, these tend to be helpful in the advancement of the art of medicine. This effect is seen directly with the establishment of robotic surgery in the field of gynecologic surgery. We have clearly seen a revolution in the armada of gynecological interventions with MIS over the last three decades.[47] The field of robotic surgery has undergone rapid advancement, especially in gynecology,[7-8], since it was originally developed for medical and surgical use in battle zones. The goal was that robotic surgery could be used by surgeons in a remote location to perform simple or complex procedures with similar skill, technique and outcomes as if done in a regular operating room.

There are earlier models that helped to pave the way for the advanced systems currently in use and lead to development in the field and technique. One such model and the first robot to assist in a surgery was a single robotic arm known as Automated Endoscopic System for Optimal Positioning (AESOP) developed by Computer Motion Inc. (Computer Motion, Inc., Santa Barbara, CA, USA).[48-49] Cleared by the Food and Drug Administration (FDA) in 1994, this device was made to hold and manipulate an endoscope and remove the need for an assistant. In addition, it was designed to give a surgeon improved control over visualization and also allow command over the laparoscope using voice-activation.[50] The first commercially available robotic system, ROBODOC, described in 1992 was a robotic arm designed for use in orthopedic hip prosthesis surgery[49], and allowed for accurate incisions in the femur bone for implant insertion. In 1998, Computer Motion Inc., marketed another model that had been in development called ZEUS Surgical System (ZSS), which had a 2-D imaging system and robotic arms made to mimic the surgeon's arms. Two arms were added to the AESOP to create the ZEUS. The arms also allowed for downscaling of movement from the surgeon's hands and elimination of tremors. The surgeon sat at a console, which helped to decrease fatigue especially in longer operations and expanded on the possibility of telesurgery or remote location surgery.

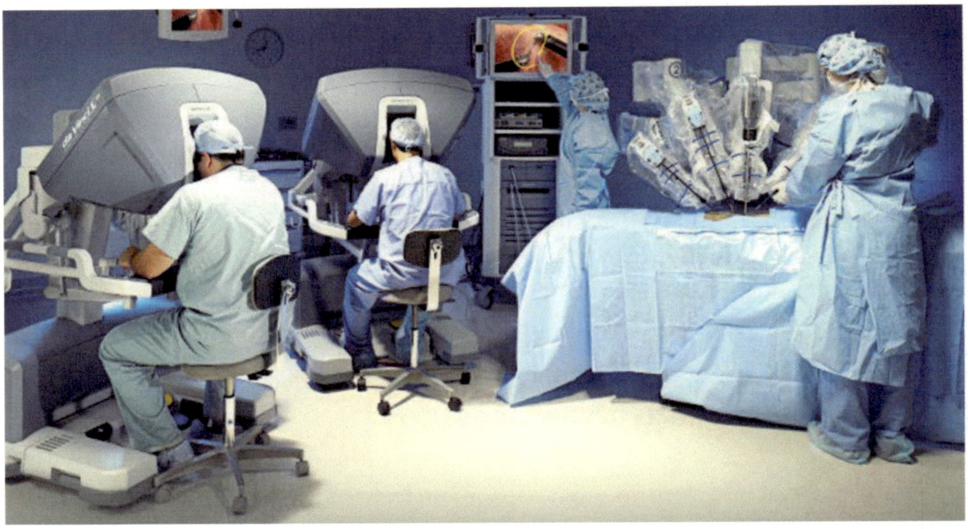

Figure 1. Da Vinci Surgical System with additional training console

Another company, Intuitive Surgical, Inc. (Intuitive Surgical, Mountain View, CA, USA) also developed a robotic surgery assist model called the Da Vinci Surgical System (DVSS) shown in Image 1.[91] Unlike the ZSS, the DVSS used a 3–D vision system produced from two endoscopes, which results in a perceptual 3–D image. It also was designed with the EndoWrist system, which offered seven degrees of freedom. This resulted in the recreation of the dexterity and range of motion of a surgeon's hand, therefore allowing a high degree of accuracy and flexibility. Instruments could thus also be rotated a full 360^0.[51] The first successful surgery was done in 1997 in Belgium.[52] The DVSS was eventually cleared by the FDA in 2005 for use in gynecologic procedures and has full regulatory clearance with the coveted Conformité Européenne (CE) mark in Europe.[53]

5. Advantages of robotic surgery

Even with the initially high cost of acquisition (estimated between 1– and 2 million U.S. dollars) of a DVSS for an institution, there are many advantages of robotic surgery that make it worthwhile. More than 7,000 peer–reviewed publications have been published on computer–enhanced robotic surgery. For example, the amount of clinical evidence and data on the robotic surgery system and technique is increasing at a rate of 100 publications per month on average.[54]

5.1. Dexterity

The invention of the ergonomic wrist instruments allowed for more accurate replication of the movement at the wrist, including rotation.

5.2. Precision

The robotic surgical system provides the ability to improve the precision with which the surgical procedure is carried out. This is due in part to different factors such as the EndoWrist concept, tremor reduction (explained below), and improved field of view.

5.3. Field and depth of view

The ability to see in a 3–D image as mentioned earlier is truly a remarkable feature. As an old adage of excellent surgical techniques, the need for adequate exposure and visualization is vital. This is also one improved quality over the laparoscopic technique, which has a limited 2–D view. In addition, robotic surgery does have the benefit of greatly increased magnification which adds ability for more precise fine microsurgery techniques. The robotic setup that includes a viewing station for the assistants and other staff in the room provides both a great interactive learning and teaching viewing option unique to this system.

5.4. Control and motion dampening

This technology was also seen in the earlier Zeus system. It gives the ability to reduce the tremors created naturally by the extension of the fingers or the resultant tension due to fatigue as operating times increase. This is somewhat similar to being on a cruise ship and not feeling the rocking of huge waves but just that gentle back and forth enough to give the calm feeling of being at sea. However, the robot is able to filter out unnecessary hand and finger motions which results in safer, more accurate intracorporeal movements.

5.5. Decreased blood loss

This can be seen as a direct result of the factors above, especially greater instrument control, viewing ability, and small entry sites.

5.6. Learning curve

Studies have looked at the required learning to be proficient in both laparoscopic and robotic techniques, with the latter often noted to be less difficult to acquire. This is due to the ergonomic setup and more counter-intuitive hand movements needed compared to a laparoscopic style. It is suggested that 20 robotic procedures are needed for proficiency.[55-56] Operative times tend to decrease and the nodal counts increase with increased surgeon's experience.

5.7. Decreased surgeon fatigue

The surgeon operator console provided on the robotic surgical system is a great enhancement, especially in longer operations. [57]

6. Techniques of robotic surgery

The use of port sites and the selection of these ports are important in MIS. As mentioned earlier, the actual technique of staging should ideally be the same regardless of type of abdominal incision.

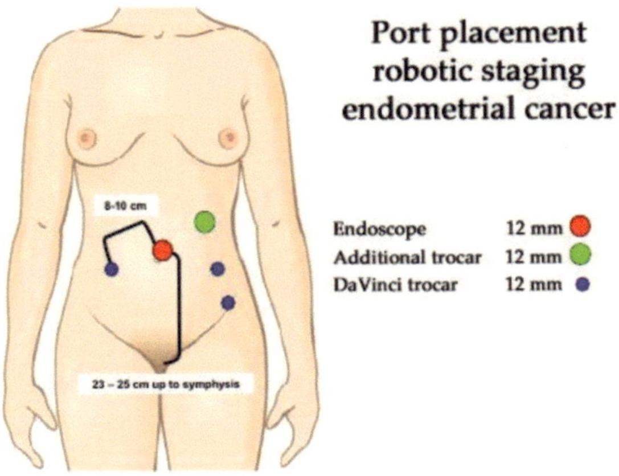

Figure 2. Schematic demonstration of the port placement in robotic assisted operation for endometrial carcinoma

Techniques include either single-site port or multiple port use and other factors play a role in determining which the best approach is used.

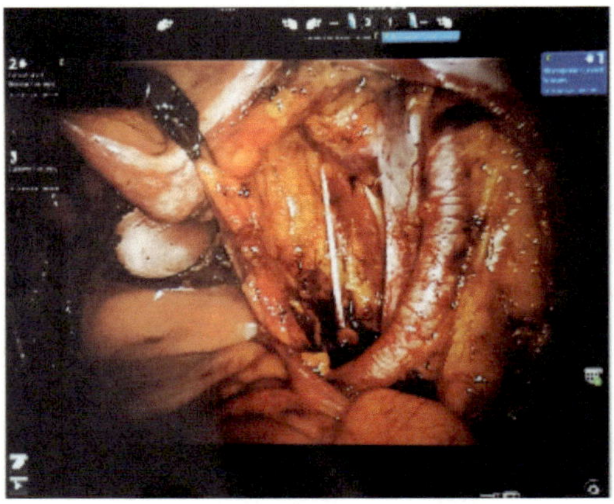

Figure 3. Pelvic lymph node retrieval

http://dx.doi.org/10.5772/60835

Our patients undergo a bowel prep regimen. Patients are positioned securely on a foam memory pad with Velcro straps placed across the breasts. This is critical for the 29^0 Trendelenburg position for the entire case. Patients are placed in lithotomy in Allen stirrups. A uterine manipulator is used in the majority of cases. Typically, 5 ports are placed as shown in the diagram, Figure 1.[58] The camera is placed approximately 25 cm above the pubic symphysis. The robot is then docked from the patient's left side. A 0^0 scope is used. The fenestrated bipolar and the monopolar hot shears are used as the operating instruments.

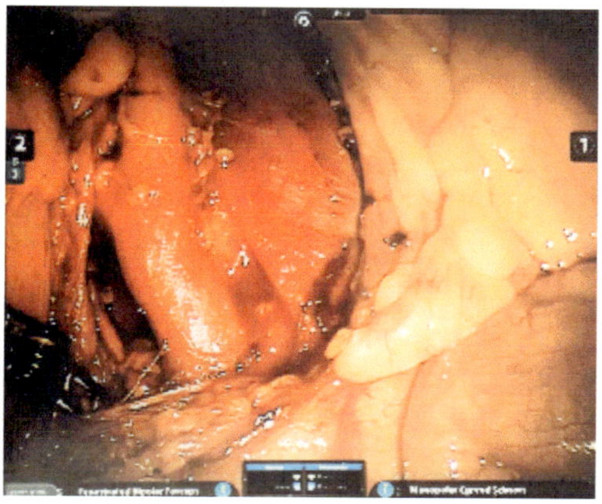

Figure 4. Para-aortic lymph node retrieval.

During indicated lymphadenectomy, pelvic and/or para–aortic, adequate dissection is essential. The robotically assisted system and technique help with improving node yield. The following images shown are during lymph node harvesting for both the pelvic and the para-aortic lymph nodes during cases at our institution. Image 2 shows the intraoperative dissection and removal of nodes in the pelvic cavity, while Image 3 shows the dissection and removal of para-aortic nodes. In Image 3, the aorta is seen on the left of the image (top-down view) branching into the right and left common iliac arteries.

7. Comparison of outcomes between open surgery and MIS

Total laparoscopic hysterectomy was compared to total abdominal hysterectomy in the LACE trial.[59] In this trial, there was notable improvement in quality of life for up to 6 months for the participants. Also, on that trial, there were more frequent serious adverse outcomes in the laparotomy versus the laparoscopy group.

The largest randomized prospective multicenter study to evaluate outcomes between open surgery and MIS is known as the Gynecologic Oncology Group (GOG) LAP2 trial, a 10-year data accrual study.[60] It compares outcomes between incidence of surgical complications, perioperative morbidity and mortality in stage I or IIa, grades I to III endometrial/uterine cancer in patients being staged with either traditional laparotomy approach versus comprehensive laparoscopic staging. The GOG in this trial aimed to evaluate the feasible role of a laparoscopic method in the primary surgical treatment of endometrial cancer in terms of staging rates, safety, recurrence, and survival. In that study, the rate of conversion to open surgery was 26%. The reasons for conversion were poor visualization, extrauterine spread and bleeding. It was noted that as the BMI increased, so did the rate of conversion. With a BMI of less than 20, the success rate was 90% compared to 34% with a BMI of 50. The median number of lymph nodes harvested was not significantly different. The complications were also evaluated. In the LAP2 study, the hospital time was 2 days in laparoscopic group compared to 4 days in the laparotomy group. The oncologic outcomes of the comparison were reassuring. The estimated 5–year survival rate was 11.6% and 13.7% for laparoscopy and laparotomy, respectively. The overall survival rate was essentially equivalent between the two groups at 89.8% at 5 years.

There have been many retrospective and other studies comparing outcomes and complications between laparotomy and robotic/laparoscopic surgery.[79-81] The key differences between the two are outlined below.

7.1. Estimated blood loss

The use of smaller multiple incisions compared to a larger incision portends to an expected decreased blood loss. In addition, the magnification and ability to control small blood vessels contributes significantly to the decreased blood loss noted. In a study by Gaia et al. comparing outcomes in laparotomy versus laparoscopic techniques, outcomes were similar except for a statistically significant reduction in blood loss favoring the laparoscopy group. However, there was no difference in transfusion rates.[61] In other studies, however, robotic surgery was associated with reduced blood loss and transfusion when compared to conventional laparoscopy.[53]

7.2. Length of operating time

Operating time has been shown in studies to be shorter in open surgery compared to MIS. Some studies suggest that operating time was on average 30 min longer for laparoscopic procedures.[59] In the LAP2 trial, operative was longer for laparoscopy by about a median of 70 min.[60] To some degree, this also is based on surgeon expertise with MIS and potential limitations with instrumentation. Some of these limitations are overcome by the robotic platform.

7.3. Increased exposure/visualization

Laparotomy may seem to have increased exposure simply due to the large abdominal incision created during the procedure. However, with the magnification obtained during laparoscopy visualization is superior, especially in the deep pelvis.

7.4. Length of Hospital Stay (LOHS)

Due to smaller incisions with minimally invasive techniques, faster expected healing and recovery time are seen in MIS compared to open surgery. This results in decreased need for prolonged admission after operation. As an example, in the LAP2 trial, hospital time was shorter, 2 days with laparoscopy compared to 4 days with laparotomy.[60] He et al. [62] in a meta–analysis noted shorter length of hospital stay (mean difference [MD], -3.42; 95% confidence interval [CI], -3.81 to -3.03; $p < 0.01$) with laparoscopy compared to laparotomy. Other studies have also demonstrated similar results regarding decreased LOHS with laparoscopy.[60, 63-65]

7.5. Lymph node yield

Various studies including the previously mentioned GOG LAP2 trial have focused on lymph node yield in either approach. Some studies have shown a similar amount of nodes sampled or retrieved while others have shown increased on either side. Also, in the 2013 meta–analysis of nine randomized controlled trials by He et al., the data showed no statistically significant difference between either approach pelvic node yield (MD, 0.45; 95% CI, -0.41 to 1.32; $p = 0.30$).[62]

7.6. Complications

In the GOG LAP2 trial, which remains the largest prospective randomized trial comparing laparoscopy to laparotomy in the management of endometrial cancer, the combined complication rate inclusive of vascular, urinary, bowel, and nerve was higher in the laparoscopy patients (10%) in comparison to the laparotomy group (8%).[60] DeNardis et al. have however shown reduced complications in robotic cohorts. In that study, major peri–operative complication was found to be 3.6% in the robotically-assisted cohort compared to 20.8% in the laparotomy group.[66]

8. Comparison of robotic surgery versus conventional laparoscopy in endometrial cancer

These two techniques are both types of MIS, although one can often think of robotic surgery as being the younger, more advanced sibling. In this way, robotic surgery in many ways has helped to enhance the techniques and outcomes involved in laparoscopic surgery. Two areas of note where this unique edge is definitely appreciated is in the treatment of both the elderly and the obese with endometrial cancer. These two conditions require additional concern due to possibility of co–morbidities, access, and post–operative survival and outcomes. Cho and Nezhat in their review of 754 case identified complication rates of 10.5%, 12.2%, and 44.6% in robotic hysterectomy, laparoscopic hysterectomy, and abdominal hysterectomy, respectively. [67] In the open cohort, the majority of complications were related to wound infections and bowel dysmotility. There was also a lower rate of conversion in the robotic group when compared to the laparoscopic group. The above–mentioned advancement in the robotic system is no doubt responsible for this observation.

8.1. Decreased Estimated Blood Loss (EBL)

Decreased blood loss is seen in many studies comparing the two techniques with robotic being associated the lesser amount. In Seamon's study, estimated blood loss was 100 and 250 mL, respectively, for robotic versus conventional laparoscopy.[68]

8.2. Decreased Length of Hospital Stays (LOHS)

Especially in the current medical climate with current societal economic situations, the trend is to improve the proper utilization of resources while, at the same time, decreasing costs wherever possible. Although robotic surgery comes with a substantial investment cost, having shorter hospital admissions especially postoperatively can help to reduce operating costs from a different angle. Studies have shown either similar in some cases or usually a slightly decreased LOHS in robotic surgery.[68]

8.3. Decreased Operating Room (OR) time

This is related to surgeon skill, experience and expertise. Since robotic surgery has been shown to have an improved learning curve, this may play a role in overall operating time. Also, coupled with the other benefits robotic surgery offers, this may result in faster times from incision to incision or from docking to incision in some studies. However, some studies have shown similar operating times between the two methods. Seamon et al. in their comparison of robotic to conventional laparoscopy reported reduced mean operative times in the robot group, 242 versus 287 min.[68]

8.4. Decreased chance of conversion to laparotomy

Some studies, both observational and retrospective comparison, have noted less chance for conversion with decreased visualization, body habitus, patient weight, and comorbidities often being reasons cited for having to do so. This occurs less in robotic than laparoscopic surgery. Gaia et al. demonstrated a 9.9% conversion rate in laparoscopy compared to 4.9% for the robotic approach.[61]

8.5. Patients with increased BMI

The prevalence of obesity is increasing. Obesity is associated with increased surgical morbidity. There is an associated increase in blood loss, operative times, wound complications, and venous thromboembolism. Hence, the development of newer techniques that will provide a comparable surgical staging with reduced morbidities is very attractive. The obesity factor affects both techniques but the qualities of the robotic surgery tend to lend toward decreased morbidity compared to laparoscopic surgery. Recall in the LAP2 trial that the success of surgical staging was decreased with increasing BMI. The robot seems to overcome this limitation associated with conventional laparoscopy. In a retrospective study by Gehrig,[69] complete surgical staging was accomplished in 92% of robotic patients in contrast to 84% in the laparoscopic group. Also notable was the shorter operative times (189 vs 215 min, $p = 0.004$, less blood loss (50 v 150 mL, $p < 0.001$) and a statistically significantly shorter hospital stay.

Another retrospective study done by Mendivil et al. comparing robotic, laparotomy, and conventional laparoscopic cohorts of morbidly obese patients (BMI > 40 kg/m^2) compared the outcomes of each procedure.[82] Robotic surgery had the longest operating time compared to laparoscopy and laparotomy (2.78 vs 1.82 and 1.35 h, $p < 0.001$) but had the least estimated blood loss respectively (100 vs 175 and 250 mL, $p = 0.002$). The length of hospital stay was significantly shorter with both minimally invasive methods compared to laparotomy (2 vs 4 days, $p = 0.002$)

8.6. Patients of advanced age

Elderly patients usually have more co–morbidities and are generally poorer surgical candidates with concomitant more advanced disease, which may require more surgical intervention. There have been studies looking at the utility of robotic surgery in this scenario, as well as laparoscopic surgeries. In a retrospective analysis by Scribner et al., laparoscopic staging was completed in 77.6% of patients. The operative time was increased for the laparoscopic group, however, there was no increased morbidity from longer anesthetic times.[70] Another study by Lavoue et al.[87] compared a population ($n = 113$) of advanced age patients (greater than or equal to 70 years) with endometrial cancer undergoing surgical staging by either robotic or traditional open surgery. The robotic group had longer operating times (244 vs 217 min, $p = 0.009$) but less estimated mean EBL (75 vs 334 mL, $p < 0.0001$), less minor adverse events (17 vs 60%, $p < 0.001$) and decreased mean LOHS (3 vs 6 days, $p < 0.0001$). However, no statistical difference ($p = 0.61$) was noted in the 2-year disease–free survival during follow-up.

A single institution retrospective chart review looked at the safety of robotic surgery in a cohort of patients with endometrial cancer ($n = 228$) compared to laparotomy.[88] The cohort was subdivided by method of surgery (robotic vs laparotomy) and age (<65 vs 65 years and older). Older patients undergoing robotic surgery had decreased estimated blood loss (131 vs 235 mL, $p = 0.03$), decreased rate of postoperative ileus (0 vs 15%, $p = 0.04$), decreased perioperative surgical complication rate (4 vs 30%, $p = 0.01$), and decreased LOHS (2.2 vs 4.4 days, $p < 0.01$) compared with laparotomy. The rate of discharge home was similar with compared to laparotomy (96 vs 91%, $p = 0.45$).

Robotic surgery with the associated advantages such as decreased EBL, decreased LOHS, and potentially decreased postoperative morbidity may show potential for improved outcomes compared to laparoscopic surgery and laparotomy. Further studies may be needed to evaluate this comparison.

8.7. Single-Port Access (SPA)

The progression from traditional open surgery toward minimally invasive methods, both robotic and conventional laparoscopic, has resulted in further innovation such as attempts at using fewer port entry sites, less trocars, and smaller abdominal incisions.

Laparoendoscopic single–site surgery (LESS), a novel technique, may lead to an additional decrease in the overall invasiveness of conventional laparoscopy. Fanfani et al.[83] in a 2012 publication of a single institution cohort trial looked at laparoendoscopic single–site surgery

(LESS) in surgical management of early–stage endometrial cancer. The results showed median age of 57 years (42–68), median BMI of 24 kg/m^2 (21–30) with median operating time of 105 min, and median EBL of 20 mL (10–180). The skin and fascial incision needed for this single-port access approach was 2.5 cm (median 2.2 cm, range of 2.0–2.5) with all patients reported being satisfied with both pain control postoperatively and the cosmetic results.

Some difficulties inherent with LESS include instrument crowding as well as clashing, decreased and/or poor visualization, loss of triangulation, and ergonomic issues.[85] The combination of robotic surgery with LESS may help to overcome some of the technical limitations noted with LESS. A retrospective case–control study by Fagotti et al. looked at the comparison outcomes between robotic and laparoendoscopic single–site hysterectomy for treatment of early endometrial cancer.[86] Although the median OR time was less in the robotic versus laparoendoscopic group (90 min vs 107 min), the data did not produce any seemingly clinically relevant differences.

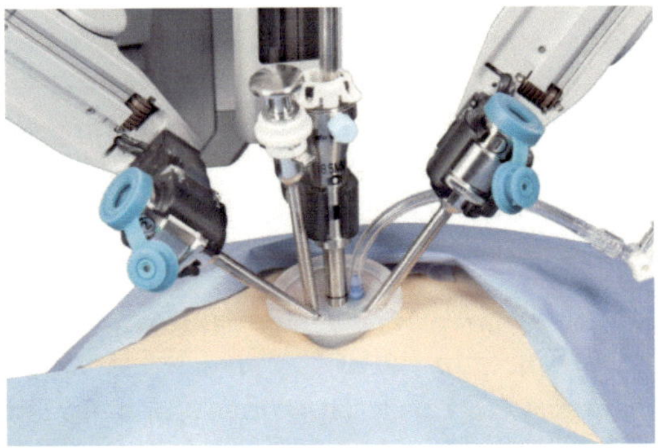

Figure 5. Single site port system

The robotic single–site port system[89] which enables operating through a small umbilical incision in common procedures such as benign hysterectomies, cholecystectomies, or salpingo–oopherectomies. The recommended size of incision needed for this five–lumen port (see Image 4[93]) is typically about 1.5 cm. As seen the port has five channels. There is a channel for the 8.5 mm scope, two robotic arms, a surgical assistant port, and an insufflation port. The instruments are semiflexible and capable of triangulation. Currently, the instruments lack the EndoWrist articulation, which might be disadvantageous. The advantages of this technique include the promise of potentially virtually scarless surgery due to the small incision, in addition to the known ones of robotic surgery such as decreased EBL and LOHS.[90] More prospective studies with larger numbers are needed to compare robotic single–site surgery with standard robotic multi-site surgery for procedures commonly done.

A pilot study published in 2013 by Vizza et al.[88] looked at the feasibility and safety of using robotic single-site hysterectomy in patients with low–risk early stage endometrial cancer. The five–lumen port described above was used with the size of the umbilical incision ranging from 2 to 2.5 cm. The median age was 64 years with a median BMI of 26.6 kg/m^2. The results showed median OR time to be 90 min, median blood loss of 75 mL with no reported conversion to laparoscopy or laparotomy, and median LOHS of 2 days. No reported complications occurred neither intra– nor postoperatively. The study concluded that robotic single–site hysterectomy was a safe and technically possible option in this patient group. Future studies with other gynecologic oncologic procedures and cases need to be carried out to evaluate the feasibility and advantages of this technique.

8.8. Cost

Any cost analysis of the different modalities of surgery and staging in endometrial cancer cannot overlook the impact of hospital stay on overall cost. Since the robot has been effective in shifting hysterectomy and staging to an essentially an outpatient procedure, there will be an anticipated decrease in overall hospital cost.

A cost effective analysis of robotically assisted management of new endometrial cancer was performed by Leitao et al.[71] The costs were inclusive of all surgical aspects of care provided up to 6 months following discharge. In that study, the total mean amortized cost per case was $20,487 for laparoscopy, 20,467 for robotically assisted, and $24, 642 for laparotomy. It was concluded that when laparotomy rates are reduced by virtue of the robot, then there is notable cost neutralization. A similar finding of laparoscopy being the least expensive approach was noted. Interestingly, if the cost of the robotic disposable instruments did not exceed $1,046, then from a societal perspective the robotic approach would be the least expensive.[46] In other studies, the utilization of the robot was deemed to be approximately 1.5 times higher than conventional laparoscopy. However, the mentioned reduction in completion of case and decreased conversion to laparotomy cannot be ignored.

Future studies will probably examine the use of the robot in debulking advanced cases of uterine cancers. Single–site surgeries will probably become more popular. Advancements in the actual technology are only expected to sky rocket. One can only imagine what the next step involves or what direction robotic computer-enhanced telesurgery would take. The important factor overall is being able to find that balance of effective patient care and management with the proper utilization of resources based on overall cost as well as reimbursement.

Author details

Mark Williams[1,2], John Villeneuve[1,2] and Bernice Robinson-Bennett[1,2*]

*Address all correspondence to: bernice.robinson-bennett@readinghealth.org

1 Department of Gynecologic Oncology, McGlinn Cancer Institute, Reading Hospital, Reading Health System, Reading, Pennsylvania, USA

2 Department of Obstetrics and Gynecology, Reading Hospital, Reading Health System, Reading, Pennsylvania, USA

References

[1] Siegel R L, Miller K D, Jemal A. Cancer statistics, 2015. CA: A Cancer Journal for Clinicians. 2015; 65: 5–29. doi:10.3322/caac.21254.

[2] American Cancer Society. Cancer Facts & Figures 2015. Atlanta: American Cancer Society; 2015.

[3] National Cancer Institute. What You Need to Know About Cancer of the Uterus. Bethesda: National Cancer Institute; 2012. Endometrial Cancer.

[4] Jemal A, Bray F, Center MM, et al. Global cancer statistics. CA: A Cancer Journal for Clinicians. 2011; 61:69.

[5] Münstedt K, Grant P, Woenckhaus J, Roth G, Tinneberg H-R. Cancer of the endometrium: current aspects of diagnostics and treatment. World Journal of Surgical Oncology. 2004;2:24. doi:10.1186/1477-7819-2-24.

[6] American College of Obstetricians and Gynecologists. ACOG practice bulletin, clinical management guidelines for obstetrician-gynecologists, number 149, April 2015: endometrial cancer. Obstet Gynecol 2015;125:1006–26.

[7] Robotic surgery in gynecology. Committee Opinion No.628. American College of Obstetricians and Gynecologists. Obstetrics and Gynecology. 2015; 125-760-7

[8] Liu H, Lu D, Wang L, Shi G, Song H, Clarke J. Robotic surgery for benign gynecealogical disease. Cochrane Database of Systematic Reviews 2012, Issue 2, Art. No. CD008978. DOI: 10.1002/14651858.CD008978.pub2.

[9] Gallup DG, Stock RJ. Adenocarcinoma of the endometrium in women 40 years of age or younger. Obstetrics and Gynecology. 1984 Sep;64(3):417-20.

[10] Crissman JD, Azoury RS, Barnes AE, Schellhas HF. Endometrial carcinoma in women 40 years of age or younger. Obstetrics and Gynecology. 1981 Jun;57(6):699–704.

[11] Hurt, K. Joseph. Cancer of the Uterine Corpus. In: The Johns Hopkins Manual of Gynecology and Obstetrics. 4th ed. Philadelphia: Wolters Kluwer Health/Lippincott Williams & Wilkins; 2011. Print.

[12] Dunlop MG1, Farrington SM, Carothers AD, Wyllie AH, Sharp L, Burn J, Liu B, Kinzler KW, Vogelstein B. Cancer risk associated with germline DNA mismatch repair gene mutations. Human Molecular Genetics. 1997 Jan;6(1):105-10.

[13] Rock J A, Jones H W, & Te L R. Endometrial cancer. In: Te Linde's Operative Gynecology. Philadelphia: Wolters Kluwer Health/Lippincott Williams & Wilkins; 2008.

[14] Goodman MT, Hankin JH, Wilkens LR, et al. Diet, body size, physical activity, and the risk of endometrial cancer. Cancer Research. 1997; 57:5077-85.

[15] Hoskins, William J. Corpus: epithelial tumors. In: Principles and Practice of Gynecologic Oncology. 4th ed. Philadelphia: Lippincott Williams & Wilkins; 2005. Print.

[16] Arem H1, Chlebowski R, Stefanick ML, Anderson G, Wactawski-Wende J, Sims S, Gunter MJ, Irwin ML. Body mass index, physical activity, and survival after endometrial cancer diagnosis: results from the Women's Health Initiative. Gynecologic Oncology. 2013 Feb;128(2):181-6. doi: 10.1016/j.ygyno.2012.10.029. Epub 2012 Nov 2.

[17] Arem H, Irwin ML. Obesity and endometrial cancer survival: a systematic review. International Journal of Obesity (London). 2013 May; 37(5):634-9. Epub 2012 Jun 19.

[18] Park J Y, Cho J H, Min J Y, Kim D Y, Kim J H, Kim Y M, Nam, J H. Impact of body mass index on the prognosis of Korean women with endometrioid adenocarcinoma of the uterus: A cohort study. Obstetrics and Gynecology Science. 2014; 57(2), 115–120. doi:10.5468/ogs.2014.57.2.115.

[19] Terry P, Baron JA, Weiderpass E, Yuen J, Lichtenstein P, Nyrén O. Lifestyle and endometrial cancer risk: a cohort study from the Swedish Twin Registry. International Journal of Cancer. 1999 Jul 2; 82(1):38-42.

[20] Key TJA, Pike MC. The dose–effect relationship between unopposed oestrogens and endometrial mitotic rate: its central role in explaining and predicting endometrial cancer risk. British Journal of Cancer. 1988; 57: 205-12.

[21] Beresford SAA, Weiss NS, Voigt LF, McKnight B. Risk of endometrial cancer in relation to use of oestrogen combined with cyclic progestagen therapy in postmenopausal women. Lancet 1997; 349: 458-61.

[22] Creasman WT, Morrow CP, Bundy BN, et al. Surgical pathologic spread patterns of endometrial cancer. (a Gynecologic Oncology Group study). Cancer. 1987; 60:2035–41.

[23] Patsner B, Tenhoppen DJ, Mann WJ. Use of serum CA-125 levels to monitor therapy of patients with advanced or recurrent endometrial carcinoma. European Journal of Gynaecological Oncology 1989;10:322–5.

[24] Patsner B, Orr JW Jr, Mann WJ Jr. Use of serum CA 125 measurement in posttreatment surveillance of early-stage endometrial carcinoma. American Journal Obstetrics and Gynecology. 1990;162: 427–9.

[25] International Federation of Gynecology and Obstetrics: classification and staging of malignant tumors in the female pelvis. International Journal of Gynaecology and Obstetrics. 1971; 9:172.

[26] Boronow R, Morrow C, Creasman W, et al. Surgical staging in endometrial cancer: clinical-pathological findings of a prospective study. Obstetrics and Gynecology. 1984; 63:825-32.

[27] Morrow CP, Bundy BN, Kurman RJ, et al. Relationship between surgical-pathological risk factors and outcome in clinical stage I and II carcinoma of the endometrium: A Gynecologic Oncology Group study. Gynecologic Oncology. 1991; 40:55-65.

[28] Abeler VM, Kjordstad K, Berle E. Carcinoma of the endometrium in Norway: a histopathological and prognostic survey of a total population. International Journal of Gynecological Cancer. 1992; 2:9-22.

[29] Mutch DG. The new FIGO staging system for cancers of the vulva, cervix, endometrium, and sarcomas. Gynecologic Oncology. 2009; 115:325–8.

[30] Pecorelli S. Revised FIGO staging for carcinoma of the vulva, cervix, and endometrium. International Journal of Gynaecology and Obstetrics. 2009; 105(2):103-4, 2009.

[31] Tan J, Chetty N, Kondalsamy-Chennakesavan S, et al. Applying the FIGO 2009 staging system for carcinoma of the vulva to patients previously staged with the FIGO 1988 staging system. Gynecologic Oncology. 2010; 116:S21-2.

[32] Nezhat CR, Burrell MO, Nezhat FR, Benigno BB, Welander CE. Laparoscopic radical hysterectomy with paraaortic and pelvic node dissection. American Journal of Obstetrics and Gynecology. 1992; 166(3), 864–5.

[33] Dargent D, Mathevet P. [Radical laparoscopic vaginal hysterectomy]. Journal de Gynécologie, Obstétrique et Biologie de la Reproduction. (Paris). 1992; 21(6), 709–10.

[34] Querleu D, Leblanc E, Castelain B. Laparoscopic pelvic lymphadenectomy in the staging of early carcinoma of the cervix. American Journal of Obstetrics and Gynecology. 1991; 164(2), 579–81.

[35] Doll KM, Suri A, Gehrig PA. Minimally invasive surgery in endometrial cancer. Expert Review of Obstetrics & Gynecology. 01/2014; 8(3). DOI: 10.1586/eog.13.14.

[36] Childers JM, Surwit EA. Combined laparoscopic and vaginal surgery for the management of two cases of stage I endometrial cancer. Gynecologic Oncology. 1992; 45(1): 46–51.

[37] Childers JM, Brzechffa PR, Hatch KD, Surwit EA. Laparoscopically assisted surgical staging (LASS) of endometrial cancer. Gynecologic Oncology. 1993; 51(1): 33–38.

[38] Eltabbakh GH, Shamonki MI, Moody JM, Garafano LL. Laparoscopy as the primary modality for the treatment of women with endometrial carcinoma. Cancer. 2001; 91(2): 378–87.

[39] Scribner DR Jr, Walker JL, Johnson GA, McMeekin SD, Gold MA, Mannel RS. Surgical management of early-stage endometrial cancer in the elderly: is laparoscopy feasible? Gynecologic Oncology. 2001; 83(3): 563–568.

[40] Barnett JC, Havrilesky LJ, Bondurant AE, et al. Adverse events associated with laparoscopy vs laparotomy in the treatment of endometrial cancer. American Journal of Obstetrics and Gynecology. 2011; 205(2): 143.e1–143.e6.

[41] Wright JD, Burke WM, Wilde ET, et al. Comparative effectiveness of robotic versus laparoscopic hysterectomy for endometrial cancer. Journal of Clinical Oncology. 2012; 30(8): 783–91.

[42] Venkat P, Chen LM, Young-Lin N, et al. An economic analysis of robotic versus laparoscopic surgery for endometrial cancer: costs, charges and reimbursements to hospitals and professionals. Gynecologic Oncology. 2012; 125(1): 237–240.

[43] Barnett JC, Judd JP, Wu JM, Scales CD Jr, Myers ER, Havrilesky LJ. Cost comparison among robotic, laparoscopic, and open hysterectomy for endometrial cancer. Obstetrics and Gynecology. 2010; 116(3): 685–693.

[44] Fader AN, Escobar PF. Laparoendoscopic single-site surgery (LESS) in gynecologic oncology: technique and initial report. Gynecologic Oncology. 2009; 114(2): 157–61.

[45] Fagotti A, Boruta DM 2nd, Scambia G, Fanfani F, Paglia A, Escobar PF. First 100 early endometrial cancer cases treated with laparoendoscopic single-site surgery: a multicentric retrospective study. American Journal of Obstetrics and Gynecology. 2012; 206(4): 353.e1–353.e6.

[46] Holub Z. The role of laparoscopy in the surgical treatment of endometrial cancer. Clinical and Experimental Obstetrics and Gynecology. 2003; 30(1): 7–12.

[47] Csorba R. Robotic Surgery in gynecology. Orvosi Hetilap. 2012 Jun 24;153(25):967-72. doi: 10.1556/OH.2012.29373 [Article in Hungarian].

[48] Satava RM. Robotic surgery: from past to future-a personal journey. Surgical Clinics of North America. 2003;83:1491-500, xii.

[49] Bann S, Khan M, Hernandez J, Munz Y, Moorthy K, Datta V, et al. Robotics in surgery. Journal of the American College of Surgeons. 2003; 196:784-95.

[50] Robotics: the future of minimally invasive heart surgery. Biomed.brown.edu. Retrieved April 19, 2011.

[51] Yim GW, Kim YT. Robotic surgery in gynecologic cancer. Current Opinion in Obstetrics and Gynecology. 2012 Feb;24(1):14-23. doi: 10.1097/GCO.0b013e32834daebc.

[52] Himpens J, Leman G, Cadiere GB. Telesurgical laparoscopic cholecystectomy. Surgical Endoscopy. 1998;12:1091.

[53] Reza M, Maeso S, Blasco JA, Andradas E. Meta-analysis of observational studies on the safety and effectiveness of robotic gynaecological surgery. British Journal of Surgery. 2010 Dec;97(12):1772-83. doi: 10.1002/bjs.7269.

[54] Intuitive Surgical: Welcome to Intuitive Surgical. Available at http://www.intuitivesurgical.com/company/. Retrieved March 11, 2015.

[55] Seamon LG, Cohn DE, Richardson DL, Valmadre S, Carlson MJ, Phillips GS, et al. Robotic hysterectomy and pelvic-aortic lymphadenectomy for endometrial cancer. Obstetrics and Gynecology. 2008;112(6):1207–13.

[56] Seamon LG, Fowler JM, Richardson DL, Carlson MJ, Valmadre S, Phillips GS, et al. A detailed analysis of the learning curve: robotic hysterectomy and pelvic-aortic lymphadenectomy for endometrial cancer. Gynecologic Oncology. 2009;114(2):162–67.

[57] Fourman MM, Saber AA. Robotic bariatric surgery: a systematic review. Surgery for Obesity and Related Diseases. 2012 Jul;8(4):483-8. Epub 2012 Mar 29.

[58] Malgorzata, L, Verena, B, Kati, H, Achim, S, Simone, M and Christhardt, K. Surgical Treatment of Endometrial Cancer. Journal of Cancer Therapy. 2010; 1 (4); 181-91. doi: 10.4236/jct.2010.14028.

[59] Janda M, Gebski V, Brand A, et al. Quality of life after total laparoscopic hysterectomy versus total abdominal hysterectomy for stage I endometrial cancer (LACE): a randomised trial. Lancet Oncology.2010;11(8):772–80.

[60] Walker JL, Piedmonte MR, Spirtos NM, et al. Laparoscopy compared with laparotomy for comprehensive surgical staging of uterine cancer: Gynecologic Oncology Group Study LAP2. Journal of Clinical Oncology. 2009; 27(32), 5331–6.

[61] Gaia G, Holloway RW, Santoro L, Ahmad S, Di Silverio E, Spinillo A. Robotic-assisted hysterectomy for endometrial cancer compared with traditional laparoscopic and laparotomy approaches: a systematic review. Obstetrics and Gynecology. 2010 Dec; 116(6):1422-31. doi: 10.1097/AOG.0b013e3181f74153.

[62] He H, Zeng D, Ou H, Tang Y, Li J, Zhong H. Laparoscopic treatment of endometrial cancer: systematic review. Journal of Minimally Invasive Gynecology. 2013 Jul-Aug; 20(4):413-23. Epub 2013 Mar 15.

[63] Malzoni M, Tinelli R, Cosentino F, et al. Total laparoscopic hysterectomy versus abdominal hysterectomy with lymphadenectomy for early-stage endometrial cancer: a prospective randomized study. Gynecologic Oncology. 2009; 112 (1):,126–33.

[64] Tozzi R, Malur S, Koehler C, Schneider A. Laparoscopy versus laparotomy in endometrial cancer: first analysis of survival of a randomized prospective study. Journal of Minimally Invasive Gynecology. 2005; 12 (2): 130–6.

[65] Zullo F, Palomba S, Falbo A, et al. Laparoscopic surgery vs laparotomy for early stage endometrial cancer: long-term data of a randomized controlled trial. American Journal of Obstetrics and Gynecology. 2009; 200 (3):,296–e1.

[66] DeNardis SA, Holloway RW, Bigsby GE 4th, Pikaart DP, Ahmad S, Finkler NJ. Robotically assisted laparoscopic hysterectomy versus total abdominal hysterectomy and lymphadenectomy for endometrial cancer. Gynecologic Oncology. 2008 Dec; 111(3):412-7. doi: 10.1016/j.ygyno.2008.08.025. Epub 2008 Oct 1.

[67] Cho JE, Nezhat FR. Robotics and gynecologic oncology: review of the literature. Journal of Minimally Invasive Gynecology. 2009 Nov-Dec;16(6):669-81. doi: 10.1016/j.jmig.2009.06.024.

[68] Seamon LG, Cohn DE, Henretta MS, et al. Minimally invasive comprehensive surgical staging for endometrial cancer: robotics or laparoscopy? Gynecologic Oncology. 2009;133: 36–41.

[69] Gehrig PA, Cantrell LA, Shafer A, Abaid LN, Mendivil A, Boggess JF. What is the optimal minimally invasive surgical procedure for endometrial cancer staging in the obese and morbidly obese woman? Gynecologic Oncology. 2008 Oct;111(1):41-5. doi: 10.1016/j.ygyno.2008.06.030. Epub 2008 Aug 9.

[70] Scribner DR Jr, Walker JL, Johnson GA, McMeekin DS, Gold MA, Mannel RS. Laparoscopic pelvic and paraaortic lymph node dissection in the obese. Gynecologic Oncology. 2002 Mar;84(3):426-30.

[71] Leitao MM Jr, Bartashnik A, Wagner I, Lee SJ, Caroline A, Hoskins WJ, Thaler HT, Abu-Rustum NR, Sonoda Y, Brown CL, Jewell EL, Barakat RR, Gardner GJ. Cost-effectiveness analysis of robotically assisted laparoscopy for newly diagnosed uterine cancers. Obstetrics and Gynecology. 2014 May;123(5):1031-7. doi: 10.1097/AOG.0000000000000223.

[72] Kaaks R, Lukanova A, Kurzer MS. Obesity, endogenous hormones, and endometrial cancer risk: a synthetic review. Cancer Epidemiology, Biomarkers and Prevention. 2002, 11:1531-43.

[73] National Cancer Institute. What You Need to Know About Cancer of the Uterus. Bethesda: National Cancer Institute; 2012. Endometrial Cancer.

[74] Kirby TO, Leath CA 3rd, Kilgore LC. Surgical staging in endometrial cancer. Oncology (Williston Park). 2006 Jan;20(1):45-50; discussion 50, 53-4, 63.

[75] Frumovitz M, Singh DK, Meyer L, et al: Predictors of final histology in patients with endometrial cancer. Gynecologic Oncology. 2004; 95:463- 468.

[76] Eltabbakh GH, Shamonki J, Mount SL. Surgical stage, final grade, and survival of women with endometrial carcinoma whose preoperative endometrial biopsy shows well-differentiated tumors. Gynecologic Oncology. 2005;99:309.

[77] Cowles TA, Magrina JF, Masterson, BJ, and Capen CV. Comparison of clinical and surgical staging in patients With Endometrial Carcinoma. Obstetrics and Gynecology. 1985 Sep; 66(3):413-6.

[78] Rungruang B, Olawaiye AB. Comprehensive surgical staging for endometrial cancer. Reviews in Obstetrics and Gynecology. 2012; 5(1): 28–34.

[79] Humphrey, MM., Apte SM. The use of minimally invasive surgery for endometrial cancer. Cancer Control. 2009 Jan;16(1):30-7.

[80] Ran L, Jin J, Xu Y, Bu Y, Song F. Comparison of robotic surgery with laparoscopy and laparotomy for treatment of endometrial cancer: a meta-analysis. PLoS One. 2014 Sep 26;9(9):e108361. doi: 10.1371/journal.pone.0108361. eCollection 2014.

[81] Holloway RW, Ahmad S. Robotic-assisted surgery in the management of endometrial cancer. Journal of Obstetrics and Gynaecology Research. 2012 Jan.doi:10.1111/j.1447-0756.2011.01744.x.

[82] Mendivil A A, Rettenmaier M A, Abaid L N, Brown J V, Micha J P, Lopez K L, Goldstein B H. A comparison of open surgery, robotic-assisted surgery and conventional laparoscopic surgery in the treatment of morbidly obese endometrial cancer patients. Journal of the Society of Laparoendoscopic Surgeons. 2015; 19(1): e2014.00001. doi: 10.4293/JSLS.2014.00001.

[83] Fanfani F, Rossitto C, Gagliardi ML, et al. Total laparoendoscopic single-site surgery (LESS) hysterectomy in low-risk early endometrial cancer: a pilot study. Surgical Endoscopy. 2012;26(1):41–6.

[84] Vizza E, Corrado G, Mancini E, et al. Robotic single-site hysterectomy in low risk endometrial cancer: a pilot study. Annals of Surgical Oncology.2013;20(8):2759–64.

[85] Sendağ F, Akdemir A, Oztekin MK. Robotic single-incision transumbilical total hysterectomy using a single-site robotic platform: initial report and technique. Journal of Minimally Invasive Gynecology.2013;21(1):147–151.

[86] Fagotti A, Corrado G, Fanfani F, Mancini M, Paglia A, Vizzielli G, Sindico S, Scambia G, Vizza E. Robotic single-site hysterectomy (RSS-H) vs. laparoendoscopic single-site hysterectomy (LESS-H) in early endometrial cancer: A double-institution case–control study. Gynecologic Oncology. 2013 Jul; 130 (1): 219-23.

[87] Lavoue V, Zeng X, Lau S, Press JZ, Abitbol J, Gotlieb R, How J, Wang Y, Gotlieb WH. Impact of robotics on the outcome of elderly patients with endometrial cancer. Gynecologic Oncology. 2014 Jun;133(3):556-62. doi: 10.1016/j.ygyno.2014.03.572. Epub 2014 Apr 4.

[88] Doo DW, Guntupalli SR, Corr BR, Sheeder J, Davidson SA, Behbakht K, Jarrett MJ, Guy MS. Comparative surgical outcomes for endometrial cancer patients 65 Years Old or older staged with robotics or laparotomy. Annals of Surgical Oncology. 2015 Feb 12. Epub ahead of print.

[89] Intuitive Surgical: Welcome to Intuitive Surgical. Available at http://www.intuitivesurgical.com/products/davinci_surgical_system/da-vinci-single-site/. Retrieved April 14, 2015.

[90] Cela V, Freschi L, Simi G, Ruggiero M, Tana R, Pluchino N. Robotic single–site hysterectomy: feasibility, learning curve and surgical outcome. Surgical Endoscopy. 2013 Jul;27(7):2638–43. doi: 10.1007/s00464-012-2780-8. Epub 2013 Feb 8.

[91] Image. Retrieved April 14, 2015, from http://stfrancishealthcare.org/wp-content/uploads/davinci_surgical_system_1.jpg.

[92] Fu YS, Gambone JC, Berek JS. Pathophysiology and management of endometrial hyperplasia and carcinoma. Western Journal of Medicine. 1990;153(1):50-61.

[93] Image. Retrieved April 14, 2015 from, http://intuitivesurgical.com/company/media/images/singlesite/Final_docked_position_4205.jpg.

Chapter 13

Cervical Cancer in Human Immunodeficiency Virus (HIV) Positive Patients

Atara Ntekim

Additional information is available at the end of the chapter

http://dx.doi.org/10.5772/60664

Abstract

The clinical management of cervical cancer in human immunodeficiency virus (HIV) positive patients is associated with challenges mainly due to the state of their immunity. They are managed like their HIV seronegative counterparts with surgery or chemoradiotherapy. HIV, cervical cancer, radiotherapy and chemotherapy lower immunity through reduction in CD4 cell counts.

A perspective on the management of HIV positive patients with cervical cancer is hereby provided.

Available studies were reviewed and peculiar characteristics of HIV patients with cervical cancer were examined. Strategies for managing such patients were identified.

HIV positive patients are younger and have more aggressive disease. They have more treatment related toxicities, poorer disease control with higher rates of incomplete and treatment delays than their HIV negative counterparts. Highly active anti-retroviral therapy (HAART) improves treatment outcome in such patients.

HIV positive patients with cervical cancer should be commenced on HAART at diagnosis. There should be closer monitoring of CD4 cell counts and viral load while on oncology treatment towards early recognition of need for prophylaxes against opportunistic infections. The dosage of the treatment modalities should also be adjusted according to CD4 cells count status. Possible interactions between anti-retroviral therapy (ART) with chemotherapy and radiotherapy should not be overlooked.

Keywords: HIV, cervical cancer, radiotherapy, chemotherapy

1. Introduction

Cancer of the uterine cervix is the most common gynecological malignancy and occurs worldwide [1]. Close to eighty percent of cervical cancers occur in the developing countries [2]. Chronic persistent infections with high-risk HPV subtypes play an important role in the carcinogenesis of cervical cancer. Human immunodeficiency virus (HIV) infection lowers immunity and is epidemic in some developing countries especially in sub-Sahara Africa. Cervical cancer is very common in HIV seropositive patients and is associated with an aggressive course and poor treatment outcome [3]. The associated compromise in immunity caused by HIV infection poses serious challenges to the clinical management of HIV positive patients diagnosed with cervical cancer. The main modalities of managing cervical cancer are surgery, chemotherapy and radiotherapy with most patients requiring combination therapy. These treatment modalities lead to reduced immunity in patients which is further reduced if one or two modalities are combined. In a patient with immunological challenges due to HIV infection, these treatment modalities can therefore worsen the immunological competence of the individual leading to poorer treatment tolerance, undue treatment toxicity and poor treatment outcome. At present, HIV positive patients diagnosed with cervical cancer are being managed using guidelines for managing HIV seronegative patients diagnosed with cervical cancer. The outcome of treatment in HIV positive patients are worse compared with HIV negative patients and HIV positive patients present late and are less likely to complete oncology treatment [4]. Infection with HIV has also been noted to increase mortality among cancer patients generally [5]. There is therefore need to consider additional therapeutic measures applicable to cervical cancer patients who are HIV positive.

The aim of this chapter is to highlight special features associated with HIV positive patients diagnosed with cervical cancer and provide a perspective on management strategies for these patients. This was done through a review of the evidence from basic, epidemiological and clinical studies which formed the basis for the recommendations for the management of HIV positive patients diagnosed with cervical cancer.

2. Peculiarities of cervical cancer in HIV positive patients

2.1. Epidemiology of cervical cancer

Cervical cancer occurs worldwide. The incidence of cervical cancer is still high in developing countries whereas it has decreased significantly in the developed countries over the last several decades. Close to eighty percent of cervical cancer occur in the developing countries [2]. The highest incidence is in sub-Sahara Africa especially in Eastern African countries [6]. Furthermore, the mortality due to cervical cancer is about ten times higher in the developing countries where screening and treatment modalities are neither common nor easily accessible. In developed countries, screening is the main factor responsible for the decrease in the incidence and mortality rates of cervical cancer.

2.2. Risk factors for cervical cancer

The most important risk factor for the development of cervical cancer is infection with human papilloma virus [HPV] [7]. In particular, chronic persisting infections with high-risk HPV subtypes play an important role in the carcinogenesis of cervical cancer. The subtype mostly implicated in cervical cancer aetiology is types 16 followed by 18. Other subtypes are also implicated but to a lesser extent. Human Immunodeficiency Virus (HIV) infection causes low immunity in those infected. In HIV positive patients, some less carcinogenic subtypes of HPV have been reported to play an important role in the aetiology of cervical cancer (Table 1).

HIV seronegative (worldwide)		**HIV -1 seropositive** (single report)	
HPV subtype	%	HPV subtype	%
16	54.4	52	14.7
18	16.5	35	9.4
58	5.1	58	9.4
33	4.7	51	8.6
45	4.4	16	7.8
31	3.6	31	7.5
52	3.4	53	6.7
35	1.9	18	6.4
39	1.3		
59	1.3		

Table 1. Most frequent HPV types among women with invasive cervical cancer by any histology. Sources: HIV negative: ICO HPV Information Centre (2014); HIV-1 positive: [8]. Subtypes 52 and 35 that are less carcinogenic in HIV negative patients are more important in HIV positive patients.

2.3. Human Immunodeficiency Virus (HIV) infection

Immunodeficiency is an important cofactor for persisting infections with HPV. It increases the virulence and aggressiveness of HPV thereby accelerating the progression to malignant transformation of the endo-cervical epithelial cells.

Human immunodeficiency virus (HIV) lowers immunity and is epidemic in most developing countries. Cervical cancer is very common in HIV seropositive patients and has an aggressive course with poor treatment outcome [3]. Regions of high prevalence of cervical cancer corresponds with regions of high prevalence of HIV infection (Figures 1& 2).

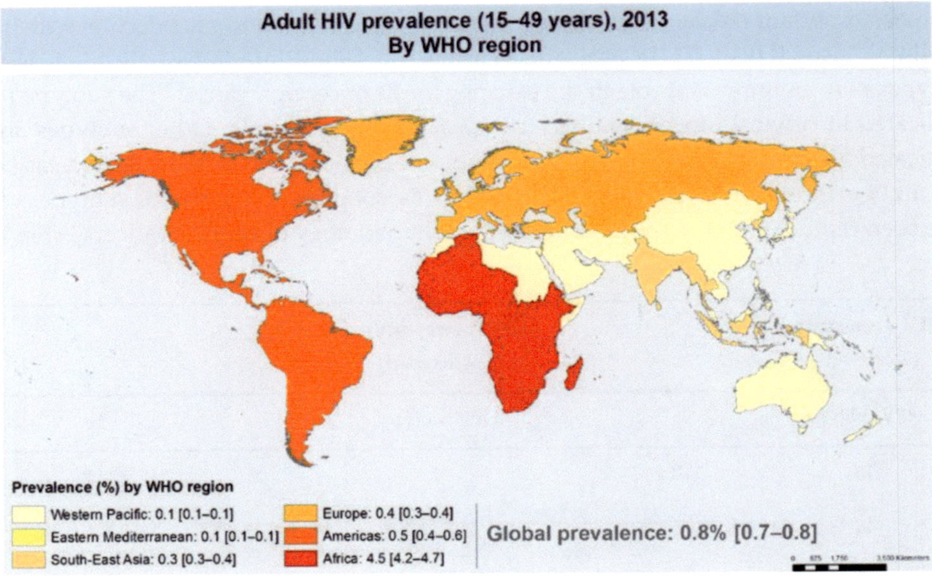

Figure 1. Adult HIV prevalence by WHO region (WHO 2013) http://www.who.int/gho/hiv/en/. Sub-Sahara Africa has the highest prevalence rate of 4.5% while Western Pacific and Eastern Mediterranean have the least with 0.1% prevalence.

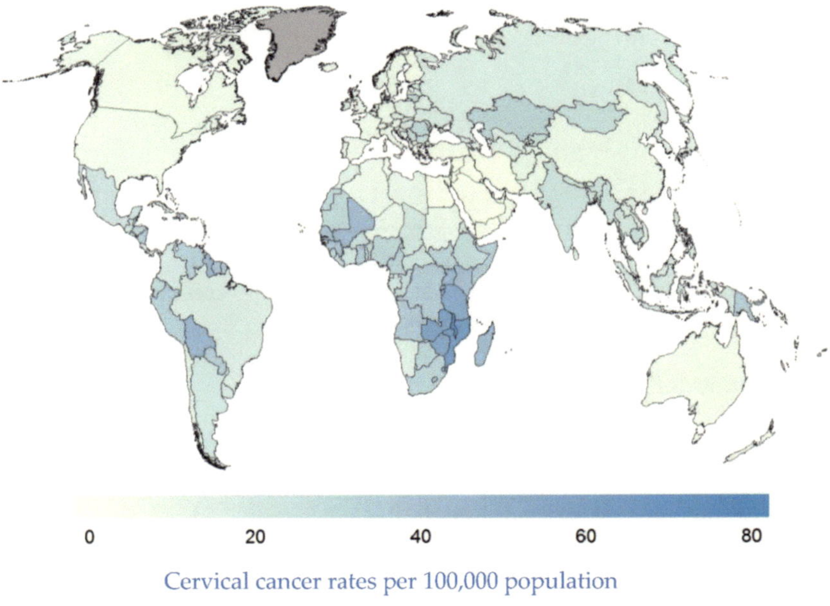

Figure 2. Estimated Cervical Cancer Incidence Worldwide in 2012 (GLOBOCAN 2012)

2.4. HIV infection and cervical cancer

Cervical cancer is one of the malignancies commonly diagnosed in people living with HIV. Other commonly associated malignancies in HIV setting include lymphomas, Kaposis' sarcoma, anal carcinoma and other HPV associated malignancies like vulval and penile cancers. Worldwide, cervical cancer incidence is higher among HIV positive women compared with HIV negative women. In a North American multi-cohort collaboration prospective study involving 13,690 HIV positive and 12,021 HIV negative women, it was found that HIV positive women had 7 times more incidence of cervical cancer than their HIV negative counterparts [9]. In a study in West Africa to assess the relationship between HIV infection and cervical cancer, HIV infected women had higher rates of 22/132 (16.7%) than controls 10/120 (8.3%) ($p = 0.048$) [10].

Cervical cancer has been observed to occur in younger age ranges among HIV positive patients than with HIV negative women (about 10 years younger) and the disease is also noted to have a more aggressive course with metastasis to unusual sites like the skin and brain. Recurrences are much earlier and frequent than in HIV negative women [11, 12]. HIV positive women are also noted to have cervical cancer at higher CD4 counts compared with the low CD4 counts associated with other AID associated malignancies like Kaposis' sarcoma and lymphomas [13].

2.5. Screening for cervical cancer

Screening for cervical cancer is an effective strategy for reducing the incidence and mortality of cervical cancer. The availability of effective screening corresponds with reduced incidence and mortality of the disease. It is the main reason why the incidence of cervical cancer in developed world is less compared with developing (poor resource countries) where screening programs are not available. The recommended schedule of screening of sexually active female populations by The American Cancer Society is summarized in Table 2.

Population	Recommended screening method
Age <21 years	No screening
Age 21-29 years	Cytology alone every 3 years
Age 30-65 years	HPV and cytology contesting every 5 years (preferred) Cytology alone every 3 years (acceptable)
Age > 65 years	No screening following adequate negative prior screening
After hysterectomy	No screening
HPV vaccinated	Follow age specific recommendations (same as unvaccinated women)

Table 2. Recommended screening scheme for cervical cancer (adapted from Saslow (2012) [14]

In HIV infected individuals the progression of HPV infection to carcinogenesis is accelerated and there is need to shorten the period of screening in women living with HIV so as to diagnose cervical squamous epithelial changes early. In a report of long term follow up of participants using cervical cytology, Massad and colleagues (2008) reported high grade squamous epithelial lesion of 4.4 in 1000 person-years in HIV positive patients against 1.3 in 1000-person years among HIV negative women. At ten years observation period, the cumulative risk of abnormal cytology was 77% in HIV positive individuals as against 50% in HIV negative individuals [15]. In another report of a cervical cytology follow up of 409 HIV positive women, progression of cervical lesions occurred in 39 cases. In 24 [61.5%) cases, the first diagnosis was benign cellular changes (BCC) and 21 out of the 24 cases had low-grade squamous intraepithelial lesion (LSIL) after one year. In 11 (28.2%) out of the 204 cases, the first diagnosis was BCC, and 9 cases had high-grade intraepithelial lesion (HSIL) after I year. In 2 (5.0%) out of the 204 cases, the first diagnosis was LSIL and the second was HSIL at one year interval. Two (5.0%) had the first diagnosis as HSIL, and the second as invasive carcinoma at 2-yr interval [16]. Cervical intraepithelial neoplasia (CIN) has also been reported to be more common in HIV positive women with CD4 cell count < 200 cells /ul [17]. Cervical cancer has also been noted to occur in younger women with HIV infection than in those without, and the peak incidence has been reported to be a decade earlier [18]. These results point to the need for shorter screening intervals for HIV positive women. In addition, the diagnosis of abnormal cervical cytology has been shown to be unrelated with current intake of highly active anti-retroviral therapy (HAART) [19]. It could therefore be beneficial to commence cervical cancer screening at an earlier age possibly at age 19 years with a screening interval of 2 years for those with CD4 count ≥ 200 cells/ul and yearly for those with CD4 count < 200 cells/ul irrespective of HAART status.

2.6. Pathophysiology of HIV infection

HIV infection lowers immunity through the destruction of CD4 lymphocytes. The first target of HIV in the host system is the CD4 T cells. The HIV cell envelope binds to the CD4 cell receptor causing further activation of co-receptors that will eventually lead to the fusion of the host and viral cell membranes. The virus then gets totally into the host cell. This process leads to the destruction of CD4 cells through various mechanisms as the virus multiplies in the host system [20, 21].

The level of destruction is related to the level of HIV viral load in the patients system. CD4 cell count and viral load are the recommended tests to measure HIV positive patients' immune status which can also indicate the rate of destruction of immune cells [22]. Progressive reduction in CD4 cell population reduces the ability of the body to ward off infective agents leading to occurrence of opportunistic infections in HIV infected individuals. Dormant infections such as Herpes zoster can also be reactivated under conditions of depressed immunity. These opportunistic infections add to the deterioration of the clinical states of HIV infected patients leading to poor treatment outcome. Opportunistic infections are common if CD4 cells count is below 200 cells/ul [23]. The list of common infections associated with depressed immunity is presented in Table 3.

Infective Agents	Species
Viral	Human Herpes viruses (Herpes simplex types 1 & 2, varicellazoster virus, Epstein-Barr virus, Cytomegalovirus), Measles, Respiratory syncytial virus, Influenza, Adenovirus
Bacterial	Legionella pneumophila, Listeria monocytogenes, Salmonella typhimurium, Mycobacterium tuberculosis, Atypical mycobacterium
Parasitic	Pneumocystis pneumonia, Toxoplasma gondii, Cryptosporidia spp,
Fungal	Candida spp, Cryptococcus neoformans, Histoplasma capsulatum, Coccidioides immiti

Table 3. Common opportunistic infections associated with depressed T cell immunity Adapted from Mackall (2000) [23].

2.7. Clinical aspects of HIV infection and cervical cancer

The higher the HIV viral load, the more likely the compromise in the immune status. Cervical cancer patients with HIV have been reported as having lower levels of CD4 cells count than HIV sero positive patients without cervical cancer. In a report by Leitao and colleagues (2008) comparing the CD4 cells count and viral load in 15 HIV positive cases with cervical cancer with 60 HIV positive patients without cervical cancer controls, the median CD4 count for cases was 208 cells/lL (range, 18-1102 cells/lL) while that for controls was 445 cells/lL (range, 20-1201 cells/lL) ($p = 0.03$). The median viral load was 16,918 copies/mL (range, 50-214,915 copies/mL) for cases while that for control was 1430 copies/mL (range, 50-571,000 copies/mL) for controls ($p= 0.15$ [24]). In the WHO staging of HIV, the association of HIV with cervical cancer is classified under stage IV as with other AIDS defining malignancies indicating severity and warrants the commencement of anti-retroviral therapy [25]. HIV infection is also noted to be associated with high grade cervical cancer which leads to rapid progression of the disease.

2.8. Management of cervical cancer

The management of cervical cancer follows a multimodality approach. Relevant clinical examinations and investigations to assess the stage of the disease and the suitability of the patient for the modes of therapy have to be done. The choice of treatment depends on the stage of the disease and the performance status of the patient. The treatment choice usually involves surgery, radiotherapy and chemotherapy either alone or in combinations.

The treatment is usually chosen based on the stage of the disease. Treatment follows guidelines that operate in various countries and regions. The European Society for Medical Oncology (ESMO) guidelines (2012) is outlined in Table 4. [26]

2.9. CD4 cell count and cervical cancer treatment

Chemotherapy leads to suppressed immunity especially through the reduction of CD4 and CD8 cell counts in HIV positive patients. The effect is more marked on CD4 cells. The recovery is slow and better with CD8 than CD4 cells. The recovery of CD4 cells depends on the state of the thymus gland as they are thymus dependent. The thymus gland undergoes involution in the adults and hence recovery of CD4 cells count is usually very slow in those with involute thymus gland. The effect of chemotherapy is more marked with

Stage	Treatment	Issue
IA1	Conization or simple hysterectomy ± salpingo-ophorectomy and PLND if LVSI	Conservative surgery
IA2	Conization/radical trachelectomy or modified radical hysterectomy and PLND	Adjuvant CT/RT if risk factors (LVSI, G3, positive resection margins, multiple nodes)
IB1, IIA	Radical hysterectomy and PLND	Adjuvant CT/RT if risk factors (LVSI, G3, positive resection margins, multiple nodes)
IB2, IIB–IV	Combination CT/RT with cisplatin	NACT to large bulky tumors prior to CT/RT

PLND- pelvic lymphadenectomy; LVSI- lymphovascular space invasion; CT- computed tomography; NACT- neoadjuvant chemotherapy; RT- radiation therapy

Table 4. Cervical cancer treatment according to Stage (ESMO guideline 2012).

alkylating agents, purine nucleoside analogues and steroids [23]. In a study to assess the activity of the thymus gland after chemotherapy, it was reported that in younger patients aged between 18-49 years, the thymus function was evident in 63% of the participants compared with 0% of their counterparts aged 70-91years three months post treatment [27]. Pelvic radiotherapy has been reported to lower immune cells significantly in HIV sero negative patients. These cells include CD4 T- lymphocytes, B cells and Helper T cells. The reduction could be up to 50% in some instances [28, 29].

The advent of highly active anti-retroviral therapy (HAART) has improved the immunological status of HIV positive patients and control the increase in viral load [30]. HAART leads to rapid reduction in HIV viral load and sometimes to clinically undetectable level [31]. In a study to assess the effects of combination chemotherapy on immune status of HIV associated lymphoma patients, Powles (2002) reported that there was a significant drop in CD4 T cells. Following completion of treatment, the recovery of CD4 T-cells was faster in patients receiving HAART than in those without HAART [32]. The treatment with HAART does not however prevent the development of cervical cancer in HIV positive patients [33].

Patients with compromised immunity usually suffer more treatment toxicities as well. Chemoradiotherapy used in the treatment of cervical cancer affect the immune status of patients. Chemotherapy leads to immune cells suppression and the toxicity following radiotherapy is increased in patients with compromised immunity [18]. HIV positive patients not on HAART are therefore more likely to experience compromised immunity than those on HAART. With decreasing immune status among HIV positive patients, the rate of decrease of CD4 cells can be unpredictable and such patients can suffer from opportunistic infections that will further complicate their conditions.

2.10. Management of cervical cancer in HIV positive patients

Decisions on the management of cervical cancer in HIV positive patients are not straight forward. This is because of the immune concerns about such patients. Contributory factors to immune compromise in such patients include the cancer, the HIV infection and the modalities of treatment – chemotherapy and radiotherapy. There is the fear that oncology treatment will worsen the immune status of treatment. Standard treatment as with HIV seronegative patients are recommended. Radiation treatment of HIV positive patients with cervical cancer however, has been reported to be associated with a seven fold increase in multi-systemic toxicities compared with HIV sero-negative patients [18]. HIV patients with malignancy have also been reported to have impaired ability of the mucosa to repair radiation damage. In treating oropharyngeal tumour with radiation, it was reported that HIV positive patients had mucosal reaction with lesser doses of radiation than HIV negative patients [34]. With regards to cervical cancer, it is likely that the tissues with mucosal lining close to the treatment fields like urinary bladder and gastro intestinal tract (GIT) might be affected in a similar way. This pattern of mucosal reaction is attributable to low immune status of the patients.

Close to about 10% of HIV positive patients are also reported to be co-infected with hepatitis B virus (HBV) or hepatitis C virus (HCV) or with both [35]. HIV positive patients diagnosed with cervical cancer should therefore be routinely screened for HBV and HCV. A study in sub-Sahara Africa reported that among HIV-infected individuals, mean HBV and HCV prevalence rates were 15% and 7%, respectively [36]. Such co-infections have been reported to accelerate the progression of HIV infection [37]. Such infections also warrant extra caution in using HAART drugs that are metabolised in the liver to minimise liver toxicity that may occur [38]. Chemotherapy and radiotherapy may also activate viral hepatitis in such patients leading to complications of therapy [39].

Essential measures to improve treatment tolerance and optimal outcome in HIV positive patients with cervical cancer include early commencement of HAART (at diagnosis) based on WHO recommendation of commencement of anti- retroviral therapy (ART) in WHO HIV stage IV patients. Other studies have also recommended the commencement (at diagnosis) of ART in all patients diagnosed with cancer based on the study results that show better outcome of treatment in such patients. Such patients are noted to have better CD4 cell count and viral load responses compared with those not on ART and are more likely to complete oncology treatment on schedule [40, 41, 42]. Generally, early commencement of ART in HIV positive individuals has been recently shown to be of benefit. In a randomized trial in Cote d'Ivore West Africa, in which 2,056 participants with HIV-1 infection were included in the analysis (Temprano Trial), it was reported that ART reduced the possibility of severe illness by 44% in people starting treatment immediately at diagnosis, as compared to those starting ART only when their CD4 levels drop to below 500/mm^3. The study also reported that prophylaxis against tuberculosis with isoniazid initiated among people living with HIV with a CD4 count greater than 500/mm^3 reduced the risk of severe illness by 35%, compared with those without such treatment. Early initiation of isoniazid was also not associated with increase in the development of resistance to isoniazid [43].

Regular monitoring of CD4 cell count and viral load assay is needed towards early intervention in case of derangements below critical levels. Msadabwe (2009) reported the CD4 cells count trend during treatment and up to three months after treatment of HIV positive patients with cervical cancer treated with chemoradiotherapy. The average initial CD4 cells count was 321.06 cells /mm^2 at commencement of treatment. This gradually dropped to 62.56 cells/mm^2 at the end of treatment giving a mean difference of 258.2 cells /mm^2. There was however, gradual rise after treatment but by 3 months which was the end of the follow up period of the study, the pre-treatment level was not reached. The average count at the end of three months was one third of the pre-treatment value [44]. Significant drop in CD4 cells following radiotherapy applies to both HIV negative and HIV positive patients especially if the radiation fields are around areas with large lymphoid tissues such as the chest and pelvis. In HIV seronegative patients treated for early stage breast cancer and stage I seminoma with radiotherapy, it was reported that the CD4 cells count dropped by about 200 cells/ul and that pre-treatment levels could not be attained after six years follow up [45]. Monthly CD4 cells count assay is therefore needed to monitor the trend in CD4 cells count during treatment and at three monthly intervals after treatment to ensure adequate CD4 count levels. This practice will enable the early commencement of prophylaxis against opportunistic infections if CD4 cells count is below critical levels so as to reduce morbidity in the patients. The recommended CD4 levels for commencement of appropriate prophylaxis are presented in Table 5.

Pathogen	Initiate Prophylaxis	Preferred agent	Discontinuation of Prophylaxis
Mycobacterium avium complex (MAC)	CD4 <50 cells/mm3	Azithromycin 1200mg orally once weekly or Clarithromycin 500mg orally twice weekly	CD4 count increase to >100 cells/mm3 for ≥3 months in response to ART
Toxoplasma gondii encephalitis (TE)	CD4 <100 cells/mm3 and Positive serology for Toxoplasma (IgG+)	Trimethoprim/ Sulfamethoxazole (TMP/SMX) double strength daily	Patient receiving ART with increase in CD4 count to >200 cells/mm3 for ≥3 months
Pneumocystis pneumonia (PCP)	CD4 <200 cells/mm3 or a history of oropharyngeal candidiasis	Trimethoprim/ Sulfamethoxazole (TMP/SMX) Single strength daily or double strength three times weekly.	CD4 count >200 cells/mm3 for >3 months in response to ART · Adequate viral suppression · If PCP occurred with CD4 >200 cells/mm3, prophylaxis should be maintained

Table 5. Criteria for initiating and discontinuing prophylaxis for opportunistic infections in HIV positive patients [adapted from NIH- AIDS Information 2015]. [46]

Other steps include testing for viral load every six months. This will ensure early diagnosis of drug resistances as increasing viral load while patient is on ART may indicate onset of drug resistance which should be promptly investigated and appropriate ART changes made.

External beam radiation therapy should be delivered at a daily dose of 1.8Gy per fraction to HIV positive patients to minimize toxicity [47]. Patients with CD4 cells count less than 200 cells/ul should be treated with 1.5Gy per fraction while the dose of weekly cisplatin should be given at a reduced dose of 30-35mg/m². These modifications have been reported to result in treatment tolerance similar to HIV negative patients [45]. Patients with CD4 cells count less than 150 cells /ul may however, not be able to withstand long course of radiation therapy and should be given short course treatments depending on performance status. The rate of completion of chemotherapy has been reported to be 30-45% among HIV positive patients compared with 64-89% among HIV negative patients[48, 49].

The above measures could help in improving the rate of completion of treatment in HIV positive patients. Renal dysfunction not myelo- suppression or gastrointestinal toxicity has been reported in a retrospective study, to be the main cause of chemotherapy suspension in HIV positive patients treated for cervical cancer and that chemotherapy was the most difficult section to be completed in HIV positive patients [4]. Carboplatin chemotherapy may be preferred to cisplatin in order to improve chemotherapy completion rate in HIV positive patients. Patients with CD4 cells count less than 200 cells/ul should however, not receive chemotherapy.

2.11. Drug interactions between chemotherapy and anti-retroviral agents

Platinum compounds commonly used in the chemotherapy of cervical cancer are cisplatin and carboplatin. Patients with persistent or recurrent and metastatic disease can have paclitaxel added to their treatment regimen [50]. On the other hand, anti-retroviral therapy in HIV treatment consists of combinations of three different drugs from at least two different drug classes (Table 6).

Nucleoside Reverse Transcriptase Inhibitors (NRTIs)	**Non-Nucleoside Reverse Transcriptase Inhibitors (NNRTIs)**	**Protease Inhibitors**	**Entry and Integrase Inhibitors**
Abacavir (ABC)	Delavirdine (DLV)	Atazanavir (ATV)	Dolutegravir (DTG)
Didanosine (ddI)	*Efavirenz (EFV)	Darunavir (DRV)	Elvitegravir (EVG)
Emtricitabine (FTC)	Etravirine (ETR)	Fosamprenavir (FPV/ FOS-APV)	Maraviroc (MVC)
*Lamivudine [3TC)	Nevirapine (NVP)	Indinavir (IDV)	Raltegravir (RAL)
*Stavudine (d4T)	Rilpivirine (RPV)	Lopinavir	
*Tenofovir (DF/TDF)		Nelfinavir (NFV)	
Zidovudine AZT/ZDV		Ritonavir (RTV)	
		Saquinavir (SQV)	
		Tipranavir (TPV)	

*Drugs commonly used for first line treatment of HIV infections.

Table 6. Major HIV drug classes. At least three drugs from two drug classes are selected for the treatment of HIV when ART is indicated Sources: NIH-NIAID, 2015; hiv-druginteractions.org 2015). [51]

Commonly used first line drugs are stavudine or tenofovir, lamivudine [Nucleoside Reverse Transcriptase Inhibitors (NRTIs) and efavirenz [Non-Nucleoside Reverse Transcriptase Inhibitors (NNRTIs) [4]. Various other second line combinations are used in cases of drug resistance development or intolerable side effects of the first line combination drug regimen. Pharmacokinetic enhancers like Cobicistat [COBI] can be included with some of the combinations to increase the effectiveness of the treatment. Most HIV positive patients diagnosed with cervical cancer who are on HAART are likely to be placed on regimen containing the above drugs [52, 53].

Possibilities of drug interactions and potentiation of toxicities exist among these chemotherapy and ART drugs and these can affect treatment outcome. Paclitaxel is metabolized mainly by CYP 2C8 enzyme of the cytochrome P450 system to 6 alpha-hydroxypaclitaxel. Paclitaxel metabolites are inactive in comparison with the parent drug [54]. CYP 2C8 enzyme can be inhibited by some ART drugs such as Delavirdine, Ritonavir, Fosamprenavir, Atazanavir, Indinavir, Lopinavir, Nelfinavir and Saquinavir. Concomitant intake of any of these agents can lead to increased toxicity of paclitaxel. On the other hand, Nevirapine is CYP 2C8 enzyme inducer and on concomitant intake of this agent with paclitaxel can lead to accelerated clearance of the active parent drug leading to ineffectiveness of paclitaxel [55].

Drugs	**Stavudine**	**Tenofovir**	**Lamivudine**	**Efavirenz**
Cisplatin	[a] Potential interaction	[a] Potential interaction	[b] Potential interaction	No interaction
Carboplatin	[c] Potential interaction	[d] Potential interaction	[e] Potential interaction	No interaction
Paclitaxel	No interaction	No interaction	No interaction	[f] Potential interaction

[a] Might increase risk of neuropathy as both drugs could cause neuropathy.

[b] Cisplatin is eliminated through renal route via organic cation transporter 2 (OCT2) and human multidrug and toxin extrusion 1 (MATE1) enzymes. Cisplatin and lamivudine could compete for OCT2 which could slow their elimination. Lamivudine dose could be adjusted.

[c] Carboplatin and stavudine administered together can increase the risk of peripheral neuropathy due to additive toxicity.

[d]. Both have nephrotoxic potential. Dose of tenofovir may need to be adjusted appropriately.

[e]. Lamivudine may affect renal function hence dose may need to be adjusted.

[f] Efavirenz is a strong inhibitor of CYP2C8 enzyme mostly involved in the metabolism of paclitaxel. Co administration of these agents may increase the toxicity of paclitaxel.

NB. The above interactions are supported by very low levels of evidence.

Table 7. Cytotoxic and HIV drugs interactions relevant to HIV and cervical cancer (Source: HIV drugsinteraction.org. Accessed 2015 March 11).

There can be overlapping side effects between chemotherapy and ART drugs. Myelo-suppression is associated with most chemotherapeutic agents including paclitaxel and platinum compounds and this can also be induced by the ART drug zidovudine. Paclitaxel can also cause neuropathy likewise didanosine and stavudine. Care therefore has to be exercised in patients that take these drugs concomitantly or other alternatives should be given. Cisplatin and carboplatin can cause nephrotoxicity likewise the ART drug tenofovir while nausea and vomiting which is common with most chemotherapy drugs can also be induced by ART drugs in the classes of protease inhibitors, nucleoside and nonnucleoside reverse transcriptase inhibitors [50]. Patients on these agents should have effective management of nausea and vomiting with potent anti-emetics.

The possible interactions of cytotoxic drugs commonly used in cervical cancer chemotherapy with first line drugs used in the treatment of HIV infection are presented in Table 7 above.

Interactions between cytotoxic drugs used in the treatment of cervical cancer and first line ART drugs are quite favorable as contained in Table 7 with the associated levels of evidence. Combining the treatment modalities in HIV positive patients should therefore be tolerated by most patients.

3. Conclusion

The outcome of treatment in HIV positive patients diagnosed with cervical cancer is still poor especially in regions with high prevalence of HIV and cervical cancer. This could be improved through prompt commencement of such patients on ART at diagnosis. Close monitoring of the immune status (CD4 cell) and viral load is needed to ensure early diagnosis of depressed immune status and HAART treatment resistance. This could give early indication for commencement of appropriate prophylaxis against opportunistic infections and review of ART drug combinations. There is need to continue further search for other modes of treatment such as targeted therapies and radio sensitizers that can improve the effectiveness of managing HIV positive patients diagnosed with cervical cancer. Prospective studies are also needed to establish optimal radiation and chemotherapy doses in HIV positive patients diagnosed with cervical cancer.

Author details

Atara Ntekim*

Address all correspondence to: tarantekim@yahoo.com

Department of Radiation Oncology, College of Medicine/ University College Hospital, University of Ibadan, Ibadan, Nigeria

References

[1] Arbyn M, Castellsagué X, de Sanjosé S, Bruni L, Saraiya M, Bray F, et al. Worldwide burden of cervical cancer in 2008. Ann Oncol [Internet]. 2011 Dec [cited 2015 Mar 14]; 22(12):2675–86. Available from: http://www.ncbi.nlm.nih.gov/pubmed/21471563

[2] Akhtar-Danesh N, Lytwyn A, Elit L. Five-year trends in mortality indices among gynecological cancer patients in Canada. Gynecol Oncol. 2012;127(3):620–4.

[3] Prabha Devi K, Bindhu Priya N. Conventional Pap Smear Screening in HIV Seropositive Women in South India. J Obstet Gynecol India [Internet]. 2013;63(1):55–8. Available from: http://www.ncbi.nlm.nih.gov/pubmed/24431601

[4] Simonds HM, Wright JD, du Toit N, Neugut AI, Jacobson JS. Completion of and early response to chemoradiation among human immunodeficiency virus (HIV)-positive and HIV-negative patients with locally advanced cervical carcinoma in South Africa. Cancer [Internet]. 2012;118(11):2971–9. Available from: http://www.ncbi.nlm.nih.gov/pubmed/22072021

[5] Coghill AE, Newcomb P a, Madeleine MM, Richardson BA, Mutyaba I, Okuku F, et al. Contribution of HIV infection to mortality among cancer patients in Uganda. AIDS [Internet]. 2013;27(April):2933–42. Available from: http://www.ncbi.nlm.nih.gov/pubmed/23921614

[6] GLOBOCAN. Global Cancer Statistics [Internet]. Global Cancer Statistics. 2012 [cited 2015 Feb 21]. Available from: http://globocan.iarc.fr/Pages/fact_sheets_cancer.aspx

[7] Crow JM. HPV: The global burden. Nature [Internet]. 2012 Aug 30 [cited 2015 Mar 14];488(7413):S2–3. Available from: http://www.ncbi.nlm.nih.gov/pubmed/22932437

[8] Didelot-Rousseau M-N, Nagot N, Costes-Martineau V, Vallès X, Ouedraogo A, Konate I, et al. Human papillomavirus genotype distribution and cervical squamous intraepithelial lesions among high-risk women with and without HIV-1 infection in Burkina Faso. Br J Cancer. 2006;95(3):355–62.

[9] Abraham AG, D'Souza G, Jing Y, Gange SJ, Sterling TR, Silverberg MJ, et al. Invasive cervical cancer risk among HIV-infected women: A North American multicohort collaboration prospective study. J Acquir Immune Defic Syndr [Internet]. 2013;62(4): 405–13. Available from: http://www.embase.com/search/results?subaction=viewrecord&from=export&id=L368753963

[10] Adjorlolo-Johnson G, Unger ER, Boni-Ouattara E, Touré-Coulibaly K, Maurice C, Vernon SD, et al. Assessing the relationship between HIV infection and cervical cancer in Côte d'Ivoire: a case-control study. BMC Infect Dis. 2010;10:242.

[11] Maiman M. Management of cervical neoplasia in human immunodeficiency virus-infected women. J Natl Cancer InstituteMonographs. 1998;(23)(23):43–9.

[12] Amit A, Edwards CL, Athey P, Kaplan AL. Extensive subcutaneous metastases from squamous cell carcinoma of the cervix in patient with HIV. Int J Gynecol Cancer. 2001;11(1):78–80.

[13] Klevens RM, Fleming PL, Mays MA, Frey R. Characteristics of women with AIDS and invasive cervical cancer. Obstet Gynecol. 1996;88(2):269–73.

[14] Saslow D, Solomon D, Lawson HW, Killackey M, Kulasingam SL, Cain J, et al. American Cancer Society, American Society for Colposcopy and Cervical Pathology, and American Society for Clinical Pathology screening guidelines for the prevention and early detection of cervical cancer. Am J Clin Pathol. 2012;137(4):516–42.

[15] Massad LS, Seaberg EC, Wright RL, Darragh T, Lee YC, Colie C, et al. Squamous cervical lesions in women with human immunodeficiency virus: long-term follow-up. Obs Gynecol [Internet]. 2008;111(6):1388–93. Available from: http://www.ncbi.nlm.nih.gov/entrez/query.fcgi?cmd=Retrieve&db=PubMed&dopt=Citation&list_uids=18515523

[16] Calore EE, Pereira SMM, Cavaliere MJ. Progression of cervical lesions in HIV-seropositive women: A cytological study. Diagn Cytopathol. 2001;24(2):117–9.

[17] Ahr A, Rody A, Cimposiau C, Faul-Burbes C, Kissler S, Kaufmann M, et al. Cervical cancer screening of HIV-positive women: is a prolongation of the screening interval meaningful? Zentralbl Gynakol. 2006;128(5):242–5.

[18] Gichangi P, Bwayo J, Estambale B, Rogo K, Njuguna E, Ojwang S, et al. HIV impact on acute morbidity and pelvic tumor control following radiotherapy for cervical cancer. Gynecol Oncol [Internet]. 2006 Feb [cited 2014 Apr 18];100(2):405–11. Available from: http://www.ncbi.nlm.nih.gov/pubmed/16274737

[19] Firnhaber C, Van Le H, Pettifor A, Schulze D, Michelow P, Sanne IM, et al. Association between cervical dysplasia and human papillomavirus in HIV seropositive women from Johannesburg South Africa. Cancer Causes Control. 2010;21(3):433–43.

[20] Siliciano RF. The role of CD4 in HIV envelope-mediated pathogenesis. Curr Top Microbiol Immunol. 1996;205:159–79.

[21] Wilen CB, Tilton JC, Doms RW. HIV: Cell binding and entry. Cold Spring Harb Perspect Med. Cold Spring Harbor Laboratory Press; 2012;2(8).

[22] Simon V, Ho D, Karim QA. HIV/AIDS epidemiology, pathogenesis, prevention, and treatment. Lancet [Internet]. 2006;368(9534):489–504. Available from: http://www.sciencedirect.com/science/article/pii/S0140673606691575

[23] Mackall CL. T-cell immunodeficiency following cytotoxic antineoplastic therapy: a review. Stem Cells. 2000;18(1):10–8.

[24] Leitao MM, White P, Cracchiolo B. Cervical cancer in patients infected with the human immunodeficiency virus. Cancer. 2008;112(12):2683–9.

[25] WHO. WHO HIV staging for African region [Internet]. WHO. 2007 [cited 2015 Mar 2]. Available from: http://www.who.int/hiv/pub/guidelines/clinicalstaging.pdf

[26] Colombo N, Carinelli S, Colombo A, Marini C, Rollo D, Sessa C. Cervical cancer: ESMO Clinical Practice Guidelines for diagnosis, treatment and follow-up. Ann Oncol [Internet]. 2012 Oct [cited 2015 Mar 13];23 Suppl 7:vii27–32. Available from: http://www.ncbi.nlm.nih.gov/pubmed/22997451

[27] Sfikakis PP, Gourgoulis GM, Moulopoulos LA, Kouvatseas G, Theofilopoulos AN, Dimopoulos MA. Age-related thymic activity in adults following chemotherapy-induced lymphopenia. Eur J Clin Invest. 2005;35(6):380–7.

[28] Lissoni P, Meregalli S, Bonetto E, Mancuso M, Brivio F, Colciago M, et al. Radiotherapy-induced lymphocytopenia: Changes in total lymphocyte count and in lymphocyte subpopulations under pelvic irradiation in gynecologic neoplasms. J Biol Regul Homeost Agents. 2005;19(3-4):153–8.

[29] Kahn S, Jani A, Edelman S, Rossi P, Godette K, Landry J, et al. Matched cohort analysis of outcomes of definitive radiotherapy for prostate cancer in human immunodeficiency virus-positive patients. Int J Radiat Oncol Biol Phys [Internet]. 2012 May 1 [cited 2015 Mar 13];83(1):16–21. Available from: http://www.ncbi.nlm.nih.gov/pubmed/22104362

[30] April MD, Wood R, Berkowitz BK, Paltiel AD, Anglaret X, Losina E, et al. The survival benefits of antiretroviral therapy in South Africa. J Infect Dis [Internet]. 2014 Feb 15 [cited 2015 Mar 14];209(4):491–9. Available from: http://www.pubmedcentral.nih.gov/articlerender.fcgi?artid=3903379&tool=pmcentrez&rendertype=abstract

[31] Sedaghat AR, Siliciano RF, Wilke CO. Low-level HIV-1 replication and the dynamics of the resting CD4+ T cell reservoir for HIV-1 in the setting of HAART. BMC Infect Dis [Internet]. 2008 Jan [cited 2015 Mar 14];8:2. Available from: http://www.pubmedcentral.nih.gov/articlerender.fcgi?artid=2254415&tool=pmcentrez&rendertype=abstract

[32] Powles T, Imami N, Nelson M, Gazzard BG, Bower M. Effects of combination chemotherapy and highly active antiretroviral therapy on immune parameters in HIV-1 associated lymphoma. AIDS [Internet]. 2002 Mar 8 [cited 2015 Mar 14];16(4):531–6. Available from: http://www.ncbi.nlm.nih.gov/pubmed/11872995

[33] Adler DH. The impact of HAART on HPV-related cervical disease. Curr HIV Res [Internet]. 2010 Oct [cited 2015 Mar 14];8(7):493–7. Available from: http://www.pubmedcentral.nih.gov/articlerender.fcgi?artid=3108243&tool=pmcentrez&rendertype=abstract

[34] Watkins EB, Findlay P, Gelmann E, Lane HC, Zabell A. Enhanced mucosal reactions in AIDS patients receiving oropharyngeal irradiation. Int J Radiat Oncol Biol Phys [Internet]. 1987 Sep [cited 2015 Mar 13];13(9):1403–8. Available from: http://www.ncbi.nlm.nih.gov/pubmed/3624048

[35] Tremeau-Bravard A, Ogbukagu IC, Ticao CJ, Abubakar JJ. Seroprevalence of hepatitis B and C infection among the HIV-positive population in Abuja, Nigeria. Afr Health Sci. 2012;12(3):312–7.

[36] Barth RE, Huijgen Q, Taljaard J, Hoepelman AIM. Hepatitis B/C and HIV in sub-Saharan Africa: an association between highly prevalent infectious diseases. A systematic review and meta-analysis. Int J Infect Dis [Internet]. 2010 Dec [cited 2015 Mar 13]; 14(12):e1024–31. Available from: http://www.ncbi.nlm.nih.gov/pubmed/20870439

[37] Nikolopoulos GK, Paraskevis D, Hatzitheodorou E, Moschidis Z, Sypsa V, Zavitsanos X, et al. Impact of hepatitis B virus infection on the progression of AIDS and mortality in HIV-infected individuals: a cohort study and meta-analysis. Clin Infect Dis. 2009;48(12):1763–71.

[38] Hu J, Ludgate L. HIV-HBV and HIV-HCV coinfection and liver cancer development. Cancer Treat Res. 2007;133:241–52.

[39] Musyoki AM, Msibi TL, Motswaledi MH, Selabe SG, Monokoane TS, Mphahlele MJ. Active co-infection with HBV and/or HCV in South African HIV positive patients due for cancer therapy. J Med Virol [Internet]. 2015 Feb [cited 2015 Mar 13];87(2):213–21. Available from: http://www.ncbi.nlm.nih.gov/pubmed/25156907

[40] Ntekim AI, Folasire AM. Clinical Medicine Insights: Oncology CD4 Count and Anti Retroviral Therapy for HIV Positive Patients With Cancer in Nigeria -A Pilot Study. : 61–6.

[41] Munkukpa H. Acute toxicity in cervical cancer HIV positive versus HIV negative patients treated by radical chemo-radiotherapy in Zambia [Internet]. Dissertation University of Witswatersrand, Johannesburg,South Africa. 2012 [cited 2015 Mar 11]. Available from: https://ujdigispace.uj.ac.za/bitstream/handle/10210/8344/Munkupa.pdf;jsessionid

[42] Musyoki AM, Msibi TL, Motswaledi MH, Selabe SG, Mphahlele MJ. Sustained favourable HIV viral load response in South African patients during concomitant HAART and cancer therapy. J Med Virol [Internet]. 2015 Feb [cited 2015 Mar 13]; 87(2):192–8. Available from: http://www.ncbi.nlm.nih.gov/pubmed/25156795

[43] Christine Danel, Delphine Gabillard, Jerome Le Carro, Xavier Anglaret1, Raoul Moh, Serge Eholie, Hervé Ménan, Anani Badje, Gerard Kouame JBN. Early ART and IPT in HIV-Infected African Adults With High CD4 Count (Temprano Trial) (2015). Conference on Retroviruses and Opportunistic Infections (CROI) [Internet]. Seattle, Washington, USA; Available from: http://www.croiconference.org/sessions/early-art-and-ipt-hiv-infected-african-adults-high-cd4-count-temprano-trial.

[44] Msadabwe S. A randomized study to compare radical concurrent chemoradiotherapy against radical radiotherapy, as treatment of cancer of the cervix in HIV infected patients (dissertation) [Internet]. Dissertation. 2009 [cited 2015 Feb 2]. Available from: http://wiredspace.wits.ac.za/bitstream/handle/10539/7468/MMed R

[45] Housri N, Yarchoan R, Kaushal A. Radiotherapy for patients with the human immunodeficiency virus: are special precautions necessary? Cancer [Internet]. 2010 Jan 15 [cited 2015 Mar 14];116(2):273–83. Available from: http://www.pubmedcentral.nih.gov/articlerender.fcgi?artid=3409663&tool=pmcentrez&rendertype=abstract

[46] HIH. AIDS information [Internet]. 2015 [cited 2015 Feb 23]. Available from: http://aidsinfo.nih.gov/contentfiles/lvguidelines/adultoitablesonly.pdf

[47] Simonds HM, Wright JD, Du Toit N, Neugut AI, Jacobson JS. Completion of and early response to chemoradiation among human immunodeficiency virus (HIV)-positive and HIV-negative patients with locally advanced cervical carcinoma in South Africa. Cancer. 2012;118(11):2971–9.

[48] Oehler-Jänne C, Huguet F, Provencher S, Seifert B, Negretti L, Riener M-O, et al. HIV-specific differences in outcome of squamous cell carcinoma of the anal canal: a multicentric cohort study of HIV-positive patients receiving highly active antiretroviral therapy. J Clin Oncol [Internet]. 2008 May 20 [cited 2015 Mar 13];26(15):2550–7. Available from: http://www.ncbi.nlm.nih.gov/pubmed/18427149

[49] Hammad N, Heilbrun LK, Gupta S, Tageja N, Philip PA, Shields AF, et al. Squamous cell cancer of the anal canal in HIV-infected patients receiving highly active antiretroviral therapy: a single institution experience. Am J Clin Oncol [Internet]. 2011 Apr [cited 2015 Mar 13];34(2):135–9. Available from: http://www.pubmedcentral.nih.gov/articlerender.fcgi?artid=3908654&tool=pmcentrez&rendertype=abstract

[50] Kitagawa R, Katsumata N, Shibata T, Kamura T, Kasamatsu T, Nakanishi T, et al. Paclitaxel Plus Carboplatin Versus Paclitaxel Plus Cisplatin in Metastatic or Recurrent Cervical Cancer: The Open-Label Randomized Phase III Trial JCOG0505. J Clin Oncol [Internet]. 2015 Mar 2 [cited 2015 Mar 13]; Available from: http://www.ncbi.nlm.nih.gov/pubmed/25732161

[51] University of Liverpool. HIV drug interactions [Internet]. 2015 [cited 2015 Mar 11]. Available from: http://www.hiv-druginteractions.org/Interactions.aspx

[52] NIH. HIV drugs [Internet]. Understanding HIV treatment. 2015 [cited 2015 Mar 10]. Available from: http://www.niaid.nih.gov/topics/HIVAIDS/Understanding/Treatment/Pages/arvDrugClasses.aspx

[53] NIH. Approved HIV medicines [Internet]. AIDS information. 2015 [cited 2015 Mar 11]. Available from: http://aidsinfo.nih.gov/education-materials/fact-sheets/19/58/fda-approved-hiv-medicines#

[54] Vaclavikova R, Soucek P, Svobodova L, Anzenbacher P, Simek P, Guengerich FP, et al. Different in vitro metabolism of paclitaxel and docetaxel in humans, rats, pigs, and minipigs. Drug Metab Dispos. 2004;32(6):666–74.

[55] Rubinstein PG, Aboulafia DM, Zloza A. Malignancies in HIV / AIDS: from epidemiology to therapeutic challenges. 2014;(September 2013).

Chapter 14

Sentinel Lymph Node Detection in Early Stage Cervical Cancer

Elisa Moreno-Palacios, Elsa Delgado,
Javier De Santiago and Ignacio Zapardiel

Additional information is available at the end of the chapter

http://dx.doi.org/10.5772/61099

Abstract

Worldwide, cervical cancer is the fourth most common malignancy among women. Radical hysterectomy and pelvic lymphadenectomy is the standard treatment for early stage cervical cancer. If lymph node metastasis is present at the time of diagnosis, 5-year survival rate drops from 90% to 57%. The risk of lymph node metastases in women with early stage cervical cancer is approximately 15%, and determines the use of adjuvant treatment. Over 80% of patients do not benefit from pelvic lymphadenectomy, but may suffer from adverse complications or sequelae such as lymphedema, lymphocyst formation, and neurovascular and ureteral injury. The sentinel lymph node is the first node to which metastatic disease will spread from a primary tumor. The clinical benefits of biopsy of only the sentinel lymph node includes a significant reduction in the adverse effects of complete lymphadenectomy. The specific benefits of sentinel lymph node detection in early stage cervical cancer includes improved identification of metastatic lymph nodes through ultrastaging and identification of alternate lymph node drainage sites, as well as the possibility of intraoperative frozen section analysis, which may be used to guide surgical management. Sentinel lymph node detection in early stage cervical cancer could become the standard of care in the near future.

Keywords: Cervical cancer, sentinel lymph node, lymphadenectomy, ultrastaging, micrometastasis

1. Introduction

Worldwide, cervical cancer is the fourth most common cancer among women, after breast, colorectal, and lung cancers. Almost 70% of the global burden occurs in developing countries, where it accounts for almost 12% of all female malignancies, being a major public health problem in many developing countries [1]. It is well known that the most important cause of cervical cancer is the presence of a persistent papillomavirus infection [2]. The risk factors for developing cervical cancer are the same as those for acquiring the human papillomavirus (HPV) infection, such as early age intercourse, multiple sexual partners, and sexual contact with high-risk men. HPV type 16 and 18 are responsible for approximately 70–75% of all cervical tumors [3].

However, long-term (1992-2010) cancer incidence trends for all racial and ethnic groups show that cervical cancer has experienced the largest decrease in incidence among women [4]. This decrease in incidence is related mostly to cervical cancer screening programs with Papanicolaou smears and HPV DNA cervical detection. Moreover, cervical cancer screening programs are associated with a potentially significant reduction in the diagnosis of advanced cervical cancers and death. Cervical cancer screening is well established in developed countries, but it is still taken of in developing countries.

Most developed countries have introduced HPV vaccination in their vaccination calendar, expecting to lower the incidence of cervical cancer. However, cervical cancer still represents a health problem in developed countries with 54,517 new cases diagnosed and 24,874 deaths from this disease every year in Europe [5].

2. Diagnosis

Early stage cervical cancer is commonly asymptomatic, diagnosed by pathological Papanicolaou smears. Advanced cervical cancer can present with symptoms such as abnormal vaginal bleeding, intercourse bleeding, dyspareunia, or pelvic plain.

The diagnosis of cervical cancer requires histological confirmation in all cases. If the patient presents with a macroscopic cervical lesion, a direct biopsy ought to be performed. If changes are shown in the cytological study but there is no macroscopic lesion in the cervix a colposcopy should be carried out. If the colposcopy findings are suspicious of malignancy directed biopsies ought to be taken, on the other hand if the colposcopy doesn't present any alterations, an endocervical curettage is indicated. If microscopic cervical invasive lesions are present a conization is required for tumor staging.

There are three categories of epithelial tumor of the cervix recognized by the WHO: squamous, glandular (adenocarcinoma), and other epithelial tumors including neuroendocrine tumors and undifferentiated tumors. Squamous cell carcinoma accounts for approximately 70–80% of all cervical cancers, and adenocarcinoma for 10–15%. Neuroendocrine tumors of the cervix are highly aggressive, rare tumors with a prognosis worse than stage-comparable undifferentiated squamous cell carcinoma of the cervix, and have a different therapeutic management [6]. In this chapter we will be referring to squamous and adenocarcinomas of the cervix exclusively.

The histological report of the biopsy and/or conization of the cervix should include the following information: histological type, differentiation grade, tumor size, length of stromal invasion, and the presence or absence of lymph-vascular space invasion (LVSI). Pathological information is very important for the tumor risk assessment.

3. Tumor staging

Cervical cancer FIGO classification is based on clinical examination, considering the tumors size, vaginal and parametrial involvement, bladder/rectum extension and distant metastasis. If the clinical examination is difficult or uncertain considering vaginal and/or parametrial involvement, it should be performed under anesthesia.

To determine the tumor's extension, various imaging tests are helpful, such as computed tomography (CT) scan, magnetic resonance imaging (MRI), and positron emission tomography (PET-CT). CT scan, to detect pathological loco-regional lymph nodes. While MR imaging is suited for examining soft tissue alterations, helping to determine the size, degree of stromal invasion, possible parametrial involvement, possible vaginal infiltration, and pelvic extension of the tumor. PET-CT imaging is known to determine accurately the extent of the disease, mainly by detecting possible metastatic lymph nodes and distant metastatic disease.

Cervical cancer FIGO stages IA, IB, and IIA are considered early stage tumors (Table 1). Approximately 44% of all cervical cancers are diagnosed in the early stages. Stage IA tumors are defined as invasive carcinomas that present with a stromal invasion of less than 5mm, and a horizontal extension of less than 7mm. Stage IB tumors are defined as invasive carcinomas limited to the cervix that present with a stromal invasion and a horizontal extension greater than 5mm and 7mm, respectively. Stage IIA tumors are defined as invasive carcinomas that invade beyond the uterus but do not involve the parametrium or the lower third of the vagina.

The lymph node status is not included in the FIGO staging system (Table 1), although it is the most important independent prognostic factor in early stage cervical cancer. If lymph node metastases are present at the time of diagnosis, the 5-year survival rate drops substantially. In stages IB-IIA, the 5-year survival rate drops from 88%–95% without lymph node metastasis to 51–78% with lymph node metastasis [7].

To determine the lymph node status, several imaging tests have been used, including CT and MRI. The major problem of the CT scan and the MRI is that these imaging tests only detect changes in the size and form of the lymph nodes and are not able to distinguish between metastasis and inflammation of the lymph nodes, presenting both low sensitivity and specificity. More recently, PET-CT has been seen to accurately determine the extent of the disease, particularly determining the lymph node status, with a sensitivity of 53–73% and a specificity as high as 90–97% [8,9]. Although, PET-TC presents higher sensitivity and specificity than CT and MRI, it is known to detect only lymph node metastases larger than 6mm, possibly not

International Federation of Gynecology and Obstetrics Staging of Carcinoma of the Cervix	
Stage O	Carcinoma in situ, intraepithelial carcinoma; Cases of stage O should not be included in any therapeutic statistics for invasive carcinoma.
Stage I	The carcinoma is strictly confined to the cervix (extension to the corpus should be disregarded.)
Stage IA	Invasive cancer identified only microscopically. All gross lesions, even with superficial invasion, are stage IB cancers. Invasion is limited to measured stromal invasion with a maximum depth of 5 mm and no wider than 7 mm. (The depth of invasion should not be more than 5 mm taken from the base of the epithelium, either surface or glandular; from which it originates. Vascular space involvement, either venous or lymphatic, should not alter the staging.)
Stage IAl	Measured invasion of stroma no greater than 3 mm in depth and no wider than 7 mm.
Stage IA2	Measured invasion of stroma greater than 3 mm and rio greater than 5 mm in depth and no wider than 7 mm.
Stage IB	Clinical lesions confined tothe cervix or preclinical lesions greater than IA.
Stage IBl	Clinical lesions no greateithan 4 cm in size.
Stage IB2	Clinical lesions greater than 4 cm in size.
Stage II	The carcinoma extends beyond the cervix, but has not extended onto the pelvic wall; the carcinoma involves the vagina but not far as the lower third.
Stage IIA	No obvious parametrial involvement.
Stage IIB	Obvious parametrial involvement. The carcinoma has extended onto the pelvic wall; on rectal examination there is no cancer-free space between the tumor and the pelvic wall; the tumor involves the lower third of the vagina; all cases with a hydronephrosis or nonfunctioning kidney should be included, unless they are known to be due to another cause.
Stage III	No extension onto the pelvic wall, but involvement of the lower third of the vagina.
Stage IIIA	Extension onto the pelvic wall or h:ydronephrosis or nonfunctioning kidney.
Stage IIIB	The carcinoma has extended beyond the true pelvis or has clinically involved the mucosa of the bladder or rectum.
StageIV	The carcinoma has extended beyond the true pelvis or has clinically involved the mucosa of the bladder or rectum.
Stage IVA	Spread of the growth to adjacent organs.
Stage IVB	Spread to distant organs.

Table 1. FIGO stage classification.

accurately detecting lymph node metastases in a high percentage of patients. Until the present moment, pelvic lymphadenectomy has been the standard surgical procedure for the assessment of the lymph node status in early stage cervical cancer, being an integral component of the definitive surgical management.

4. Treatment

There are several treatment options for cervical cancer, depending on the stage, the prognostic factors, and the wish to preserve fertility of the patient.

In early stage cervical cancer, surgery is considered the standard treatment, although radiotherapy is equally effective, only differing in terms of morbidity and complications. Surgery offers benefits over radiotherapy in early stage cervical cancer, such as ovarian function preservation, maintenance of a more functional vagina, and facilitation of the knowledge of

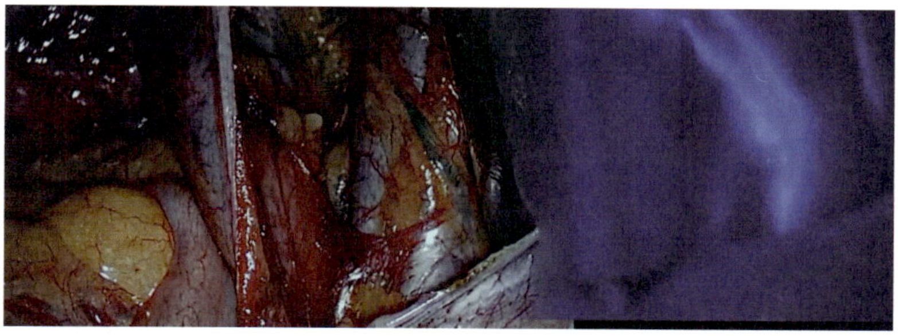

Figure 5. Lymphatic channels with fluorescein.

pathological prognostic factors. In locally advanced stages, a combination of radiotherapy and chemotherapy is the standard treatment.

Fertility-preserving surgery, consisting of radical or simple trachelectomy can be offered to young patients with early stage cervical cancer with a strong wish to preserve their fertility [10].

The goal of radical hysterectomy or radical trachelectomy is to remove the tumor with free margins by excising the uterus, cervix, and parametrium. Pelvic lymphadenectomy is performed to determine the presence or absence of lymph node metastasis, for both prognostic and therapeutic planning. Pelvic lymphadenectomy is a mere staging surgical procedure. In the absence of lymph node metastasis, pelvic lymphadenectomy has no therapeutic effect, with potential complications and associated sequelae.

There are different possible surgical approaches such as laparotomy, laparoscopy, or vaginal surgery. All surgical approaches are considered comparable in terms of oncological results when carried out by experienced surgeons. Minimally invasive surgery (laparoscopy) shows the same efficiency as conventional laparotomy, with lesser blood loss, shorter hospital stay, and lower perioperative morbidity [11].

The risk of lymph node metastasis in early stage cervical cancer is approximately 15%. Consequently, 85% of patients with early stage cervical cancer not only do not benefit from the pelvic lymphadenectomy, but can also suffer complications and morbidity. Pelvic lymphadenectomy is associated with a 4% risk of intraoperative complications such as vascular and neurological lesions, as well as long-term complications, especially lymphocyst formation and lymphedema [12]. Lymphocyst formation occurs in up to 30% of the patients subjected to a pelvic lymphadenectomy. Lymphedema of the lower abdomen, pubis, and lower extremities occurs in 25% of the patients, more frequently in those patients that receive adjuvant radiotherapy after surgery [13]. These complications are very hard to treat and can produce an important impact in the patient's quality of life [14].

Surgery is not recommended in patients with early stage cervical cancer who present with poor prognostic factors. There are pathological factors associated with high risk of relapse such as positive or close margins, metastatic lymph nodes, or microscopic parametrial involvement. If one or more of these poor prognostic factors are present at the time of diagnosis, chemoradiotherapy is indicated. Chemo-radiation therapy in high-risk patients is associated with better 4-year overall survival and progression-free survival [15].

Patients with metastatic pelvic lymph nodes are at risk of having para-aortic metastatic lymph nodes. In order to determine the fields of radiation, a para-aortic lymphadenectomy ought to be performed [16]. Radiotherapy administration after radical hysterectomy increases the risk of radiotherapy-related complications, especially intestinal complications by adhesion formation.

A correct pre-therapeutic evaluation is needed to select patients who will benefit from receiving radio-chemotherapy. Radical hysterectomy is not recommended in early stage cervical cancer that presents poor prognostic factors, such as lymph node metastasis, due to the fact that adjuvant radiotherapy and chemotherapy are required in an attempt to improve survival. The objective of avoiding surgery is to prevent the addition of morbidity caused by the association of radiotherapy and surgery.

5. Sentinel lymph node biopsy

Sentinel lymph node (SLN) is defined as the first node to which metastatic disease will spread from a primary tumor. Consequently, in the absence of metastasis in the sentinel lymph node, all other lymph nodes will also be free of disease. Therefore, if the sentinel lymph node has no trace of disease, lymphadenectomy can be avoided, reducing the morbidity associated with a complete lymphadenectomy.

Sentinel lymph node detection was first described by Cabanas in penile cancer [17]. Since then it has been described in multiples tumors, being the standard of care in melanoma, breast, and vulvar cancer, reducing significantly the morbidity associated with the performance of a complete lymphadenectomy in these patients.

Sentinel lymph nodes are identified by the injection of dye and/or a radioactive tracer around the tumor site. In cervical cancer, the sentinel lymph node is detected by injecting Technetium (Tc-99), blue dye, or both into the cervix. Protocols of detection vary in different studies, reporting that the highest detection rate is found when the combination of Tc-99 and blue dye is used [18]. The cervix point of injection varies in different studies. In some studies, the tracer is injected submucosally into the four quadrants of the cervix, and in others the tracer is injected submucosally into the 3 and 9 o'clock of the cervix; no significant differences have been found between these two techniques [9, 18].

After the radiotracer is injected, a lymphoscintigraphic localization imaging can be conducted. Lymphoscintigraphy is an imaging technique used to identify the lymph drainage basin, the sentinel lymph node, the location of the sentinel lymph node, the number of sentinel lymph nodes, and possible secondary drainage. Lymphoscintigraphy helps the surgeon to identify and localize the sentinel lymph node during the surgical procedure [19].

Different protocols of radiotracer injection and subsequent lymphoscintigraphic imaging have been described in the literature. Protocols differ in the time frame from which the radiotracer is injected till the surgery is performed, defining long and short protocols. In the long protocols the radiotracer is injected the day before surgery and lymphoscintigraphy is performed 1h after the injection [20]. In the short protocol the radiotracer is injected between 2 and 4 hours before surgery, and the lymphoscintigraphy is performed 20 minutes after the injection [9].

The blue dye is injected to the cervix in the surgery room after the anesthetic induction is performed, with the same technique as the radiotracer was injected.

The first step of the surgery is to look for the sentinel lymph node. The sentinel lymph nodes are identified by tracing the lymphatic chains with the gamma probe, identifying nodes with radioactive counts greater than five times the background count (Figure 1). The pelvic sidewalls, presacral, and para-aortic lymph chains should be scanned to identify "hot spots" by the gamma probe and/or by identifying blue-stained lymphatic channels and lymph nodes (Figures 2 and 3). Lymph nodes that appear "hot", blue, or both are identified as sentinel lymph nodes, and are removed (Figures 4 and 5). The sentinel lymph nodes are sent for intraoperative pathological review. Lymph nodes that appear to be grossly abnormal should be also removed, whether "hot", blue, or not, since the lymphatic channels may be obstructed by tumor, and the lymphatic drainage and tracer may be bypassing such nodes.

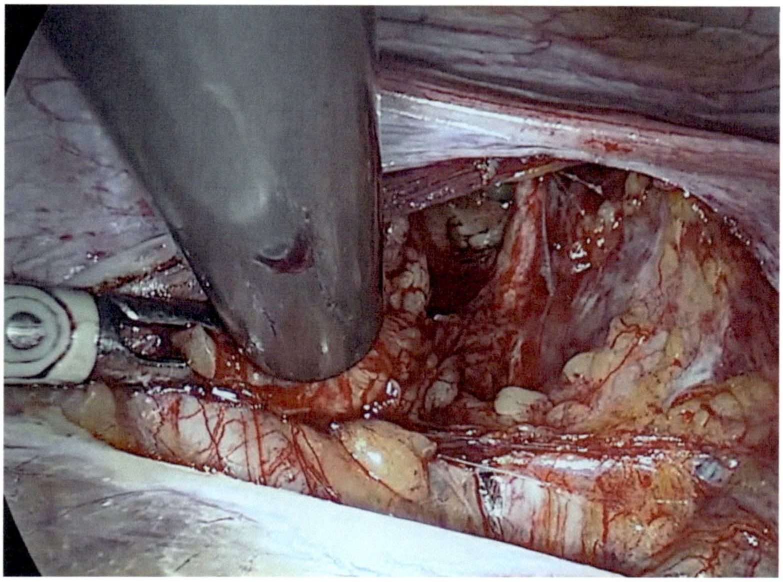

Figure 1. Detection of the sentinel lymph node with the gamma probe.

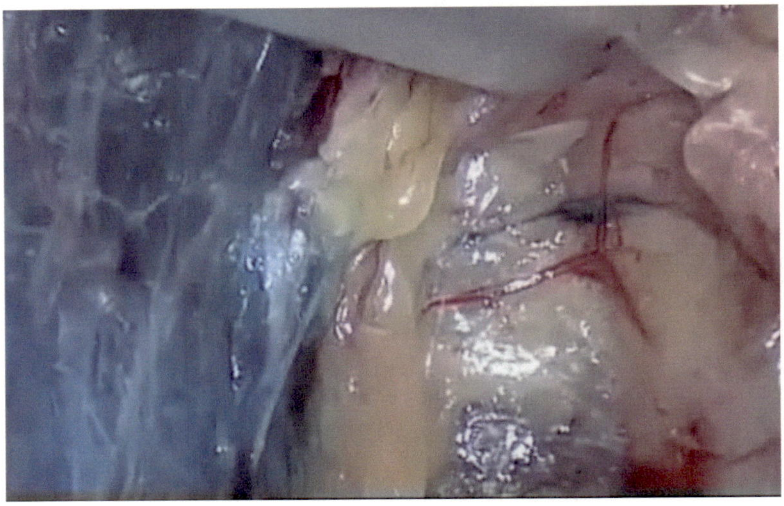

Figure 2. Blue chain of a sentinel lymph node.

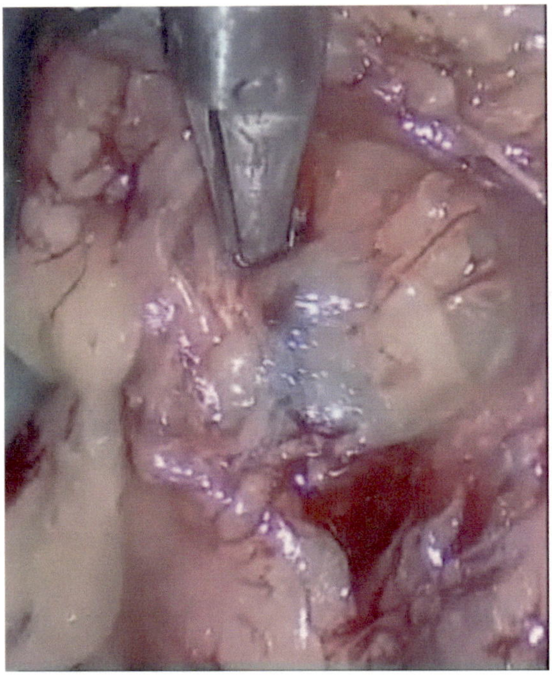

Figure 3. Blue sentinel lymph node.

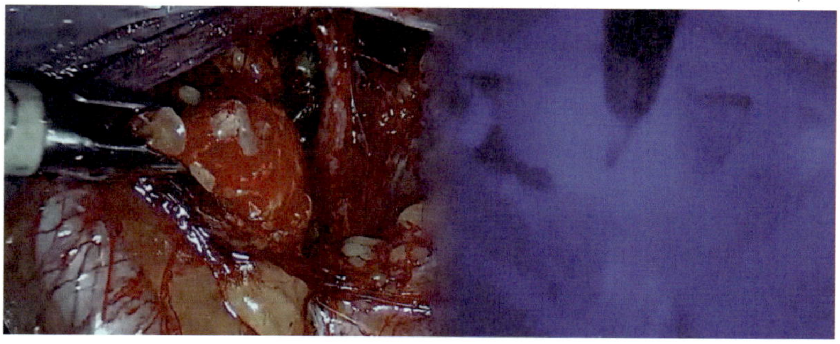

Figure 4. Resection of a blue and "hot" sentinel lymph node.

The cervix is a midline structure presenting a bilateral lymphatic drainage. The sentinel lymph node must be detected bilaterally in order to reduce the false negative rate. If no sentinel node is detected on one side, a complete lymphadenectomy must be performed on that side.

Sentinel lymph node detection in early stage cervical cancer presents several advantages over common pelvic lymphadenectomy [21]. First, it permits an intraoperative analysis of the node. Second, this technique can detect aberrant lymphatic drainage. And third, it permits ultra-staging of the sentinel lymph node and detection of micrometastasis and isolated tumor cells (ITCs).

As mentioned earlier, the association of radiotherapy and radical hysterectomy causes a higher risk of radiotherapy-related complications. To avoid the increase of morbidity caused by the association of treatments, a possibility is to perform the complete surgery in two phases instead of one. First, the pelvic lymphadenectomy can be carried out, waiting one or two weeks to obtain the definitive pathological report. If the lymph nodes are reported as negative a second surgery, a radical hysterectomy or trachelectomy, is performed. With the sentinel lymph node technique, information on the lymph node status is available in the operating room during the surgical procedure, permitting changes in the therapeutic management of the patient if necessary. If the sentinel lymph node is informed as metastatic, it is possible to complete the para-aortic lymphadenectomy as one procedure, not perform the hysterectomy, and avoid increased morbidity. Sentinel lymph node detection permits triaging patients toward surgery or chemo-radiation therapy, as well as selecting candidates for fertility-preserving surgery.

Aberrant lymphatic drainage or unusual locations of metastatic lymph nodes are due to those sentinel lymph nodes that are detected in lymphatic chains, which are not typically removed with the standard pelvic lymphadenectomy, as can be the presacral nodes or the common iliac nodes. Consequently, if a standard pelvic lymphadenectomy were to be performed without the sentinel lymph node detection technique, these metastatic nodes would not be detected. Bats et al. detected metastatic sentinel lymph nodes in an unexpected territory in up to 15% of the patients in which the sentinel lymph node technique was performed, and they concluded that the sentinel lymph node detection technique contributed to improved nodal staging [22].

Ultrastaging is the pathological process of studying the sentinel lymph nodes, consisting of a multiple serial sectioning with immunohistochemical assessment. Pathological ultrastaging permits the detection of low volume disease, which includes micrometastasis and ITC, as defined for breast cancer by the American Joint Committee of Cancer (AJCC). Macrometastasis was defined as tumor deposit greater than 2mm in diameter, micrometastasis was defined as tumor deposit between 0.2 to 2mm in diameter, and isolated tumor cells were defined as tumor deposits no larger than 0.2mm [23]. The importance of the detection of low volume disease in cervical cancer is its relationship with poor prognosis. In a study published in 2012 by Cibula et al. [24] that included 645 patients, it was observed that the presence of micrometastasis was associated with a significant reduction in the overall survival similar to those patients that presented macrometastasis, while no increased risk was found in those patients that presented ITC. Micrometastases are being detected in the sentinel lymph node in 4–15% of the patients, depending on the study [25].

Ultrastaging is a time-consuming and costly technique, not feasible for the analysis of all the lymph nodes obtained after a pelvic lymphadenectomy, but it is possible if only two to four nodes are studied with this technique. Detection of SLN and subsequent ultrastaging may detect a group of patients that would be overlooked with the standard pathological study of the pelvic lymphadenectomy nodes, although they present prognosis similar to those patients with macrometastasis. These findings highlight the importance of the SLN detection in early stage cervical cancer.

The presence of non-diagnosed micrometastasis or aberrant metastatic lymph nodes could explain the 15% of patients with an early stage cervical cancer with apparently no poor prognosis factors at diagnosis, that recur in the follow-up.

The sentinel lymph node detection has the potential to increase sensitivity in the detection of lymph node metastasis by detecting aberrant lymphatic drainage and micrometastasis [26]. Data of more than 2000 patients have been subjected to the sentinel node technique In a review published by Eiriksson et al. [9], sentinel lymph node detection in tumors of less than 2 cm presents a sensitivity of 98.2% and a negative predictive value of 99.6%, with a false negative rate of less than 5% when each hemipelvis is interpreted independently.

6. Conclusion

Sentinel lymph node detection permits minimizing surgical morbidity while maximizing the pathologic information of nodal status in patients with cervical cancer. Sentinel lymph node detection could become the standard of care in early stage cervical cancer in a close the future.

Author details

Elisa Moreno-Palacios*, Elsa Delgado, Javier De Santiago and Ignacio Zapardiel

*Address all correspondence to: elimorepal@gmail.com

Gynecologic Oncology Unit, La Paz University Hospital, Madrid, Spain

References

[1] Ferlay J, Soerjomataram I, Dikshit R, et al. Cancer incidence and mortality worldwide: sources, methods and major patterns in GLOBOCAN 2012. Int J Cancer. 2015;136:E359–E386.

[2] Kane MA. Preventing cancer with vaccines: progress in the global control of cancer. Cancer Prev Res (Phila). 2012 Jan;5(1):24–29.

[3] Cuschieri KS, Whitley MJ, Cubie HA. Human papillomavirus type specific DNA and RNA persistence- implications for cervical disease progression and monitoring. J Med Virol. 2004 May;73(1):65–70.

[4] Edwards BK, Noone AM, Mariotto AB, et al. Annual report to the nation on the status of cancer, 1975–2010, featuring prevalence of comorbidity and impact on survival among persons with lung, colorectal, breast, or prostate cancer. Cancer. 2014 May 1;120(9):1290–1314.

[5] Sankaranarayanan R, Nene BM, Shastri SS, et al. HPV screening for cervical cancer in rural India. N Engl J Med. 2009 Apr 2;360(14):1385–1394.

[6] Gardner GJ, Reidy-Lagunes D, Gehrig PA. Neuroendocrine tumors of the gynecologic tract: a society of gynecologic oncology (SGO) clinical document. Gynecol Oncol. 2011 Jul;122(1):190–198.

[7] Kim SM, Choi HS, Byun JS. Overall 5-year survival rate and prognostic factors in patients with stage IB and IIA cervical cancer treated by radical hysterectomy and pelvic lymph node dissection. Int J Gynecol Cancer. 2000 Jul;10(4):305–312.

[8] Patel CN, Nazir SA, Khan Z, et al. 18F-FDG PET/CT of cervical carcinoma. AJR Am J Roentgenol. 2011 May;196(5):1225–1233.

[9] Eiriksson LR, Covens A. Sentinel lymph node mapping in cervical cancer: the future? BJOG. 2012 Jan;119(2):129–133.

[10] Rob L, Skapa P, Robova H. Fertility-sparing surgery in patients with cervical cancer. Lancet Oncol. 2011 Feb;12(2):192–200.

[11] Wright JD, Herzog TJ, Neugut AI, et al. Comparative effectiveness of minimally invasive and abdominal radical hysterectomy for cervical cancer. Gynecol Oncol. 2012 Oct;127(1):11–17.

[12] Querleu D, Leblanc E, Cartron G, et al. Audit of preoperative and early complications of laparoscopic lymph node dissection in 1000 gynecologic cancer patients. Am J Obstet Gynecol. 2006 Nov;195(5):1287–1292.

[13] Kim HS, Sardi JE, Katsumata N, et al. Efficacy of neoadjuvant chemotherapy in patients with FIGO stage IB1 to IIA cervical cancer: an international collaborative meta-analysis. Eur J Surg Oncol. 2013 Feb;39(2):115–124.

[14] Gonçalves V. Long-term quality of life in gynecological cancer survivors. Curr Opin Obstet Gynecol. 2010 Feb;22(1):30–35.

[15] Peters WA, Liu PY, Barrett RJ, et al. Concurrent chemotherapy and pelvic radiation therapy compared with pelvic radiation therapy alone as adjuvant therapy after radical surgery in high-risk early-stage cancer of the cervix. J Clin Oncol. 2000 Apr;18(8): 1606–1613.

[16] Stryker JA, Mortel R. Survival following extended field irradiation in carcinoma of cervix metastatic to para-aortic lymph nodes. Gynecol Oncol. 2000 Dec;79(3):399–405.

[17] Cabanas RM. An approach for the treatment of penile carcinoma. Cancer. 1977 Feb; 39(2):456–466.

[18] Selman TJ, Mann C, Zamora J, et al. Diagnostic accuracy of tests for lymph node status in primary cervical cancer: a systematic review and meta-analysis. CMAJ. 2008 Mar 25;178(7):855–862.

[19] Diaz JP, Gemignani ML, Pandit-Taskar N et al. Sentinel lymph node biopsy in the management of early-stage cervical carcinoma. Gynecol Oncol. 2011 Mar;120(3):347–352.

[20] Bats AS, Frati A, Froissart M, et al. Feasibility and performance of lymphoscintigraphy in sentinel lymph node biopsy for early cervical cancer: results of the prospective multicenter SENTICOL study. Ann Nucl Med. 2015 Jan;29(1):63–70.

[21] Altgassen C, Hertel H, Brandstädt A, et al. Multicenter validation study of the sentinel lymph node concept in cervical cancer: AGO Study Group. J Clin Oncol. 2008 Jun 20;26(18):2943–2951.

[22] Bats AS, Mathevet P, Buenerd A, et al. The sentinel node technique detects unexpected drainage pathways and allows nodal ultrastaging in early cervical cancer: insights from the multicenter prospective SENTICOL study. Ann Surg Oncol. 2013 Feb;20(2): 413–422.

[23] Schwartz GF[1], Giuliano AE, Veronesi U. Proceedings of the consensus conference on the role of sentinel lymph node biopsy in carcinoma of the breast, April 19–22, 2001, Philadelphia, Pennsylvania. Cancer. 2002 May 15;94(10):2542–2551.

[24] Cibula D, Abu-Rustum NR, Dusek L, et al. Prognostic significance of low volume sentinel lymph node disease in early-stage cervical cancer. Gynecol Oncol. 2012 Mar; 124(3):496–501.

[25] Daraï E, Rouzier R, Ballester M, et al. Sentinel lymph node biopsy in gynaecological cancers: the importance of micrometastases in cervical cancer. Surg Oncol. 2008 Sep; 17(3):227–235.

[26] Gortzak-Uzan L, Jimenez W, Nofech-Mozes S, et al. Sentinel lymph node biopsy vs. pelvic lymphadenectomy in early stage cervical cancer: is it time to change the gold standard? Gynecol Oncol. 2010 Jan;116(1):28–32.

Chapter 15

Adenocarcinoma of the Endometrium — The Art of Its Diagnosis

Manoel Afonso Guimarães Gonçalves and Fernando Anschau

Additional information is available at the end of the chapter

http://dx.doi.org/10.5772/61578

Abstract

The diagnostic process begins at the first meeting with the patient, where we must relate the symptoms and signs associated with endometrial disease. Communication skills are fundamental for excellence in medical care. Even with the development and improvement of new technologies in recent decades, be it endoscopy, ultrasound, computed tomography or magnetic resonance imaging, the communication is also essential. We must have skills to recognize and elucidate a wide variety of signs and symptoms when we take a history and do a physical examination of the patient, where abnormal uterine bleeding is the first main sign that can lead to an early diagnosis of endometrial cancer. The endometrium, as every target organ of steroid hormones, shows involutional changes during ovarian failure. In peri-menopause, however, tissue hyperactivity stages occur with some frequency, showing a marked endometrial sensitivity to hormonal fluctuations, whether on an absolute or relative level. Irregular blood loss occurs in many women during this period, and although being most times of functional origin, it requires investigation. It is noteworthy that the most frequent cause of abnormal bleeding of organic origin in menopause is endometrial. Endometrial pathologies appear with advancing age. Therefore an appropriate workup should diagnose or rule out disease at this site. Thus, preventive measures should be adopted, such as screening and early diagnosis, and the best treatment for the patient should be established.

Keywords: Endometrial cancer, diagnosis, new technologies, staging, prognosis, treatment

1. Introduction

The diagnostic process begins at the first meeting with the patient, where we must relate the symptoms and signs associated with endometrial disease.

Communication skills are fundamental for excellence in medical care. Even with the development and improvement of new technologies in recent decades, be it endoscopy, ultrasound, computed tomography, or magnetic resonance imaging, the communication is also essential.

We must have skills to recognize and elucidate a wide variety of signs and symptoms when we take a history and do a physical examination of the patient, where abnormal uterine bleeding is the first main sign that can lead to an early diagnosis of endometrial cancer.[1]

The endometrium, as every target organ of steroid hormones, shows involutional changes during ovarian failure. In perimenopause, however, tissue hyperactivity stages occur with some frequency, showing a marked endometrial sensitivity to hormonal fluctuations, whether on an absolute or relative level. Irregular blood loss occurs in many women during this period, and although being most times of functional origin, it requires investigation. It is noteworthy that the most frequent cause of abnormal bleeding of organic origin in menopause is endometrial. Endometrial pathologies appear with advancing age. Therefore an appropriate workup should diagnose or rule out disease at this site. Thus, preventive measures should be adopted, such as screening and early diagnosis, and the best treatment for the patient should be established.[2]

The annual incidence of endometrial carcinoma is 2 in 100,000 women under 40 years and 40 to 50 per 100,000 women between the sixth and eighth decades, and it is expected to gradually increase due to obesity and increased longevity, especially in North America and Western Europe. In Brazil, the highest incidences are in the South and Southeast regions.[3, 4] In the United States, endometrial cancer is the most common gynecologic malignancy, and it accounted for about 39,080 new cases and 7,400 deaths from cancer in 2007.[5] The signs are early and the most common is vaginal bleeding after menopause. When diagnosed early, about 80% are confined to the uterus, in the early stages, with good outcome and low mortality. In Brazil, it is the second most frequent pelvic malignancy, with an incidence of 5.7 per 100,000 women and mortality estimated at 1.6 per 100,000 women.[6] Staging of the International Federation of Gynecology and Obstetrics (FIGO), introduced in 1988 and updated in 2009, is defined by total abdominal hysterectomy, bilateral salpingo-oophorectomy, pelvic lymphadenectomy, and periaortic and peritoneal cytology, where prognostic factors include age, grade and histological type of tumor, depth of invasion into the myometrium, cervical involvement, and the presence of lymph node metastases.

2. Diagnosis

The diagnosis is histological but should be considered based on the symptoms and physical examination. The main symptom is abnormal uterine bleeding. Other findings associated with the disease are: heaviness in the lower abdomen, pelvic pain, presence of pyometra, hematometra, presence of atypical glandular cells in cervical Pap smear, menorrhagia, and intermenstrual bleeding. Later symptoms are pain in the lower abdomen, foul-smelling secretion, urinary or intestinal disorders, and weight loss.

In postmenopausal women with uterine bleeding, premenopausal women with abnormal uterine bleeding and before hematometra and pyometra especially in older women, it is imperative to evaluate the endometrial cavity. This evaluation can be performed by blind endometrial biopsy or through hysteroscopy or curettage after gynecological examination. Endometrial biopsy is simple to perform and should be considered of value only when positive for malignancy, because it could give false-negative results. Hysteroscopy has better performance, which surpasses curettage in the diagnosis, where possible visualization of the uterine cavity leads to fewer false-negative results as curettage. If the diagnostic biopsy is atypical hyperplasia, it is necessary to evaluate the whole endometrial cavity to rule out carcinoma.

Transvaginal ultrasound in postmenopausal women, taking into account a cutoff of 5 mm endometrial thickness, has a 96% sensitivity for endometrial cancer detection. However, there is no evidence showing that the use of ultrasound in screening asymptomatic women decreases mortality.[7]

A cervical Pap smear should not be considered a screening method or diagnosis of endometrial cancer.[8] There is no indication for screening for endometrial carcinoma by any method in asymptomatic women with or without medium or high risk factors for endometrial carcinoma, such as hormone therapy with estrogen, tamoxifen users, late menopause, nulliparity, infertility or chronic anovulation, obesity, diabetes, hypertension, or metabolic syndrome. It is recommended to inform these women about the risk factors and symptoms of endometrial carcinoma, such as abnormal uterine bleeding in premenopause and any bleeding after menopause, and to advise them to seek immediate medical attention.[4, 6]

Annual screening tests by endometrial biopsy should be indicated only in women ≥35 years old, with Lynch syndrome (hereditary nonpolyposis colorectal cancer, HNPCC-II) and/or a family history of carrying the mutation in the absence of confirmation of the mutation genetics, or family history with suspicion of autosomal dominant genetic predisposition.[3, 4]

Any postmenopausal bleeding should be investigated because it is the main symptom of endometrial carcinoma, and the assessment should start with ultrasound and/or endometrial biopsy, depending on the choice and ease in carrying out the procedure. The accuracy of ultrasound as to the measurement of normal endometrial thickness of ≤4–5 mm in postmenopausal women to exclude endometrial disease is very high. If the thickness is ≤4 mm, the negative predictive value (NPV) is 99.79%, and if ≤5 mm, it is 99.47%. It is rare that a woman with endometrial thickness of <4 cm has carcinoma of the endometrium, but in the presence of endometrial thickening, there are difficulties in differentiating between benign and malignant disease. Prospective studies have shown that the risk of cancer in women with bleeding and endometrial thickness of ≤4 mm is about 1 in 1,000 women.[11, 12, 13]

Endometrial aspiration biopsy (Pipelle being the most common) has been widely used because it is done on an outpatient basis and causes little discomfort to the patient. However, there are important limitations, such as small endometrial area evaluated and very variable diagnostic sensitivity. Studies have shown a rate of false-negative results of 2.5–32.4% in Pipelle biopsies for endometrial carcinoma, especially in tumors occupying <50% of the endometrial cavity, such as polyps.[13, 14]

Women with abnormal uterine bleeding should be investigated with ultrasound (US) and/or biopsy. In menopausal women, ultrasonographic endometrial thickness of ≤4–5 mm, and/or result in a negative aspiration biopsy for endometrial cancer or hyperplasia can be followed up, but should be targeted for further tests in the persistence of any bleeding.

The endoscopic hysteroscopy examination was introduced in 1864 by the English physician Pantaleoni, and with improvements mainly in optics, proved to be since the 1980s an excellent procedure for the diagnosis of diseases of the cervical canal and the uterine cavity.

Hysteroscopy is a procedure that every day reaches a greater importance in medical examination and therapeutic arsenals of gynecologists. This is because the necessary equipment has evolved systematically and quickly toward making the procedure more and more delicate and less traumatic. Among the many changes, we can highlight the wide use of hysteroscopic instrumental with 2.0- and 2.9-mm optics.[15]

Hysteroscopy allows the complete examination of the uterine cavity: its distention, morphology, and size; anterior and posterior wall, cones, and tubal ostia; and color, appearance, surface, vascularization, and thickness of the endometrial mucosa. Endometrial sampling is targeted, where the biopsy can be performed via hysteroscopy or immediately after the procedure.

In symptomatic patients, hysteroscopy combined with histological sampling is considered first-line in the diagnostic process; it is also for asymptomatic patients with abnormal endometrial cytology or ultrasound, or even with normal endometrial cells in cervicovaginal cytology.

A randomized study showed that women with abnormal uterine bleeding can start the investigation with ultrasound and endometrial Pipelle biopsy and only use hysteroscopy and/or curettage in a second option. A systematic review showed high diagnostic accuracy of hysteroscopy for cancer, with a sensitivity of 86.4% (95% CI, 84.0–88.6%) and specificity of 99.2% (95% CI, 99.1–99.3%). The sensitivity for diagnosis of benign endometrial pathology was 78.0% (95% CI, 76.3–79.6%), while specificity was 95.8% (95% CI, 95.6–96.1%), which would correspond to moderate accuracy. It is a safe procedure, with few complications and good diagnostic performance for endometrial carcinoma in women with abnormal uterine bleeding.[16] Another systematic review compared endometrial biopsy or hysteroscopy and dilatation and curettage (D&C) combined with endometrial cytology and demonstrated high diagnostic sensitivity of hysteroscopy with cytology, but cytology was more associated with sub-staging of the disease, compared with the biopsy or D&C. If the diagnostic biopsy revealed a precursor lesion, that is, atypical hyperplasia, it is necessary to evaluate the whole endometrial cavity to rule out carcinoma. The endometrial cavity should be examined in elderly women in the presence of hematometra and pyometra and in premenopausal women with abnormal uterine bleeding. Later symptoms are pain in the lower abdomen, foul-smelling secretion, urinary or intestinal disorders, and weight loss.[17]

http://dx.doi.org/10.5772/61578

Curettage and hysteroscopy have high diagnostic accuracy, but hysteroscopy is the method of choice for small and focal lesions such as polyps and can be performed on an outpatient basis. The diagnostic procedure chosen should be in accordance with its accessibility and the surgeon's experience. Hysteroscopy is considered by many authors as the gold standard for evaluation of the uterine cavity. This examination provides enormous benefits with hits in macroscopic visual information, especially when it identifies organic changes in polyps, submucosal fibroids, complete inactivity states, or atrophic endometrium (figure 1); it also shows a high success in states of high endometrial activity: complex hyperplasia with atypia or endometrial cancer (figure 2).

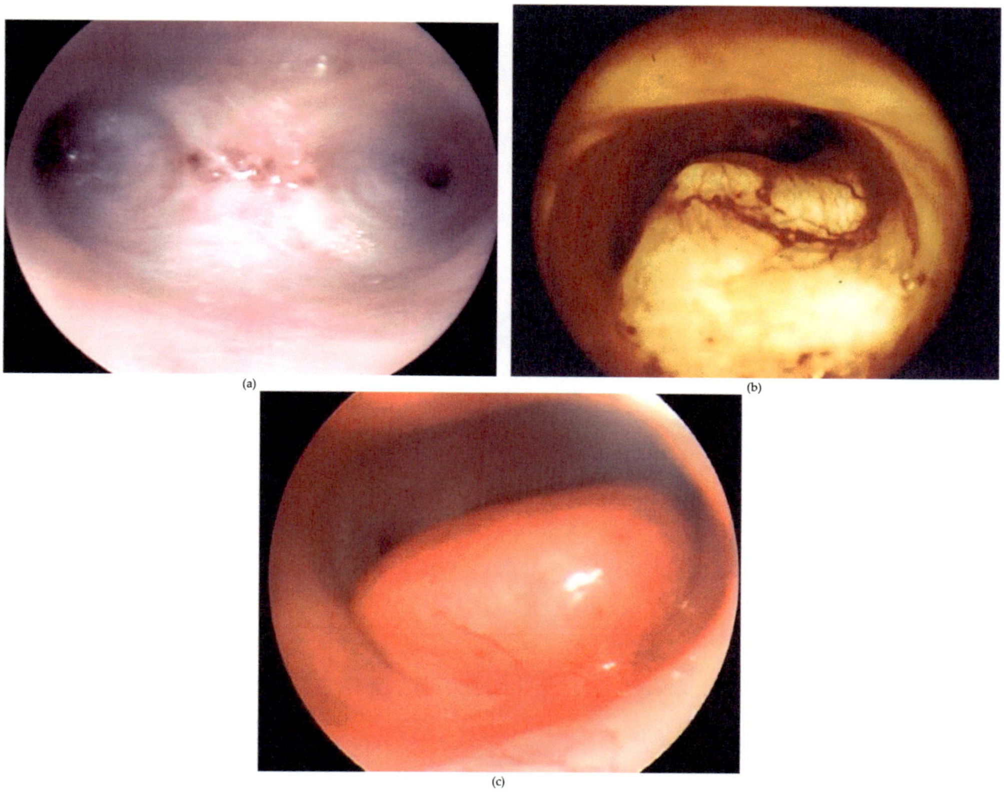

Figure 1. (a) Atrophic endometrium, (b) Submucosal fibroids, (c) Polyp

With regard to histological types, the most common is endometrioid adenocarcinoma (75–80%), where it is the most common variant of squamous differentiation. It is related to hyperestrogenism and the precursor lesion is atypical hyperplasia. Serous papilliferous (10%) and clear-cell (4%) adenocarcinomas are similar to those of the ovary and tube and may show peritoneal spread. These tumors are associated with p53 gene mutation will occur in older women, are often diagnosed at more advanced stages and have a worse prognosis. The other histological types are rarer: mucinous, squamous, and undifferentiated.[18, 19]

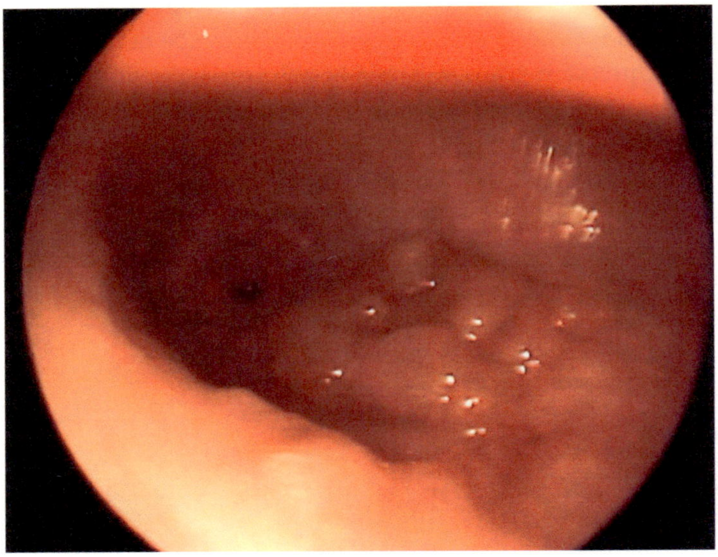

(a)

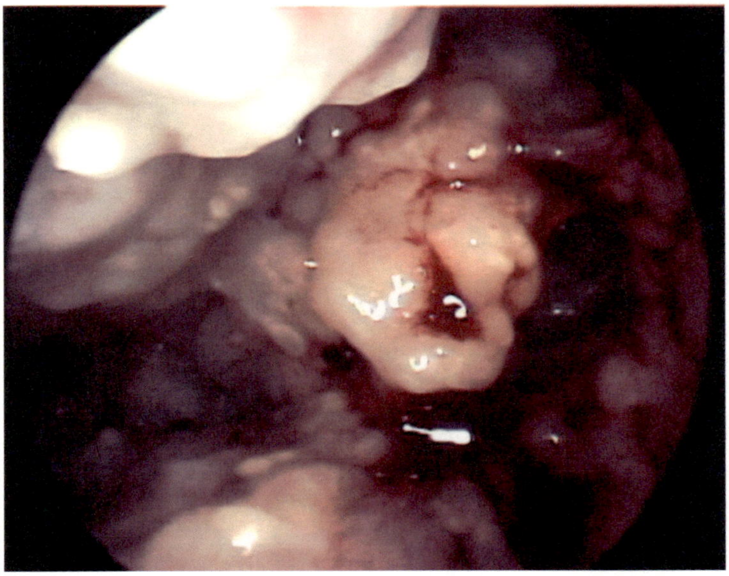

(b)

Figure 2. (a) Complex hyperplasia with atypia, (b) Endometrial cancer

Histological types

i. Endometrioid (70–80%)

- **a.** Ciliated adenocarcinoma
- **b.** Secretory adenocarcinoma

http://dx.doi.org/10.5772/61578

    c. Papillary or villoglandular adenocarcinoma

    d. Adenocarcinoma with squamous differentiation:

        1. Adenoacanthoma

        2. Adenosquamous

ii. Serous papilliferous (<10%)

iii. Mucinous (1%)

iv. Clear cells (4%)

v. Squamous cells (<1%)

vi. Mixed (10%)

vii. Undifferentiated

Adenocarcinomas should be grouped according to histopathological differentiation grade:

G1 (well differentiated); 5% or less with nonsquamous growth pattern

G2 (moderately differentiated); 6–50% with nonsquamous growth pattern

G3 (undifferentiated); more than with nonsquamous growth pattern

When nuclear atypia is inappropriate for architectural grade, increase G1 to G2 and G2 to G3.

Adenocarcinoma with squamous component is graded by the glandular component.

3. Staging

Staging begins with a general physical examination, palpation of supraclavicular and inguinal lymph nodes, vaginal examination, and digital rectal examination, eventually done under analgesia. Sampling for cervical cancer cytology, blood tests, and chest X-ray are routine. In suspected cases of bladder or rectal invasion, cystoscopy and rectosigmoidoscopy with biopsy are indicated. If the parametrium and vagina do not show neoplastic changes, surgical staging is indicated, according to the International Federation of Gynecology and Obstetrics (FIGO) (established in 1988, revised in 2009; Table 1).[8, 9] For women undergoing radiation therapy as initial treatment, FIGO clinical staging (1971) can be used, correlating with the current. The diagnostic biopsy defines the type and histological grade (Table 2); total hysterectomy with adnexectomy defines myometrial, cervical, and adnexal invasion; and peritoneal lavage defines the presence of neoplastic cells. Endometrial ablation can be performed intraoperatively, along with a biopsy of the omentum. It is only possible to prove lymph node metastasis by conducting a pelvic and para-aortic retroperitoneal lymphadenectomy in patients with poor prognostic factors. A lymph node biopsy is indicated in the presence of enlarged lymph nodes. Retroperitoneal lymphadenectomy can increase perioperative morbidity, depending on the clinical conditions of the patient and the training of the surgical team.[10, 11]

Stage	Postoperative pathological findings
I*	Tumor confined to uterine corpus
IA*	No invasion or myometrial invasion less than 50%
IB*	Myometrial invasion less than or equal to 50%
II*	Tumor invading cervical stroma, but without extending beyond uterus**
III*	Tumor local and/or regionally spreading
IIIA*	Tumor invading serosa and/or adnexa#
IIIB*	Tumor invading vagina and/or parametrium#
IIIC*	Metastasis to pelvic and/or para-aortic lymph nodes #
IIIC1*	Positive pelvic lymph nodes
IIIC2*	Positive para-aortic lymph nodes with or without positive pelvic lymph nodes
IV*	Tumor invading bladder and/or rectal mucosa and/or distant metastases
IVA*	Tumor invading bladder and/or rectal mucosa
IVB*	Distant metastases, including intra-abdominal and/or inguinal lymph node metastases

FIGO Staging – 1988, revised in 2009 [9, 10]

* G1, G2 or G3.

** Only endocervical gland involvement should be considered as stage I and no longer as stage II.

Positive cytology should be reported separately without changing the stage.

Table 1. Surgical staging of endometrial carcinoma

Clinical examination	General physical examination Examination of lymphatic drainage with palpation of supraclavicular and inguinal lymph nodes Gynecological examination Rectovaginal examination with or without analgesia
Radiological examinations	Chest X-ray
Specific examinations	Endometrial biopsy Hysteroscopy with biopsy or curettage Cystoscopy* Rectosigmoidoscopy*
Other examinations that are not considered for staging but can be done for treatment planning	Ultrasound Computed tomography Magnetic resonance Positron emission tomography Bone scintigraphy Laparoscopy Serum CA-125

*Examinations to be requested according to symptoms and clinical signs

Table 2. Examinations to be done for staging of endometrial carcinoma

A meta-analysis did not find significant differences in comparing the diagnostic accuracy of ultrasound, CT, and MRI in the staging of endometrial carcinoma, noting that the use of contrast during MRI significantly improves the performance of the method. The advantage of MRI is that it can demonstrate myometrial invasion and later stages of the disease, such as extra-uterine disease. MRI and PET/CT in patients with endometrial carcinoma were similar in the diagnosis of the primary lesion (sensitivity of 91.5 vs. 89.4%, specificity of 33.3% vs. 50.5%, accuracy of 84.9 vs. 84.9%, PPV of 91.5 vs. 93.3%, and VPN of 33.3 vs. 37.5%) and also for the detection of lymph node metastasis. The main benefit of F18-FDG PET/CT is the detection, localization, and characterization of distant metastases, including extraperitoneal metastases, and in the follow-up of recurrence. Due to the high negative predictive value in detecting lymph node metastases, it may be useful in patients with surgical contraindication. Its low positive predictive value can be related to the difficulty in differentiating reactive lymph nodes after endometrial biopsy, so PET/CT cannot replace surgical staging. While PET only demonstrates the existence of the lesion, PET/CT adds anatomic location to study. Endometrial carcinoma, similar to other tumors, has a high rate of glycolysis and uptake of FDG, a radioactive glucose analogue. There is a need for prospective studies comparing the methods, including cost-benefit assessment, so as to define the true benefits of these procedures.[7, 12, 13]

It should not be routinely used in the staging and follow-up considering the need for additional studies of the method and its high cost. Consider the use in cases of surgical and high contraindication risk of distant metastases, evaluating value for money.

4. Factors associated with prognosis

Poor prognostic factors include: serous papilliferous and clear-cell histological types; GH III tumors (poorly differentiated), which have deep myometrial invasion; cervical invasion; invasion of the vascular space; positive peritoneal cytology; and adnexal invasion. The IA G1 stage shows <5% lymph node metastases and IB G2/3 shows 5–9% positive pelvic lymph nodes and 4% para-aortic lymph nodes. However, G3 tumors, deep myometrial invasion, and/or extra-uterine disease show 20–60% pelvic lymph node metastases and 10–30% of para-aortic lymph nodes. Non-endometrioid tumors account for >50% of deaths and recurrences among endometrial carcinomas.[10, 11]

The value of lymphadenectomy is to determine the patient's prognosis and to guide adjuvant therapy, but since FIGO introduced the lymphadenectomy in 1988, there have been questions about the extent of lymphadenectomy, indications, and its risk-benefit ratio. Lymphadenectomy is performed extensively in Australia and North America. A randomized study (ASTEC) by the UK Medical Research Council found no significant differences in disease-free survival and overall survival, comparing stage I – FIGO patients who underwent pelvic lymphadenectomy or just total hysterectomy with bilateral salpingo-oophorectomy without lymphadenectomy. Those subjected to lymphadenectomy had a higher rate of postoperative complications, higher incidence of advanced disease, and IIIc stage disease. It is known that the invasion of the vascular space and positive pelvic lymph nodes are independent risk factors for metastasis in para-aortic lymph nodes (30–50% of para-aortic lymph nodes are positive in these conditions). The US National Cancer Institute's database (Surveillance, Epidemiology, and End Results program) evaluated 39,306 patients in a retrospective study comparing 12,333 with lymphadenectomy and 27,063 without lymphadenectomy and found no increase in survival in women with endometrial carcinomas of medium and high risk subjected to the procedure.[14, 17, 18]

Since FIGO staging was established in 1988 (updated in 2009), in which lymph node metastasis was categorized as IIIC, which was subdivided into IIIC1 for pelvic and lymph nodes and IIIC2 for para-aortic lymph nodes, it was suggested that pelvic lymphadenectomy be performed in patients in the early stages and the para-aortic lymphadenectomy in women with tumors with high risk of lymph node metastases, especially in the presence of positive pelvic lymph nodes, since they had clinical conditions of operability for proper staging and indication of adjuvant therapy.

Randomized studies comparing laparoscopy with laparotomy in patients with different stages of disease and variable follow-up demonstrated that the safety and efficacy of the procedures were similar and showed no significant differences in disease-free survival. However, despite not observing differences in pelvic recurrences in both groups, some reported more vaginal recurrences and laparoscopic port sites, perhaps because of increased uterine manipulation. Laparoscopy had advantages: smaller incision, better visibility of the operative field, less blood loss, less postoperative pain, faster postoperative recovery with shorter hospital stay, and faster return to normal activities without surgical limitations for obese and elderly patients. The Gynecologic Oncology Group is evaluating quality of life, disease-free survival, and overall survival in a long-term monitoring of 2616 patients, but the results of this randomized study are not yet available.[15, 16]

Laparoscopic hysterectomy is not the standard surgery for endometrial cancer. It is suggested to wait for results on survival in studies comparing laparoscopic with open surgery. It is recommended to perform laparoscopic surgeries linked to research protocols and by professionals trained in high complexity surgeries.

5. Treatment of endometrial cancer

The conventional surgical treatment of endometrial cancer is the extrafascial hysterectomy with bilateral lymphadenectomy combined or not with pelvic adnexectomy (Table 3 and Appendix). However, in the early stages, with disease limited to the uterine corpus, the role of lymphadenectomy is controversial. The results of two randomized clinical studies with patients with endometrial carcinoma in early stages showed no difference in overall survival and disease-free survival between the groups who did or did not undergo pelvic lymphadenectomy. In view of the increased morbidity that pelvic lymphadenectomy can provide and the lack of improvement in survival, this is not indicated in patients with endometrial carcinoma in early stages.[17, 30]

1. Stages I and II (occult)

IA G1: Only surgery. No indication of adjuvant radiotherapy.

IA G2: Surgery and high-dose brachytherapy in vaginal vault.

IA G3, IB G1/2/3, occult II, and serous papilliferous and clear-cell types: surgery and radiotherapy – pelvic teletherapy and vaginal vault brachytherapy.

The most important treatment is surgery: extensive longitudinal or wide transverse Maylard type incision, lavage sample for peritoneal cytology, inventory of the abdominal cavity with extrafascicular palpation of the pelvic and para-aortic lymph nodes, total hysterectomy (TH), bilateral salpingo-oophorectomy (BSO), and in some cases (Table 4) retroperitoneal lymph node biopsy and assessment of the omentum. Selective biopsy of lymph nodes routine is controversial, and a complete lymphadenectomy is indicated in the presence of poor prognostic factors and in women ≤70 years and only if there is no clinical or technical contraindication. The presence of metastases contraindicates extensive surgery, vaginal and/or laparoscopic, avoiding the risk of implants in the portals. The MRC ASTEC randomized study did not demonstrate therapeutic benefits in stage I patients subjected or not to pelvic lymphadenectomy.[17, 18] Biopsy of enlarged lymph nodes and discontinuation of the procedure are indicated if the trans-surgical pathology result is positive.

Adjuvant RT: in tumors with a good prognosis, the more frequent recurrence, that is vaginal, decreases.[19] The PORTEC randomized study of two groups after surgery without lymphadenectomy, pelvic RT compared with follow-up showed that RT decreased vaginal recurrences without survival benefits, and that survival after recurrence was significantly higher in the control group, that is, there was no benefit with external RT in tumors of low and intermediate risk.[19] Another randomized study was started of vaginal vault brachytherapy (brachy) in these cases.[20] RT decreases the incidence of local and regional recurrences but causes undesirable effects in 1–10% of patients, about 4% with intestinal complications, which can be greater than in those subjected to resection of lymph nodes.[21]1

2. Stage II

II G1/2/3: Surgery and radiotherapy – pelvic teletherapy and vaginal vault brachytherapy.

Surgery: TH + BSO or radical hysterectomy with BSO in selected cases, pelvic and para-aortic lymphadenectomy, peritoneal cytology, and biopsy of the omentum. The performance of MRI in the preoperative period may assist in the evaluation of resectability and rule out bladder invasion, especially in cases of indication for radical hysterectomy.

Adjuvant radiotherapy: pelvic teletherapy and high dose rate brachytherapy.

Intracavitary neoadjuvant radiotherapy and external radiotherapy: it may be indicated in cases of extensive cervical invasion and surgery should be performed 4–6 weeks after the end of radiotherapy to reduce intraoperative and postoperative complications: TH + BSO, peritoneal cytology, and biopsy of para-aortic lymph nodes and omentum.

3. **Stage III**

III: Surgery and radiotherapy

Only radiotherapy

Chemotherapy or hormone therapy

Surgery: If the entire tumor is resected, para-aortic lymph nodes and omentum should be biopsied.

Adjuvant RT:

IIIA: Extending to serosa or tumor implants – Pelvic teletherapy and vaginal vault brachytherapy.

IIIB: Pelvic teletherapy and brachytherapy in the entire vagina.

IIIC: Pelvic and para-aortic lymph node teletherapy and vaginal vault brachytherapy.

Only RT:

If disease unresectable: pelvic teletherapy and brachytherapy with complementation if parametrium compromised.

Chemotherapy (CT) or hormone therapy (HT):

Hormone therapy:

- Medroxyprogesterone acetate
- Megestrol acetate
- Tamoxifen

Chemotherapy:

- Doxorubicin (60 mg/m2)
- Doxorubicin + cisplatin (50 mg/m2)
- Doxorubicin + cisplatin (50 mg/m2) + paclitaxel (170 mg/m2)

It is the main treatment for extrapelvic metastases.

G1/G2 hormone receptor positive: HT with progestins (medroxyprogesterone acetate at 50–100 mg/day or megestrol acetate at 160 mg/day). Randomized studies have not shown benefits in the use of hormone therapy in overall survival.[21] G3 or serous papillary and clear-cell tumors: GOG randomized studies demonstrated antiblastic activity with doxorubicin. Adding cisplatin to doxorubicin increases the response rate and the disease-free interval but not overall survival.[22]

A randomized trial comparing doxorubicin + cisplatin with total abdomen RT demonstrated increased overall survival in III/IV patients with ≤2 cm postoperative residual disease and no parenchymal involvement of organs (overall survival of 5 years: 55% x 42%).[1] Doxorubicin, paclitaxel, and cisplatin + bone marrow stimulator produced 57% response compared to 34% responding with cisplatin and doxorubicin. The disease-free interval was 8.3 months vs. 5.3 months and overall survival 15.3 vs. 12.3 months. However, 39% moderate to severe neuropathy occurred.[24]

4. Stage IV and recurrent or refractory disease

IVA: Only radiotherapy

Chemotherapy or hormone therapy

IVB: Palliative radiotherapy

Chemotherapy or hormone therapy

Treatment is individualized depending on the patient's performance, location, and size of metastatic disease in addition to symptoms presented.

Radiation therapy can be used with symptomatic goal, such as for analgesic, decompressive, or hemostatic purposes. In extrapelvic metastases: chemotherapy (see stage III) or hormone therapy. In patients with G1/2 tumors, progestogens show response in 25–30% and a significant increase in survival, especially in those with pulmonary metastases. Tamoxifen (20 mg/day) may be indicated in the absence of response to progestogens.

Palliative RT is indicated in pelvic, lymph node, brain, or bone recurrence, and may be curative in isolated vaginal recurrences.

5. Special conditions

Diagnosis after hysterectomy: It is more frequent after vaginal prolapse surgeries and the greatest problem is usually not the removal of adnexa, where in these cases, the removal of adnexa and surgical staging are indicated. The adjuvant will be given in accordance with the protocol.

Inoperable patients: The most common causes of surgical contraindication are morbid obesity or severe cardiopulmonary disease. Brachytherapy can be successful in local control and can be combined with radiotherapy in the presence of recurrence or poor prognostic factors. Patients with hormone receptor-positive, G1/2 tumors, and contraindications for radiotherapy can be candidates for treatment with progestogens at high doses.

Young women: Endometrial carcinoma is unusual and is associated with hyperestrogenism, obesity, polycystic ovary syndrome, estrogen-producing tumors, or genetic mutations. A careful histological diagnosis is needed due to difficulty in differential diagnosis between atypical hyperplasia and well-differentiated endometrioid carcinomas. In the case of nulliparous patients ≤35 years and wishing to preserve fertility, there must be interdisciplinary discussion with psychological evaluation and signed informed consent is essential, when conventional treatment is not done (HT + SOB). Non-surgical treatment using high doses of progestogens and subsequent pregnancy has been described in the literature.

Stage	Clinical picture	Treatment
IA G1	Tumor limited to endometrium and/or <50% myometrial invasion Well differentiated	TH + BSO + PERITONEAL CYTOLOGY, biopsy of enlarged lymph nodes
IA G2 IA G1/2	≤50% myometrial invasion Well and moderately differentiated	TH+ BSO + PERITONEAL CYTOLOGY, biopsy of enlarged lymph nodes, vaginal vault Brachy
IA G3 IB G1/2/3	Tumors poorly differentiated and limited to uterine corpus Invasion "/>50% myometrium, without invading serosa	TH + BSO + PERITONEAL CYTOLOGY, pelvic, and para-aortic lymphadenectomy or biopsy of enlarged lymph nodes and omentum RT (Tele + Brachy, only Brachy)
I A/B Non-endometrioid tumors	Serous-papilliferous and clear-cell tumors limited to uterine corpus, without invading serosa	TH + BSO + PERITONEAL CYTOLOGY, pelvic, and para-aortic lymphadenectomy or biopsy of enlarged lymph nodes and omentum RT (Tele + Brachy) CT
II	Tumor invades cervix without extra-uterine disease: involves endocervical glands	TH + BSO + PERITONEAL CYTOLOGY, pelvic and para-aortic lymphadenectomy or biopsy of enlarged lymph nodes and omentum RT (Tele + Brachy)
II	Tumor invades cervix without extra-uterine disease: involves cervical stroma	TH or radical hysterectomy + BSO + PERITONEAL CYTOLOGY, pelvic and para-aortic lymphadenectomy or biopsy of enlarged lymph nodes and omentum or TH + BSO + PERITONEAL CYTOLOGY, biopsy de para-aortic and enlarged lymph nodes and omentum RT (Tele + Brachy) If preoperative RT: RT (Tele + Brachy) + TH + BSO + PERITONEAL CYTOLOGY, biopsy of para-aortic and enlarged lymph nodes and omentum
IIIA	Involvement of serosa or adnexa or positive PERITONEAL CYTOLOGY	TH + BSO + PERITONEAL CYTOLOGY, biopsy of para-aortic and enlarged lymph nodes and omentum RT (Tele + Brachy) CT or TH
IIIB	Vaginal involvement	RT (Tele + Brachy of entire vagina) CT or hormone therapy
IIIC (1 and 2)	Metastases to pelvic and/or para-aortic lymph nodes and/or parametria	If tumor resectable: surgery and RT If tumor resectable: RT only

http://dx.doi.org/10.5772/61578

Stage	Clinical picture	Treatment
		CT or hormone therapy
IVA/B	Rectal/vaginal or distant metastases	RT CT or palliative hormone therapy

High-dose vaginal vault brachytherapy (Brachy): 5 fractions of 700 cGy.

Teletherapy (Tele): 4500 cGy and high-dose brachy: 4 X 400 cGy.

Preoperative RT-intracavitary Brachy: 2 X 750 cGy and Tele: 4500 cGy

Brachy: 4 X 500 cGy of entire vagina.

IIIC – Tele: 4500 cGy pelvic, 4500 cGy/180 cGy para-aortic + Brachy: 4 X 400 cGy.

Only RT: Tele 4500 cGy pelvic, Brachy 4 X 700 cGy and complementation if parametria compromised 1440/180 cGy.

IVA – Only Tele: 5040 cGy pelvic and "boost" 1980 cGy/180 cGy.

Table 3. Treatment algorithm for endometrial carcinoma

6. Radiotherapy

The PORTEC1 study showed that patients with early carcinomas undergoing RT had significantly more complications than those without RT (25% vs. 6%) and that 1/3 of complications were severe. The recurrence rate was significantly higher in the control group (14% vs. 4%), with only vaginal in 73%, and overall survival was similar in the two groups. There is no indication of RT in women with low-risk carcinomas undergoing surgery. The results of a systematic review and meta-analysis by ASTEC/EN.5 contraindicate routine adjuvant RT in endometrial carcinomas of medium and high initial risk: (FIGO 2009) IA G3, IB G1/2/3, serous papillary and-clear cell tumors, regardless of stage and histologic grade. The benefit in the prevention of isolated local recurrence was small and the side effects of treatment were not negligible. Due to the high acute toxicity and its long-term use, even compared with brachytherapy, RT must not be the treatment of choice only for preventing local recurrence. In the study, women after surgery were randomized into two groups, with and without RT, and each group was randomized to receive brachytherapy or not, which was applied in 53% of them. Disease-free survival (R 1.05; 95% CI 0.75–1.48; p = 0.77) and overall survival after 5 years (R 1.04; 95% CI 0.84–1.29) was similar and 5-year survival was 84%. The cumulative incidence of vaginal recurrence was 6.1% without RT and 3.2% with RT, with an absolute difference of 2.9% (95% CI <0.1%–5.9%). Local recurrence was 6.1% among those who received brachytherapy alone, which was associated with lower toxicity and could be the treatment of choice to prevent local recurrence. RT with or without brachytherapy should be indicated for patients without clinical conditions for surgery or with incomplete surgical treatment. PORTEC2, a multicenter randomized study compares RT with brachytherapy and can advise on the best choice of adjuvant treatment in early carcinomas. Since RT does not prevent distant metastasis, women with poor prognosis tumors may be candidates for study protocols for systemic treatment.[25, 26]

RT decreases locoregional recurrences but does not affect overall survival. There is no indication for adjuvant RT in early carcinomas in the absence of risk factors for metastasis after staging surgery. In the presence of risk factors and after staging surgery, the indication for RT with or without brachytherapy or brachytherapy only should follow protocols of each service. RT with or without brachytherapy should be indicated for patients unsuitable for surgery or with incomplete surgical treatment.[25, 26]

Patients with high risk endometrial carcinoma, FIGO 2009 IBG3, IIG3 with myometrial invasion >50%, and III receive adjuvant therapy after surgery, but it is not clear which is better: CT or RT. A randomized study compared chemotherapy (cisplatin, doxorubicin, and cyclophosphamide) and RT for high-risk tumors and failed to show any difference between treatments with respect to increase in disease-free survival and overall survival. RT delayed local recurrences and CT distant recurrences, but without significant differences, and both treatments were well tolerated. It is expected that randomized trials combining pelvic RT with CT can demonstrate better results. The systematic review compared chemotherapy with other treatments in patients with advanced disease, recurrent or metastatic, and demonstrated that there was a significant increase in disease-free survival but not overall survival when using high-dose chemotherapy compared with lower doses. Toxicity was proportional to drug dose, with high dose producing grade 3 and 4 myelosuppression and increased gastrointestinal toxicity. The addition of anthracyclines (e.g., doxorubicin) or taxanes (e.g., paclitaxel) to cisplatin increased the response rate and are still the most promising drugs. Stage III/IV patients undergoing cytoreductive surgery, who were treated with cisplatin with doxorubicin, showed a significant increase in disease-free survival and overall survival compared with total abdominal RT with reinforcement in the pelvis. A randomized phase III study with paclitaxel combined with cisplatin and doxorubicin after surgery and RT showed no increase in disease-free survival and increased toxicity. Studies are needed evaluating the effect of chemotherapy on symptoms and its impact on quality of life in these women.[27, 28, 29]

Adjuvant CT in the early stages should be indicated according to research protocols of services, and there is indication in and stages III and IV, considering risk-benefit ratio.

7. Hormone therapy

There is no indication for adjuvant hormone therapy in early endometrial carcinomas. There may be indication for progestational agents for tumors that are advanced stage III/IV, unresectable or recurrent and hormone receptor-positive, usually histological grade 1 and 2. The most commonly used agent is medroxyprogesterone acetate at 200 mg/day. There are few studies and they show difficulties in evaluating the results because they generally involve patients with clinical conditions and contraindication for other types of treatment. The systematic review showed no increase in overall survival with progestins therapy (OR 1.05, 95% CI 0.88-1.24). There was a reduction in endometrial cancer mortality (OR 0.88, 95% CI

0.7-1.1) and recurrence of the disease (OR 0.82 95% CI 1.02-1.01), but death from other causes such as thromboembolism, stroke, and heart failure was more common in women treated with progestogens (OR 1.33 95% CI 01.02-1.73). No indication of palliative hormonal therapy in advanced tumors.[30]

There is no indication of adjuvant hormone therapy, only palliative in advanced tumors, considering risk-benefit ratio.

8. Follow-up after treatment

In the literature, there is no evidence that routine follow-up of asymptomatic patients with imaging is better than requesting it only in symptomatic patients and according to symptoms. Patients should have or do:

- Clinical, gynecological, and rectal examination 4/4 months for 2 years and every 6 months up to 5 years
- Chest X-ray and annual abdominal/vaginal US for 3 years
- Mammography (MG) and annual cancer cytology (CC)

After differentiated follow-up, all should have annual clinical and gynecological examinations, CC sampling, and MG. Other imaging tests would be requested in accordance with symptoms and/or abnormal physical examination.

- The majority of recurrences occur within the first 3 years after treatment, and it is recommended to make doctor visits quarterly or tri-annually for general history directed at symptoms of recurrence, routine physical and pelvic-rectal examinations, mainly for the diagnosis of vaginal or pelvic recurrence, which shows favorable treatment response. After this period, the visits may be semi-annual up to 5 years and then annually. Patients should be informed about the potential adverse effects of RT and the need for diagnosis if experiencing symptoms of recurrence. Further examinations should be requested in accordance with symptoms or abnormal tests, because there is no evidence that the ordering tests (cytology, chest radiography, abdominal US, CT, and Ca 125) reduce mortality. The amended CC was associated with clinical examination or suggestive of vaginal recurrence. Patients with low-risk carcinomas may have biannual routine controls, but many patients find that routine visits provide a beneficial psychological effect. The request for mammography and Pap smear should follow the screening guidelines for breast and cervical cancer. For patients at risk for colon cancer, colonoscopy should be ordered and the need for upper digestive endoscopy assessed.[31, 32]

There is no evidence that follow-up with supplementary tests in asymptomatic women and normal examination reduce mortality. Periodic doctor visits up to 3 years with anamnesis directed according to symptoms and abnormal examination are recommended. Some services suggest chest X-ray and annual abdominal/vaginal US for up to 3 years.

9. Conclusion

The period in which the endometrial mucosa should be under close and careful vigilance is menopause, both in regard to prevention and early diagnosis of its pathologies. At this stage, it is a frequent site of pathologies causing abnormal bleeding, and while myometrial changes decrease in frequency with age after menopause, endometrial changes increase, reaching a plateau or decreasing after 80 years.

The search for early diagnosis starts with a detailed history and physical examination, assessing the differentially symptomatic and asymptomatic patients with risk factors. Transvaginal ultrasound can help in this step, but we preferably use hysteroscopy combined with endometrial sampling when there is indication for evaluation of the uterine cavity.

Most tumors are diagnosed in early stages and have a good outcome because of early symptoms. The standard treatment is surgery including lymph node evaluation, combined with radiotherapy. Considering that radiotherapy decreases local recurrence but does not influence survival, chemotherapy has been used in study protocols for tumors with poorer prognosis.

Author details

Manoel Afonso Guimarães Gonçalves[1,2,3*] and Fernando Anschau[2,3,4]

*Address all correspondence to: mafonsog@terra.com.br

1 Universidade Federal de São Paulo, UNIFESP, Brazil

2 Faculty of Medicine at the Pontifical Catholic University of Rio Grande do Sul, Brazil

3 Gynecologic Oncology Sector of Gynecology Service at São Lucas Hospital, Rio Grande do Sul, Brazil

4 Conceição Hospital Group, Brazil

References

[1] Swartz MH, Physical diagnosis: history and examination, 5th edn. Philadelphia: Elsevier, 2006, 3–33.

[2] Pessini SA, Almeida SB. O endométrio no climatério. In: Áurea Beirão de Almeida e colaboradores. (Org.). Climatério. Porto Alegre: Editora Artes Médicas, 1993, 62–76.

[3] Amant F, Moerman P, Neven P, et al. Endometrial cancer. Lancet 2005; 366: 491–505.

[4] Smith RA, Cokkinides V, Brawley OW. Cancer screening in the United States, 2009: A review of current American Cancer Society guidelines and issues in cancer screening. CA: A Cancer Journal for Clinicians 2009; 59: 27–41.

[5] American Cancer Society. Cancer facts and figures 2009. Atlanta, GA: American Cancer Society, 2009. Available at: www.cancer.org. Accessed on March12, 2010.

[6] International Agency for Research on Cancer (IARC). Cancer incidence, mortality and prevalence worldwide. Disponível em: http://www.iarc.fr. Accessed on March 7, 2010.

[7] Smith-Bindman R, Kerlikowske K, Feldstein VA, Subak L, Schreidler J, Segal M, et al. Endovaginal ultrasound to exclude endometrial cancer and other endometrial abnormalities. JAMA 1998; 280(17): 1510–1517.

[8] Fung MFK, Reid A, Faught W, et al. Prospective longitudinal study of ultrasound screening for endometrial abnormalities in women with breast cancer receiving tamoxifen. Gynecologic Oncology 2003; 91: 154–159.

[9] Mitchel H, Gilles G, Medley G. Accuracy and survival benefit of cytological prediction of endometrial carcinoma on routine cervical smears. International Journal of Gynecological Pathology 1993; 12: 34–40.

[10] Fleisher AC, Wheeler JE, Lindsay II, et al. An assessment of the value of ultrasonographic screening for endometrial disease in postmenopausal women without symptoms. American Journal of Obstetrics & Gynecology 2001; 184: 70–74.

[11] Tahir MM, Bigrigg MA, Browning JJ, Brookes ST, Smith PA. A randomised controlled trial comparing transvaginal ultrasound, outpatient hysteroscopy and endometrial biopsy with inpatient hysteroscopy and curettage. British Journal of Obstetrics and Gynaecology 1999; 106(12): 1259–1264.

[12] Gupta JH, Chien PFW, Voit D, Clark TJ, Khan KS. Ultrasonographic endometrial thickness for diagnosing endometrial pathology in women with postmenopausal bleeding: a meta-analysis. Acta Obstetricia et Gynecologica Scandinavica 2002; 81: 799–816.

[13] Goldstein SR. The role of transvaginal ultrasound or endometrial biopsy in the evaluation of menopausal endometrium. American Journal of Obstetrics & Gynecology 2009; 201(1): 5–11.

[14] Goldstein RB, Bree RL, Benson CB, et al. Evaluation of the woman with postmenopausal bleeding: society of radiologists in ultrasound-sponsored consensus conference statement. Journal of Ultrasound in Medicine 2001; 20(10): 1025–1036.

[15] Crispi, CP, Oliveira, FMM, Damian, JC, Oliveira, MA, Ribeiro, PA, Tratado de Endoscopia Ginecológica, 2012, 496, 3ª edição, Editora Revinter.

[16] Clark TJ, Voit D, Gupta JK, Hyde K, Song F, Khan KS. Accuracy of hysteroscopy in the diagnosis of endometrial cancer and hyperplasia. A systematic quantitative review. JAMA 2002; 288: 1610–1621.

[17] Bradley WH, Boente MP, Brooker D, Argenta PA, Downs LS, Judson PL, Carson LF. Hysteroscopy and cytology in endometrial cancer. Obstetrics & Gynecology 2004; 104(5 Pt 1): 1030–1033.

[18] Kurman RJ, Norris HJ. Endometrial and related cellular changes. In: Kurman RJ (ed) Blaustein's Pathology of the Female Genital Tract, 4th edn. Spring-Verlag, New York, 1995, 411–437.

[19] Kinkel K, Forstner R, Danza FM, et al. Staging of endometrial cancer with MRI: guidelines of the european society of urogenital imaging. European Radiology 2009; 16(7): 1565–1574.

[20] FIGO staging for corpus cancer. British Journal of Obstetrics and Gynaecology 1992; 99(5): 440.

[21] FIGO Committee on Gynecologic Oncology. Revised FIGO staging for carcinoma of the vulva, cervix, and endometrium. International Journal of Gynecology & Obstetrics 2009; 105: 103–104.

[22] Morrow CP, Bundy BN, Kurman RJ, et al. Relationship between surgical-pathological risk factors and outcome in clinical stage I and II carcinoma of the endometrium: a Gynecologic Oncology Group study. Gynecologic Oncology 1991; 40(1): 55–65.

[23] Lurain JR, Rice BL, Rademaker AW, et al. Prognostic factors associated with recurrence in clinical stage I adenocarcinoma of the endometrium. Obstetrics & Gynecology 1991; 78(1): 63–69.

[24] Kinkel K, Kaji Y, Yu KK, Segal MR, Lu Y, Powell CB, Hricak H. Radiologic staging in patients with endometrial cancer: a meta-analysis. Radiology 1999; 212(3): 711–718.

[25] Park JY, Kim EN, Kim DY, et al. Comparison of the validity of magnetic resonance imaging and positron emission tomography/computed tomography in the preoperative evaluation of patients with uterine corpus cancer. Gynecologic Oncology 2008; 108: 486–492.

[26] Panici PB, Basile S, Maneschi F, et al. Efficacy of systematic pelvic lymphadenectomy in endometrial cancer (MRC ASTEC trial): a randomised study. Lancet 2009; 373(9658): 125–136.

[27] Kalogiannidis I, LambrechtsS, Amant F, Neven P, Van Gorp T, Vergote I. Laparoscopic surgery vs. laparotomy for early stage endometrial cancer: long-term data of a randomized controlled trial. American Journal of Obstetrics & Gynecology 2009; 200(3): 296–299.

[28] Bijen CBM, Briët JM, de Bock GH, et al. Total laparoscopic hysterectomy versus abdominal hysterectomy in the treatment of patients with early stage endometrial cancer: a randomized multi center study BMC Cancer 2009; 9: 23.

[29] Kitchener H, Swart AM, Qian Q, Amos C, Parmar MK. Efficacy of systematic pelvic lymphadenectomy in endometrial cancer (MRC ASTEC trial): a randomised study. Lancet 2009; 373: 125–136.

[30] Benedetti Panici P, Basile S, Maneschi F, Alberto Lissoni A, Signorelli M, Scambia G, et al. Systematic pelvic lymphadenectomy vs. no lymphadenectomy in early-stage endometrial carcinoma: randomized clinical trial. Journal of National Cancer Institute 2008; 100: 1707–1716.

[31] Creutzberg CL, van Putten WL, Koper PC, et al. Surgery and postoperative radiotherapy versus surgery alone for patients with stage-1 endometrial carcinoma: multicentre randomised trial. PORTEC Study Group. Post Operative Radiation Therapy in Endometrial Carcinoma. Lancet 2000; 355(9213): 1404–1411.

[32] Scholten AN, van Putten WL, Beerman H, et al. Postoperative radiotherapy for Stage 1 endometrial carcinoma: long-term outcome of the randomized PORTEC trial with central pathology review. International Journal of Radiation Oncology, Biology, Physics 2005; 63(3): 834–838.

[33] Greven KM, Lanciano RM, Herbert SH, et al. Analysis of complications in patients with endometrial carcinoma receiving adjuvant irradiation. International Journal of Radiation Oncology, Biology, Physics 1991; 21(4): 919–923.

[34] Martin-Hirsch PL, Lilford RJ, Jarvis GJ. Adjuvant progestagen therapy for the treatment of endometrial cancer: review and meta-analyses of published randomised controlled trials. European Journal of Obstetrics & Gynecology and Reproductive Biology 1996; 65(2): 201–207.

[35] Randall ME, Filiaci VL, Muss H, et al. Randomized phase III trial of whole-abdominal irradiation versus doxorubicin and cisplatin chemotherapy in advanced endometrial carcinoma: a Gynecologic Oncology Group study. Journal of Clinical Oncology 2006; 24(1): 36–44.

[36] Fleming GF, Brunetto VL, Cella D, et al. Phase III trial of doxorubicin plus cisplatin with or without paclitaxel plus filgrastim in advanced endometrial carcinoma: a Gynecologic Oncology Group study. Journal of Clinical Oncology 2004; 22(11): 2159–2166.

[37] ASTEC/EN.5 Study Group, Blake P, Swart AM, et al. Adjuvant external beam radiotherapy in the treatment of endometrial cancer (MRC ASTEC and NCIC CTG EN.5 randomised trials): pooled trial results, systematic review, and meta-analysis. Lancet 2009; 373(9658): 125–136.

[38] Creutzberg CL, van Putten WL, Koper PC, et al. Surgery and postoperative radiotherapy versus surgery alone for patients with stage-1 endometrial carcinoma: multi-

centre randomized trial. POTEC Study Group. Post Operative Radiation Therapy in Endometrial Carcinoma. Lancet 2000; 355(9213): 1404–1411.

[39] Maggi R, Lissoni A, Spina F, et al. Adjuvant chemotherapy vs. radiotherapy in high-risk endometrial carcinoma: results of a randomised trial. Cancer. 2006; 95(3): 266–271.

[40] Humber CE, Tierney JF, Symonds RP, et al. Chemotherapy for advanced, recurrent or metastatic endometrial cancer: a systematic review of Cochrane collaboration. Annals of Oncology 2007; 18(3): 409–420.

[41] Homesley HD, Filiaci V, Gibbons SK, et al. A randomized phase III trial in advanced endometrial carcinoma of surgery and volume directed radiation followed by cisplatin and doxorubicin with or without paclitaxel: a Gynecologic Oncology Group study. Gynecol Oncol 2009; 112(3): 543–552.

[42] Baekelandt MM and Castiglione M. Endometrial carcinoma: ESMO clinical recommendations for diagnosis, treatment and follow-up. Annals of Oncology 2008; 19 (Supplement 2): ii19–ii20.

[43] Fung-Kee-Fung M, Dodge J, Elit L, Lukka H, Chambers A, Oliver T and On behalf of the Cancer Care Ontario Program in Evidence-based Care Gynecology Cancer Disease Site Group. Follow-up after primary therapy for endometrial cancer: A systematic review. Gynecologic Oncology 2006; 101(3): 520–529.